AF412365

The Persisting Osler—II

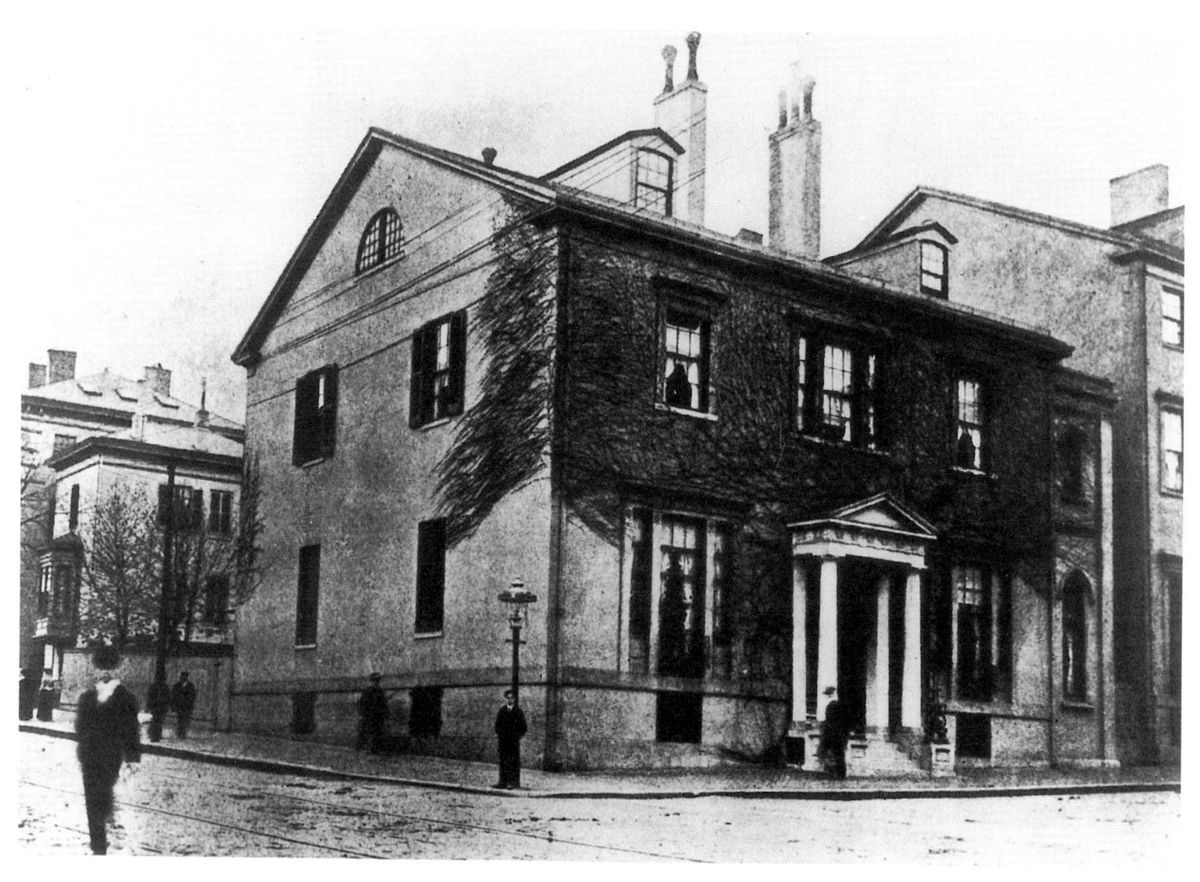

The Osler home, 1 West Franklin Street, Baltimore

# The Persisting Osler—II

Selected Transactions of the
American Osler Society 1981–1990

Edited by

Jeremiah A. Barondess, M.D.
Charles G. Roland, M.D.

Krieger Publishing Company
Malabar, Florida
1994

Original Edition 1994

Printed and Published by
KRIEGER PUBLISHING COMPANY
KRIEGER DRIVE
MALABAR, FLORIDA 32950

Copyright © 1994 by Krieger Publishing Company

Library of Congress Cataloging-In-Publication Data

The Persisting Osler, II / edited by Jeremiah A. Barondess, Charles G. Roland.
    p.   cm.
    "A selection from presentations at the annual meetings of the American Osler Society."
    Includes bibliographical references and index.
    ISBN 0-89464-856-X (alk. paper)
    1. Osler, William, Sir, 1849–1919—Congresses. 2. Physicians—Canada—Biography—Congresses. 3. American Osler Society—Congresses. I. Barondess, Jeremiah A., 1924– . II. Roland, Charles G. III. American Osler Society. Meeting. IV. Title: Persisting Osler, two. V. Title: Persisting Osler, 2.
    [DNLM: 1. Osler, William, Sir, 1849–1919. 2. American Osler Society. 3. Physicians—history—congresses. WZ 100 082p 1994]
R464.08P472   1994
610′.92—dc20
[B]
DNLM/DLC
for Library of Congress   93-23472
                                                             CIP

10 9 8 7 6 5 4 3 2 1

🍂 Contents

Appendix   363

Index   369

❦ Contributors

Robert Austrian, M.D.
Professor and Chairman Emeritus, John Herr
Musser Department of Research Medicine,
University of Pennsylvania School of
Medicine

Jeremiah A. Barondess, M.D.
President, The New York Academy of
Medicine; Professor of Clinical Medicine,
Emeritus, Cornell University Medical College

Steven L. Berk, M.D.
Professor and Chairman, Department of
Medicine, East Tennessee State University
College of Medicine

Dee J. Canale, M.D.
Associate Clinical Professor, Department of
Neurosurgery, University of Tennessee Center
for Health Sciences

George C. Ebers, M.D.
Professor, Department of Clinical Neurological
Sciences, University Hospital, London, Ontario

W. Bruce Fye, M.D.
Chairman, Cardiology Department, Marshfield
Clinic; Adjunct Professor, History of
Medicine, University of Wisconsin

Richard L. Golden, M.D.
Assistant Professor of Clinical Medicine, State
University of New York, Stonybrook; Curator,
The Osler Library, McGill University

George T. Harrell, M.D.
Vice President for Medical Sciences, Emeritus,
The Milton S. Hershey Medical Center of The
Pennsylvania State University; Dean Emeritus,
The University of Florida School of Medicine

Thomas A. Horrocks, M.A., M.S.L.S.
Director, The Francis C. Wood Institute for the
History of Medicine; Director, The Library for
Historical Services, College of Physicians of
Philadelphia

Albert R. Jonsen, Ph.D.
Professor of Ethics in Medicine, Department of
Medical History and Ethics, University of
Washington School of Medicine

Jack D. Key, M.A., M.S.
Professor of Biomedical Communications,
Mayo Medical School; Director, The Section
of Mayo Medical Center Libraries, Rochesler,
Minnesota

E. Carwile LeRoy, M.D.
Professor of Medicine, Director, Division of
Rheumatology and Immunology, Medical
University of South Carolina, Charleston

Lawrence D. Longo, M.D.
Head, Division of Perinatal Biology
Professor of Physiology and Obstetrics
 and Gynecology
Loma Linda University

Earl F. Nation, M.D.
Associate Professor of Urology, Emeritus,
University of Southern California

Edmund D. Pellegrino, M.D.
John Carroll Professor of Medicine and
Medical Ethics, Georgetown University

Alice A. Pellegrino, A.B., M.A., J.D.
Associate, Kirkpatrick and Lockhart,
Washington, DC

Robert E. Rakel, M.D.
Chairman, Department of Family Medicine;
Associate Dean for Academic & Clinical
Affairs, Baylor College of Medicine, Houston

Alvin E. Rodin, M.D.
Professor Emeritus, Department of Pathology,
Wright State University School of Medicine

Charles G. Roland, M.D.
The Jason A. Hannah Professor for the History
of Medicine, McMaster University, Hamilton,
Ontario.

Alex Sakula, M.D., F.R.C.P.
Formerly Consultant Physician, Surrey and
Sussex Hospitals, England; Past President,
Section of History of Medicine, Royal Society
of Medicine, London

Leon Z. Saunders, D.V.M.
Adjunct Professor of Pathology, School of
Veterinary Medicine, University of Pennsylvania

Warren A. Sawyer (Deceased)
Librarian, Medical University of South
Carolina, Charleston

William B. Spaulding, M.D. (Deceased)
Fellow of the Royal College of Physicians of
Canada; Master, American College of
Physicians.

E.A. Vastyan, B.A., B.D., L.H.D.
University Professor of Humanities, Emeritus,
College of Medicine, Pennsylvania State
University, Milton S. Hershey Medical Center

Frederick B. Wagner, Jr., M.D.
The Grace Revere Osler Professor of Surgery,
Emeritus, Jefferson Medical College

Faith Wallis, Ph.D.
Professor, Department of Social Studies of
Medicine; Librarian, The Osler Library,
McGill University, Montreal, Canada

Lord Walton of Detchant
Former Professor of Neurology, University
of Newcastle Upon Tyne;
President, World Federation of Neurology

❦ Preface

In 1985 The American Osler Society published selections from the papers presented at its first ten annual meetings, 1971–1980. The present volume does the same for its second decade. As in the first volume, each of the papers herein was read, more or less in the form in which it appears here, at a meeting of the Society.

The degree to which Osler's career, philosophy, and inspiration continue to animate amateurs and serious historical scholars in medicine and related fields is remarkable not only by virtue of persistence, but of breadth as well. In thinking about Osler and what he meant, we are, in effect, examining a period that saw the emergence and burgeoning of scientifically based clinical medicine and of medical science on this continent and, in fact, in the western world. It seems especially appropriate, in an era in which the mandate given to medicine by the wider society is being reshaped by scientific and especially by fiscal forces, that we remind ourselves periodically of the images and ideals that drew most physicians to medicine in the first place, and recognize again the importance of seeing modern medicine as part of a lengthy and remarkable evolution. That we should see ourselves as part of a lineage characterized in part by major figures like Osler also provides for us an opportunity to feel some stability in a time of change.

The American Osler Society includes on its rolls men and women who have primary commitment to disciplines such as medicine, literature, librarianship, and history. The studies in this volume attest once again to the range of interests of these members and to the rich interlacings of their interests with broader considerations in philosophy and historiography. The Editors may perhaps be excused if they congratulate not only the members whose works are published or republished here, but the other members of the Society as well; we thank each of them for their willingness to have their work included here and for their help and support.

We continue to hope, in the words of the Preface to the first volume, that "... these essays will serve to stimulate thought and further exploration of those timeless issues that captured Sir William's energies, and that remain vital for the modern physician."

Jeremiah A. Barondess, M.D.
Charles G. Roland, M.D.

SECTION I

🍎 Ethics and Humanism

"Our Lords, The Sick"

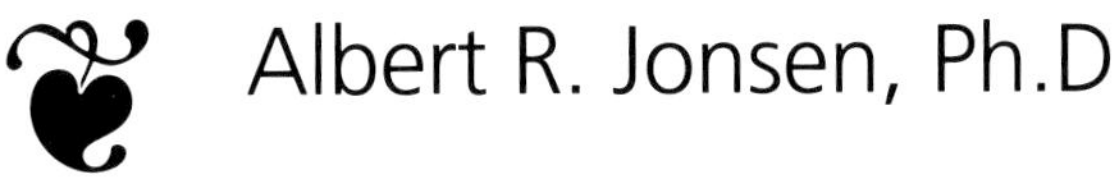 Albert R. Jonsen, Ph.D.

On Saturday, June 22, 1911, the morning post brought to 13 Norham Gardens a confidential letter from 10 Downing Street. The missive bore the news that William Osler, Regius Professor of Medicine, had been created baronet, on the occasion of the Coronation of King George V. Several days later, Dr. Osler wrote to a friend, ". . . they have put a baronetcy on me—much to the embarrassment of my democratic simplicity—but it does not seem to make any difference in my internal sensations."[1] One month later, Sir William spoke in Reading, at the unveiling of memorials to the first and last abbotts of the great medieval monastery of that city—a most uncharacteristic appearance for the Regius Professor, but one to which he had been enticed by a physician whose hobby was the history of the abbey. In his address, the new peer said, ". . . you see here in stone symbolized the beginning and the end of a great epoch—of a vast movement to the strength of which our wonderful cathedrals and many other superb ruins bear enduring testimony. Marvellous, indeed, was the faith that found expression in such works! Small wonder that the thirteenth had been called the greatest of centuries."[2]

Sir William, in accepting the baronetcy despite his "democratic simplicity," stepped into a medieval tradition. He became a knight, a peer of the realm. He accepted a title and a few prerogatives—though only a few—that came to him from one of the most powerful social institutions of our culture, the knighted nobility, an institution that came into being throughout Europe as the Roman Empire fragmented into innumerable duchies and baronies and counties, served by men sworn to fealty to liege lords.

Certainly, Sir William did not identify himself with the customs, ideals, and concepts of the vanished class—indeed, by speaking of his democratic simplicity, he repudiated them. He graciously accepted the empty honor, long shorn of its political or military might. And despite his remark of the occasion of the Reading Abbey ceremony—he was quoting the title of a book by a

Read at the annual meeting of the American Osler Society, April 12, 1986.

Based in part on and reprinted with permission from "The Nobility of Medicine," *In: The New Medicine and Old Ethics*, Cambridge, MA, *Harvard University Press*, 1990, Chapter 3 friend, physician and historian James J. Walsh, *The Thirteenth, Greatest of Centuries*[3,4]—I assume that Osler, like many of his contemporaries, had little respect or love for that era, over which still hung the cloud of the Dark Ages. Sir William was, above all, a classicist both ancient and renaissance, and, we can imagine, found something rather extreme, rather grotesque in the gothic.

But I take this entry into the titled nobility more as a symbol than as a significant fact about Osler's life and thought. Sir William was more a peer of medicine than a peer of the realm. He came to prominence at a time when a number of medical men had attained notice among their colleagues and before the public—a notice that paid respect to scientific learning and healing skills but above all to their creation of a distinctive profession, in the modern sense. Educated in universities, authors of scholarly volumes, influential in public affairs, particularly in the relatively recent public health reforms, founders and promoters of the relatively recent public hospitals—these men formed a kind of nobility. They were, in skills and in science, persons of account, far more so than their somewhat frivolous and overbearing predecessors, the jealous and sometimes vicious members of the Royal College. Many of these peers of medicine had been knighted: Sir Arthur Keith, Sir Thomas Lewis, Sir James Mackenzie, Sir Ronald Ross, Sir Thomas Allbutt, whom Osler's close friend, medical historian Charles Singer, called, "the most learned physician of the last 100 years",[5] " and above all, the great Lord Lister, Baron of Lyme Regis. In democratic America, Osler had left behind an untitled peerage of equal prestige: Oliver Wendell Holmes, William and Charles Mayo, Walter Reed, William Stewart Halsted, William Henry Welch and the young man who would become his biographer, Harvey Cushing. Sir William and his contemporaries brought to the medical profession a respect it had historically lacked. It still enjoys the trailing clouds of glory.

These peers of medicine also were nobles in their ethics toward their patients. While it is difficult to know with certainty, both because the record is not written and the motives of men cannot be easily read, I have the impression that their ethics were "noblesse oblige." Although we use this phrase with disdain today, it has a noble history. It recalls the moral obligation placed on lords to protect their vassals, or knights to protect the poor and the weak. Power, coming ultimately from God, was to be used for God's favored poor; fealty to a liege was reciprocated by the liege's duty to protect the vassal. An ethic perhaps more honored in the breach—I do not know—but certainly an ideal that made civilization out of chaos.

I estimate that the great physicians of the late 19th and 20th centuries maintained, even unknowingly, such ethics. The opening words of the paradigm book of medical ethics, penned by Thomas Percival in 1803, bear witness in elegant language to the ethic of noblesse oblige:

> Physicians and surgeons should minister to the sick, reflecting that the ease, health and lives of those committed to their charge depend on their skills, attention and fidelity. They should study, in their deportment, so to unite tenderness with steadiness, and condescension with authority, as to inspire the minds of their patients with gratitude, respect and confidence.[6]

Those words were incorporated into the Code of Ethics of the American Medical Association and stood unchanged from 1847 to 1912; their spirit lived long afterward. I am puzzled somewhat by the rarity of Sir William's allusions to the duty owed towards patients. What we call "ethical problems" are almost unseen in his voluminous writing, as best I know, nothing, for example, like the reflections on truth-telling by his distinguished younger contemporary,

Richard Cabot of Harvard. Yet everywhere there is a sense of the Hippocratic obligation "to benefit and, at least, to do no harm." There is a sense, and occasional words, that reflect an attitude of courtesy, respect, kindness. Certainly, there is the sense of dedication to the cure and comfort of the sick, even when it entailed, as it often did in those days, some personal risk.

The ethic of noblesse oblige, despite its somewhat antique formulation and dated sentiments, is, indeed, a noble one. It is rigorous in its demands and gracious in its effects. Those who lived by it did much good. What can be said in criticism of this ethic? It is difficult to criticize it without seeming either a cynic or so morally fastidious as to be foolish. Yet, I dare to do so in the name of an important principle, one which, if adopted, leads to a number of implications quite different from the principle of noblesse oblige.

As I noted Sir William's acceptance of a medieval honor, taken as a symbol, my criticism also turns on a medieval fact, taken as a symbol. Sir William most probably knew of the Knights Hospitallers of St. John of Jerusalem—indeed, he may have been inducted as an honorary member of the English Priory, although I can find no evidence of this. However, he probably paid little attention to the history of that religious-military order and knew little of its practices.

Founded in Jerusalem at the end of the 11th century, its original purpose was to provide hostels for pilgrims to the Holy Land and to care for the sick among them. It established at Jerusalem, Acre, and other places on the route from Eastern Europe to Palestine, institutions that were the precursors of the modern hospital. The famous Hotels-Dieu, which were the more immediate modern predecessors of our modern hospitals, were modelled on the Hospitals of the Knights of St. John.[7]

Within one hundred years of the founding, the order had assumed military duties as well, for it became obvious that the routes of pilgrimage needed to be protected against Moslem incursions. Many local Christian rulers deeded to them frontier castles and, not a century old, the Hospital became a mighty military force. They never abandoned their care of the sick, but this work of mercy became subordinate to the vast military and naval apparatus. The Knights themselves, who were vowed religious, with obligations to celebrate the Divine Office in choir and to live in celibacy and poverty, became soldiers, and, in the course of time, it appears that the virtues of religion were overwhelmed by the power and glory of military life.

Still, to the end of the reign of the Knights, which came at the fall of Malta to the Turks in the mid-sixteenth century, the brothers maintained their dedication to hospital work: it remained the soul of their community. Every brother, at his induction into the Knights, recited the vow found in the earliest rule of the Order.

> The brethren of the Hospital should serve our Lords, the sick, with zeal and devotion, as if they were serfs to their Lords. [Rule of 1181]

The Rule again says,

> How should Our Lords, the sick, be received and served? When the sick man shall come to the hospital, let him be received thus: let the Holy Sacrament be given him and afterwards let him be carried to bed and served there as if he were a lord. [Rule of Blessed Raymond, c. 1150]

Centuries later, the leaders of the Hospital continue to proclaim,

> We make a promise which no other people make, promising to be the serf and slave of our lords, the sick. [Chapter of 1301]

The rule bears witness to this dedication in many ways: the sick were to be served food before the brothers, were to eat off silver plates, were to be given white bread, were to have first call on bedding. "Our Lords, the sick, shall each have their own sheets and coverlet, broad and long, as well as a gown and slippers to go to the latrine." "Our Lords the Sick who die in the hospital, if they have shirts and breeches, shall be buried in the same." [Chapter of 1301] The revenues that supported the hospitals were not to be diverted to other purposes. In 1296, the officers of the Hospitals complained that the Masters had been spending improperly the resources "that should have been spent for the benefit of our Lords the Sick, to sustain them and the poor."[8]

I am sure many of the brothers left the chapel and rode off to war where they killed and maimed, as did all other knights. I am sure that, corrupted by money and power, they, like many other churchmen, made a mockery of their vows of celibacy and poverty. Yet, in those words, "My Lords, the Sick," they left to all subsequent medicine a precious heritage. They introduced, in antique language, the obligation to serve the sick regardless of risk or cost, a duty unknown to Hippocratic medicine."[9] They placed themselves at the command of those whom they treated; they subordinated, in principle, their ease and their convenience, to the patients whom they received into the Great Hospitals at Jerusalem, Acre, Cyprus and elsewhere.

It is important to realize the meaning, to a medieval man, of an oath, "to be the serf and slave of our Lords the Sick." The Knights of the Hospital, who were often born and bred of the nobility, knew clearly the social position of the serf. The serf simply had no rights and certainly had many and onerous duties. Will Durant lists seventeen obligations of the serf to the lord, ranging from taxes in money to days of labor in corvee and even including the infamous "jus primae noctis," in which the serf's right to sleep with his bride had to be redeemed by money. While in fact, as Durant says, the actual life of the serf may not have been as terrible as we imagine, it was one defined in terms of obligations and not in terms of rights or privileges.[10]

What, then, is the difference between an ethic of "noblesse oblige" and the ethic of dedication as a serf to the sick? What relevance does it have to modern medicine and contemporary practitioners? I suggest that modern medicine must ask itself whether its practitioners are a peerage in the fashion of Sir William and his colleagues, or a nobility like the Knights of the Hospital? But isn't this a foolish suggestion? Why should modern physicians think of themselves as a peerage in the fashion of Sir William and his colleagues, or a nobility at all? Is not such a metaphor outmoded, indeed even outrageous?

I would not dismiss it too quickly. First, the profession is still held high in honor, even though its prestige has slipped somewhat. Second, it is still a profession held by an obligation to compliance and to service—it alone among the professions still honors an Oath. In these features, it is somewhat like a nobility. But even more, it is held to act in concert as a barrier, a wall of protection, against the ravage of illness in individuals and in society. In this, it acts as did the medieval nobility, protectors of the realm. Sir William recognized these duties, saying, "the physicians' challenge is the curing of disease, educating the people in the laws of health and preventing the spread of plagues and pestilence."[11]

However, the knights of the realm and the knights of the Hospital differ. The former hold power and bend to protect the poor; the latter, in principle, hold no power and vow to serve the poor. In this is the modern lesson. The nobility of medicine has, in the last century, attained great power: the profession's monopoly has created great institutions and controls a vast economy. Their control lies not in the sword, but in the prescription and in admitting privileges. However, in recent years, that power is being eroded. The government, the insurance companies, the courts and legislators have whittled away at that power.

Now, as medicine begins to feel embattled, will it fight, as did the nobility of the *ancien regime* during the age of revolution, to preserve power and privilege? Will it turn, as did those same nobles, from protecting the poor, to protecting themselves and their status? The ethic of "noblesse oblige" falters when the power of the noble is attacked. It is a powerful ethic only when its adherents are safe. Recall that the Declaration of the Rights of Man declared that the Revolution had abolished the feudal state, and with it not only its dominance, but its ethic of noblesse oblige.

The dedication of the Knights of the Hospital to "Our Lords, the Sick" is quite different. It sees the relationship not as a spill-over of power, a "trickle down" ethic, a condescending compassion, flowing from power, but as a commitment of all one's energy to those who have no energy. Institutions are constructed to empower the powerless, and those who build and guard them are vigilant lest the institution serve their ends rather than the goal of healing and helping. They are even willing to make personal sacrifice so that this work goes on. When the institution is threatened they rally around their sick rather than around their treasury.

These are, I admit, exaggerated images, yet behind the rhetoric lies a real challenge: at a time when the genuine nobility of medicine, a nobility that arises from the science and compassion of men like Sir William, is compromised and threatened from within and without, at a time when many of medicine's younger practitioners either have forgotten, or have never learned, the ethic of noblesse oblige, the choice of an ethic is crucial. Beyond choice lies the continued commitment to an ethic. The Knights of the Hospital gradually fell away from their primordial ethic. They became the builders of fortresses and navies; they amassed a wealth that made them objects of envy to kings and popes. They ended their long history (though they still exist as an honorary and charitable society) as men of power and military might, who eventually fell before the onslaught of mightier power. The parallel to modern medicine is not, I think, too far-fetched. If it is to survive as a service, inspired by humane concern, it must choose its ethic and remain faithful to it. I am suggesting that the ethic of Our Lords the Sick is worthy of remembrance in these latter days. I hope Sir William, peer of medicine, would agree with me.

Notes

1. Harvey Cushing, *The Life of Sir William Osler* (Oxford: The Clarendon Press, 1925,) Vol. II, p. 275.
2. *Ibid.*, p. 281.
3. *Ibid.*, p. 391, 522.
4. James Walsh, *The Thirteenth, Greatest of Centuries* (New York: Catholic Summer School Press, 1907).
5. Charles Singer, *A Short History of Medicine* (Oxford: Oxford University Press, 1962), p. 626.
6. *Percival's Medical Ethics,* Chauncey Leake (ed.) (Huntington, New York: Krieger, 1976), p. 71.

7. Edgar Hume, *The Medical Works of the Knights Hospitallers of St. John of Jerusalem* (Baltimore: The Johns Hopkins Press, 1940).
8. Jonathan Riley-Smith, *The Knights of St. John in Jerusalem and Cyprus* (New York: Macmillan, 1976), p. 331.
9. Ludwig Edelstein, *Ancient Medicine* (Baltimore: The Johns Hopkins Press, 1967), pp. 319–348.
10. Will Durant, *The Age of Faith* (New York: Simon and Schuster, 1950), pp. 555–558.
11. Robert Bennett Bean & William Bennett Bean (ed.), *Sir William Osler's Aphorisms, From His Bedside Teachings and Writings* (Springfield, Illinois: Charles C. Thomas, 1968), #90, p. 63.

Percival's Medical Ethics: The Moral Philosophy of an Eighteenth Century English Gentleman

 Edmund D. Pellegrino, M.D.

Since its appearance in 1803, Percival's Ethics has been the dominant influence in Anglo-American medical ethics and the paradigmatic source document for the first, and subsequent, AMA Code. Its influence is exceeded only by the Oath and deontological books of the Hippocratic Corpus. Yet the moral philosophy underlying Percival's Ethics has not been well studied, and indeed, seems misunderstood in the standard account given by most contemporary commentators.

In this essay, I would like to offer some evidence contrary to the standard account: (1) that Percival's Code is mere etiquette and not ethics; (2) that it lacks philosophical substance; and (3) that it perpetuates a spirit of paternalistic condescension totally unsuited to our democratic times.

Against this view I will suggest (1) that Percival was a better moral philosopher than he is credited with being; (2) that beneath the surface of professional decorum there is a sound and definable moral theory; and (3) that we are obliged to take Percival's moral philosophy seriously today when we are in the midst of an unprecedented reappraisal of the whole of medical morality.

My contentions, which are presented more fully elsewhere,[1] are based in a reading of the whole of Percival's work edited and published in 1807 by his son Edward.[2] These texts show that Percival was a lifelong student of moral philosophy, that he produced a three-part work on this subject, and that his "Code" is built upon life-long and intellectually substantial ethical reflections. Interpreted without a knowledge of Percival's other ethical writings the Code does seem to consist mainly of rules of polite condescension for a lordly

Read at the annual meeting of the American Osler Society, May 14, 1985.

Reprinted with permission from *Archives of Internal Medicine, 146*:2265, 1986 profession. If one reads Percival's other works, however, it becomes clear that Percival grounded his Code in the classical virtue theory of ethics, as it applies to the medical profession.

I will examine first the standard account of Percival promulgated by the majority of modern commentators, then some of the actual content of his moral philosophy, and finally, Percival's expressions of that philosophy in his Code.

The Standard Account

Almost all recent ethicists and historians take Percival to task for his elitism, for a code that seems to give preeminence to the good of the medical guild, and that reeks of a demeaning paternalism repugnant to our pluralistic and participatory democracy. Each authority emphasizes some particular failing: thus, Laurence McCullough decries Percival's moralization without philosophical analysis,[3] which he contrasts with John and James Gregory, physician-colleagues of Percival. Chauncey Leake and Chester Burns in the two American editions of Percival's Ethics lament the overemphasis on intraprofessional ethics and etiquette at the expense of formal ethical considerations.[4] Waddington decries Percival's neglect of the physician-patient relationship.[5] Berlant sees most of Percival's maxims as instruments for propagating the monopolistic tendencies of the profession.[6] Veatch and King are distressed over Percival's paternalism and his condescension which they find repugnant in our more egalitarian times.[7,8] Katz stresses the neglect of communication and patient participation in the patient-physician relationship.[9]

Such unanimity of opinion among scholars is surprising, since the body of Percival's writing offers considerable evidence to the contrary. That evidence is contained in Percival's own writings in moral philosophy and in the content of his Code, once we interpret it against Percival's other moral treatises and his own life.

Percival's Ethics is clearly not a formal work of ethics but rather of medical morals, the fruit of critical moral reflection on the part of a well-educated Eighteenth Century physician. His Code, on the other hand, is not intended to be a treatise in moral philosophy. It is, rather, a set of maxims or aphorisms devised to guide the conduct of the good physician. It was composed, as we know, at a time of intense controversy in the staff of the Manchester Infirmary. The occasion called for concrete moral guidelines and an irenic spirit, not formal ethical discourse or controversy. This should not obscure the fact that Percival's Code rests on a base of ethical presuppositions explicated in Percival's other moral writings.

Percival's Moral Philosophy

Percival's most sustained effort in moral philosophy, outside his *Medical Ethics*, was a three part work (1775, 1777, 1803) entitled *A Father's Instructions: Adapted to Different Periods of Life from Youth to Maturity and Designed to Promote Virtue, a Taste for Knowledge, and Attentive Observation of the Words of Nature.*[10] This work was intended "to inspire a love of moral excellence," awaken "a knowledge of the works of God," and "instruct in the use of word and idiom."[11]

In this work, and in a *Socratic Dialogue on Truth,* Percival taught by giving examples rather than by abstract concept. "Dry precepts," he said, "are little attended and soon forgotten," paraphrasing Seneca.[12] His philosophical approach accords well with his medical philosophy in which Percival insists on observations of cases, rather than theorizing about disease. In this, Percival was an ardent exponent of the Baconian and Newtonian method applied to medicine—a method shared by the most progressive clinicians of the day. The "cases" Percival used to illustrate his moral lessons reveal a wide range of reading in Classical authors, the Bible, the history of Europe and his own country, and in the literature of his own times. All his works are interspersed with quotations apposite to his moral argument.

Percival's favorite model is Cicero, whom he calls "the Great Roman Casuist." In content and method, Percival's moral philosophy resembles Cicero's "De Officiis." It has the same practicality, use of cases and stories, and the same grounding of moral action on the old Stoic virtues. Like Cicero and the Stoics, Percival believed that the virtues were the bases for the life a moral man must live. The virtues he esteemed highest were almost identical with the Stoic virtues—veracity, faithfulness, justice, benevolence, and the cultivation of good habits. For Percival, these virtues were axiomatic for the moral life.

Percival's moral philosophy was, perhaps, less formally analytic than that of his contemporary medical moralists, John and James Gregory. They derived their medical ethics from the moral sentiment theories of David Hume and Francis Hutcheson, rather than Classical or Medieval sources.[13] That fact does not, as some commentators assume, make the Gregorys any more sophisticated as moralists than Percival.

As a matter of fact, Percival was not a stranger to Hume's thought. While a student at Edinburgh, he became acquainted with Hume. He admired him as a person, even though Hume's views on religion were uncongenial to him. Percival's son Edward underscores this fact in the following way: ". . . at an early period of his life, his faith in Christianity was staggered for a while by the perusal of Hume's essay on miracles."[14]

Another chief characteristic of Percival's life and thought was the close integration of faith and reason. Philosophy and theology were, for him, complementary and not antagonistic as they were to many Enlightenment thinkers. As he grew older, however, theology came to play a more dominant role. But Percival always understood the need to balance faith and reason: ". . . his zeal for the propagation of his doctrines was invariably guarded by the temperate spirit of his philosophy."[15] He saw clearly the dangers of both skepticism and credulity: "The fastidiousness of skepticism by an instantaneous decision rejects truth combined with adventitious falsehood. The blindness of credulity adopts falsehood even as a sanction to truth."[16]

Percival did not feel the contradiction between medicine and religion, which troubled so many physicians in his time. He quotes Thomas Browne, William Harvey, and John Gregory, to refute the charges of impiety so often made against physicians as a class. In fact, Percival states, "An intimate acquaintance with the works of nature raise the mind to the sublime conceptions of the Supreme Being.[17] In this, he was a follower of Francis Bacon, for whom the alliance of science and faith was the desired goal of serious studies. To this scientific perspective, Percival married his Christian faith. His views on suffering, illness, and the role of Divine Providence in healing were part and parcel of that Christian faith. They influenced his medical-ethical writings, which always called for a synthesis of competence and compassion.

In this respect, Percival's *Ethics* was also influenced by the work of his friend, the Rev. Thomas Gisborne, to whom he refers specifically in several places. In the preface to his Ethics, Percival notes that he sent this work to Gisborne while the latter was composing his *Enquiry into the Duties of Men in the Higher and Middle Class of Society in Great Britain, Resulting from Their Respective Stations, Professions, and Employment.*"[18] Gisborne, in turn, paid tribute to Percival's *Ethics* and included a detailed chapter in his own work defining the obligations of physicians. Percival did not feel that Gisborne's work superseded his own, but rather complemented it.[19] Just precisely how and in what order these two men influenced each other's views on medical ethics is still problematic. Both Percival and Gisborne reflected the persistent strain of theology in much of ethics in Enlightenment England. This was in contrast with the fiercer anti-religious spirit of the French Enlightenment.

Percival's writing and teachings were reflected in his own character and behavior which increased the influence of his writings among his contemporaries. To judge by the opinion of his peers, at least as expressed in their correspondence with him, he lived by the virtues he extolled. "Error," Percival said, "is most dangerous when dignified by example."[20] His son says of him that "in truth, the masterly picture so lately drawn in that volume (*The Medical Ethics*) in which he has delineated the requisites and qualifications of the medical practitioner displays the most exact portraiture of himself. . . ."[21] Allowing for the understandable adulation of a loving son, there had to be substantial truth in this assessment of Percival's character. Only such a person could have been asked by the warring factions at Manchester to write a set of rules which was so quickly accepted by both sides.

In sum, the moral philosophy undergirding Percival's *Medical Ethics* is that of a morally perceptive English physician of the Augustan age, grounded in a deep religious faith, joined to a love of learning and thinking, cognizant of the importance of character and virtue, and living out his precepts in his own personal and professional life. All of this is what Percival means to subsume under the term "Gentleman," when in his dedication of his *Ethics* to his son, he says that the purpose of *Medical Ethics* was to form him ". . . . to that propriety and dignity of conduct of a Gentleman."[22]

It is important to understand that, for Percival, a Gentleman was defined more by the virtue of his conduct, than by the purity of his patents of nobility, or the size of his estates. Percival placed his trust in the character of the physician as gentleman, as someone who by virtue of his profession voluntarily assumes uncommon responsibility, is expected to behave accordingly, and to be accountable for that behavior.

We are not necessarily the richer morally, in our day, for grounding our ethics in rules and rights rather than virtue. We have, as Percival did, good reasons to doubt the character of an unfortunate number of those who practice medicine. But, it remains to be seen whether law, rights, and duties can provide a more reassuring foundation for medical ethics than the character of a virtuous physician.[23] We still need physicians who voluntarily, consciously, and sincerely impose upon themselves a higher degree of self-effacement than is customary in other callings.

Percival's ethics was based in the principles of benevolence and beneficence to both individuals and society, as were the ethics of his Edinburgh contemporaries, John and James Gregory. The Gregorys derived the virtues (now called principles) of benevolence, beneficence and justice from the moral sense theories of Shaftesbury and Hume. Percival's virtues, however, remained virtues in the Classical sense—habits of right and good expectations of a good person.[24] His conception of virtue was a synthesis of the natural virtues taught by the Roman Stoics, joined with the supernatural virtues taught by Christian theology.

Percival practiced the virtues he preached in every aspect of his private and personal life—in his relationships with his family, friends, and colleagues, in his opposition to slavery, his espousal of religious liberty for Catholics and Quakers and of philanthropic causes like the improvement of hospital care and medical care for the poor and the mentally ill, and in the establishment of educational and cultural institutions.[25]

All of this was part of the consistent and coherent moral philosophy that undergirded the terse moral aphorisms of Percival's Code. That this philosophy does not appear explicitly stated in the Code is, therefore, not evidence for its non-existence. The purposes the Code were to serve were practical and ironic, not speculative or dialectical. Percival's rules of conduct for his confreres at the Manchester Infirmary were thoroughly consistent with his own character, his moral philosophy and his religious faith and were acted upon in his own daily life. To dissect them free of each other is to do violence to a synergistic unity of thought and action in Percival as a person. This sort of unity is easily misunderstood in our times when every effort is made to keep philosophical argument, religious faith and even personal behavior as far apart as possible.

Percival's Code: The Threads of its Moral Philosophy

Only a few examples will suffice to show how Percival's Code reflects in its necessarily brief maxims, the deeper moral philosophy that undergrids it. I will draw upon two of the four chapters in Percival's Code—those dealing with hospital practice and private and general practice. I have dealt elsewhere with the two remaining chapters—the relationships with apothecaries and the law.[26]

The principle operating and central to the maxims of Percival's Codes is beneficence—a genuine concern for the good of the individual patient and patient care in general—and by "care," Percival meant more than technical competence. He grounds the physician's moral obligations firmly in the nature of his special role as one who deals with the lives of others. On this account, Percival enjoins the virtues of "tenderness," "steadiness," "authority," and "condescension."[27] Words like those are easily misinterpreted in the more skeptical climate of our times. What they meant in Percival's moral philosophy is more clearly apparent by examining a few of the specific recommendations in his Code. Percival's regard for benevolence and beneficence are evidenced in some of the following ways:

For example, Percival is concerned with the way attending physicians were assigned in the Manchester Infirmary. The system could deprive patients of the physician of their choice. Percival urges the assigned physician to consult with the physician of the patient's preference, not for the physician's benefit, but to spare delays in treatment and to prevent the patient's lying to gain access to the physician he desires.[28]

Percival also shows a special solicitude for the effect of illness upon the patient as a person. Thus, he counsels that the patient's feelings, emotions, and anxieties be attended to as conscientiously as his physical symptoms. He proscribes discussion of the patient's illness and prognosis among physicians, visitors, or medical students in the presence of the patient. His worry is less with maintaining professional secrecy than with potential harm to the patient.

Discretion is enjoined in obtaining the patient's history on the open ward so that confidentiality and the patient's dignity can be protected, especially on the part of the "hospital pupils." When the patient is seriously ill, and in danger of dying, he should be encouraged to make a last will to do justice to his heirs.[29]

The potential conflict of economics with ethics did not escape Percival. He denounced the false economy of crowded wards.[30] He warned against unwise economies in treatment, urging physicians not to use drugs of inferior quality. Rather, Percival deemed it the physician's social obligation to society to provide the best quality medications for those who are ill: "no economy of a fatal tendency ought to be admitted into institutions founded on the principles of purest beneficence, and which, in this age and country, can never want contributions adequate to their liberal support."[31] This advice, given today's fixation on cost containment and prospective payment plans, is more pertinent than ever.

In unusual cases, and when ordinary treatments fail, Percival sanctions experimentation with new remedies and new treatments. But the physician must always be guided by "sound reason and well-authenticated facts."[32] Here his respect for the Baconian emphasis on observation and logical induction is joined with the benefits of clinical investigation to all patients. Percival was, as many of his essays on medical topics show, a clinical investigator in the best sense.

Percival made strong recommendations for the maintenance of accurate hospital registers[33] in order to chart the prevalence and incidence of disease with the aim of discovering the effects of climate, seasons, and occupations. But these registers were to serve more than epidemiologic interest. They could serve to monitor the differences between office and hospital practice of the same illness. In this way, the selection of patients who might benefit and those who might be damaged by a hospital stay could be improved. Here is an early example of patient care research.

Percival felt the medical staff had a *moral* obligation to form committees to monitor the physical context in which patient care occurred—e.g., ventilation, diet, cleanliness, and quality of medications. Those committees could, through the collective action of the staff, influence the trustees to make needed improvements. By involving physicians, the administration could avoid the resistance of physicians when they are not consulted on policies affecting the care of patients.[34] Percival's motivation was the betterment of patient care and not the protection of professional prerogatives.

Consultation was a preoccupation of Percival. It took up six articles in Chapter I (XVIII–XXIV), seven articles in Chapter II. It was a general professional concern in his time as it has been to the present. Consultations, Percival felt, should be used frequently, especially in complex cases, or when an operation is contemplated. Steps should be taken to protect the patient against anxiety. Occasionally the reasons for the consultation should be concealed from the patient. (This would be difficult to justify today.) When operations are to be done, care must be taken to avoid unnecessary delay, lest the anticipation of surgery unduly alarm the patient.[35] During the operation, a decorous silence is necessary, except to comfort and assure the patient.[36] While some of Percival's recommendations could be classified as more decorum than ethics, the most important of them are motivated by concern for the good of the patient.

Percival showed similar solicitude for the poor and the mentally impaired. He encouraged the establishment of dispensaries in small towns and in the country since they were less expensive than hospitals. He felt that physicians have a special obligation to encourage the use of dispensaries, especially to provide attendance on the poor who use them.

Percival's maxims for "Locked Hospitals" for the insane are especially revealing of that mixture of solicitude and beneficent concern that characterize his ethics.[37] He argues for the establishment of hospitals for the insane because of the special nature of their illness and because they provide accommodations even an "opulent" family cannot provide when one of its members becomes mentally ill. He is candid about how little is known about mental disorders and urges intensive study by clinical observation Here, he advises maintenance of journals recording the details of each case—age, sex, occupation, progress, treatments, and in fatal cases, post mortem examination of the brain.

Since patients in mental hospitals are secluded from observation by the public, and their complaints of ill-treatment are not likely to be heard or given much weight, physicians who attend to them are under ". . . the strictest obligation of honor, as well as humanity, to secure these unhappy sufferers all the tenderness and indulgence compatible with steady and effectual government."[38] With respect to treatment, it is better to "err on the side of caution, than of temerity" although a "boldness of practice" may well be indicated under certain circumstances.[39] Special solicitude must be shown to female patients, and care taken to assure that properly-trained nurses are in attendance upon them. On discharge, Percival advises that the patient should receive a sum of money, decent clothes, and help in finding employment.[40]

Percival's solicitude for the peculiar predicament of the mentally ill is, however, intermixed with a moralistic attitude on the origins of insanity common among his contemporaries. Like them, he felt that insanity was in part the result of a dissipated life, and thus the wages of sin. While counselling sound treatment on hygienic and humane grounds, he also advised that the insane be assisted not only in the "restoration of reason," but also in the "renewal of the image of God." "Thus on discharge and during treatment, books adapted to 'moral improvement' should be placed in their hands."[41] This sounds naive in our day, but Percival was motivated by a concern for the patient consistent with the ethos of his times. We should not judge too severely from the later vantage point of our own time.

Chapter II: Private and General Practice

The same "steadiness, attention, and humanity" prescribed in hospital practice should be observed in private practice. Confidentiality, temperance in the use of alcohol, and a scrupulous regard for fidelity and honor are requisite. The physician should, as much as possible, be a minister of hope and comfort. So much is this the case that he should have someone else inform the patient of impending danger or death![42] We could not contenance this today, of course.

While Percival was acutely sensitive to etiquette among physicians, overstressing, from our standpoint today, the guild aspects of the profession, nevertheless, he always placed the patient's good before that of professional loyalties. Thus, if a physician observed a colleague's ignorance or neglect, he had an obligation to intervene and to disclose the fact to the physician and then, if necessary, to the patient and family. The facts must, of course, be correct and the motives for disclosure must not arise from self-interest or jealousy.[43] This is a far stronger stand in the patient's interest than many physicians today would espouse.

In Chapter II, Percival devotes seven articles (II, V, VII, VIII, IX, X, XII) to the decorum of consultations, the subject whose prominent place has subjected Percival's *Ethics* most easily to the designation of medical etiquette. He also considers other "guild" matters, like the setting of fees, taking care of other physicians as patients, and the relationships of physicians with surgeons. But even in these "guild" matters, there is always an underlying concern for the welfare of the patient. For instance, Percival insists strongly on the separation of medicine and surgery. He does so not to avoid friction or territorial disputes, but because concentration of skills is required for safe practice in each specialty.[44] Likewise, he admits the intimacy of professional fees, but says they must always be subject to "knowledge, benevolence, and virtue." These virtues must regulate the physician's economic self-interests and even take precedence over them.[45]

Several other important obligations based in concern for the patient's welfare complete Chapter II. Quack medication should be discouraged, for example. But if the patient is obstinate in its use, the physician should not desert the patient or vent his displeasure. Rather he should be indulgent, carefully observing the effects of the medication, warning the patient if signs of harmful effect appear. He must be ready always to help if the patient's unwise experiment rebounds to his disadvantage.[46] The physician should not dispense secret nostrums even if they are his own invention. A new medication, if proven useful, should be revealed to others in keeping with the benevolence the physician is expected to exhibit to all who are ill.[47] Medical knowledge for Percival was not proprietary, but knowledge to which all the sick had a rightful claim.

Equally important to the patient's welfare are Percival's strong recommendations that physicians be critical of their own clinical failings. They must, he says, scrutinize their own clinical experience and avoid self-deception and easy excuses for error. In this way, they can fulfill the obligation constantly to improve their performance and avoid serious errors in clinical judgment.

This becomes a special responsibility as the physician ages and his powers of intellect and manual skills begin to waver. "Let both the physician and surgeon never forget that their professions are public trusts, properly rendered lucrative while they fulfill them, but which they are bound to relinquish as soon as they find themselves unequal to their adequate and faithful execution."[48]

Percival's maxims in the last two chapters are equally illustrative of his moral philosophy, and equally pertinent for our times. In them Percival insists on cooperation between physicians and apothecaries and between medicine and jurisprudence as moral obligations. Few things are as pertinent to our day when cooperation between health professionals and legal issues are so insistently intermingled with medical ethics.

Percival's moral philosophy and the 20th century

Percival's ethics must not be discredited because we misunderstand what was meant by the ethics of a Christian Gentleman in the Eighteenth Century.

The concept of the "gentleman" for example, which is so explicit in Percival, is also used in almost the same way by John Gregory. Thus, Gregory, speaking of the pursuit of self-interest, says that some physicians ". . . . have acted with candour, with honour, with the image of ingenuous and liberal manners of gentlemen. Conscious of their own worth, they disdained every artifice and depended for success on their merit."[49] In considering the need to use "remedies from every source," Gregory makes this a duty of a "liberal profession, whose object is the life and health of the human species, a profession to be exercised by gentlemen of honour, and ingenuous manners; the dignity of which can never be supported by means inconsistent with its ultimate object, and that only tends to increase the pride and pockets of a few individuals."[50] These sentiments are almost identical with the sense in which Percival uses the terms "gentlemen," "condescension," and "indulgence."

The pejorative sense in which we often use the word "gentleman" today does not exhaust its usages in the past. The article in the Oxford English Dictionary is a long one. It outlines the uses and meanings that define a gentleman as one who is qualified to bear arms, one of noble or genteel birth, of wealth, position, and power. But there is also a sense in which the Gentleman is one whose gentle birth is accompanied by "appropriate qualities and behavior and chivalrous instincts and fine feelings." Isaak Walton is quoted, "I would rather prove myself to be a gentleman, by being learned and humble, valiant and inoffensive, vertuous [*sic*] and communicable, then [*sic*] by a fond ostentation of riches."[51] The emphasis was not on a person's circumstances, but his behavior in them (Steele), or a readiness to be kindly, condescending, treating every person with due respect (Appleton). Steele and Appleton were Eighteenth Century writers whose meanings probably reflect Percival's use of the term most accurately.

On such a view, the virtues of benevolence and beneficence were expected of a gentleman, especially if one added the qualifier of "Christian" to it. "Condescension" then implied an obligation to disregard differences in privilege, position and power. Self-effacement became a necessary act of Christian charity.

It is easy, at this distance, to accuse Percival of propagating the profession's welfare under the guise of benevolence. But a careful reading of the *Ethics* and his other moral essays make this an unconvincing accusation. Almost always when one of Percival's rules seems to conflict with the good of the patient, Percival reminds his reader that the physician's prime dedication must be the interests of the sick. Given the times in which they were written, Percival's maxims show surprising concern for the patient's wishes. In many ways, his feeling for patient welfare was superior to some of the actual practices in our own day. For example, he is far more respectful of the patient's need to decide how and where to be treated, what medication to take, and to disagree with his physicians, than many physicians in his own time and our own.

Percival extended his ethics consideration to institutional ethics (a subject just beginning to be explored today). He prescribed for the proper governance of hospitals and reminded the trustees of their responsibility to oversee patient care. He recommended committees of physicians to carry out the professional aspects of this charge. But he also called for a trustees' committee which would have overall responsibility. On that committee, he specifically states that *no* physicians or officers of the Infirmary are to be appointed. Thus, he sought a balance between the authority of the physicians, which he deemed to be technically necessary, and the authority of the Board, which would supercede the authority of physicians. Percival's dedication to the guild of medicine, for which he is so often criticized, did not keep him from recognizing the necessity of trustee authority.[52]

Today, benevolence and beneficence have almost become vices for some medical ethicists. They equate paternalism with opposition to patient autonomy. The commitment to autonomy is so strong that many ethicists prefer a contractual to a conventional relationship. Also, they prefer to place their trust in duties and rights rather than in the physician's character.

Yet benevolence and beneficence are not intrinsically opposed to autonomy. One can argue that respect for autonomy is respect for one very important dimension of patient good. To over-ride the patient's wishes is to violate his very humanity. In this respect, the beneficent physician is one who enhances his patient's capacity to make his own choice of what is good, rather than presuming that the patient does not, or cannot know his own good.[53]

We cannot conjecture what Percival would have said about patient autonomy. That concept surfaced only briefly and intermittently before Percival's time.[54] Percival said very little about "communication" with the patient in our modern sense of that term. He would probably have subsumed this under his concept of "indulgence," another word that to our ears smacks of patronization, yet, as Percival used it, seems closer to compassionate understanding of the patient's predicament.

This review of the moral philosophy underlying Percival's ethical Code suggests that a more careful revision of the standard account of his work by today's ethicists and historians is indicated. We cannot yet tell where our contemporary scrutiny of professional medical ethics will lead us. But in the reconstruction of medical ethics underway for the last two decades, we must give respectful attention to Percival's thoughts. They were drafted in a different social and moral climate than ours, it's true. Today, rights and duty-based ethics are preferred to virtue-based ethics. But it is time to reexamine the inter-relationship of legal, duty-based, and virtue-based ethics. I have suggested elsewhere that a complete medical morality involves all three.[55]

Percival teaches us how a virtuous man of the Eighteenth Century sought to interpret his obligation to his patient, his hospital, and his society. We know how different is our cultural and social milieu from his. To suggest a resuscitation of all of Percival's axioms would be a sentimental anachronism at best, and a dangerous re-enforcement of some of medicine's less admirable tendencies.

Yet beneath the emphasis on professional etiquette, and the emphasis on how a Christian gentleman should behave, there is a viable ethic many of whose elements are neither time-, nor culture-bound. It is the lesson of this ethic and its call to personal virtue and character that an Eighteenth Century physician can teach us. To use Percival's Ethics to learn this lesson is a use of the past which we, and the future, can ignore only at considerable peril.

References

1. E.D. Pellegrino, Introduction: "Thomas Percival's Ethics: The Ethics Beneath the Etiquette," in *Medical Ethics; or, a Code of Institutions and Precepts Adapted to the Professional Conduct of Physicians and Surgeons,* Thomas Percival, Classics of Medicine Library, Birmingham, Alabama, 1985, reprinted from the 1805 edition.
2. T. Percival, *Medical Ethics: or, A Code of Institutes and Precepts Adapted to the Professional Conduct of Physicians and Surgeons* (Manchester: J. Johnson, 1803). All further references are to the text in V–II of *The Works, Literary, Moral, and Medical of Thomas Percival, M.D.* to which are prefixed memoirs of his life and writings and a selection from his literary correspondence. 4V, (London, J. Johnson, 1807).
3. L.B. McCullough, "The Legacy of Modern Anglo–American Medical Ethics," in *The Clinical Encounter,* E. Shelp, ed. (Dordrecht: D. Reidel, 1983), p. 47–63 and L.B. McCullough, "Historical Perspectives on the Ethical Dimensions of the Physician-Patient Relationship: The Medical Ethics of Dr. John Gregory," in *Ethics in Science and Medicine,* Vol V, pp. 47–53.
4. *Percival's Medical Ethics,* Chauncey D. Leake, ed., (Huntington, NY: Robert E. Krieger, 1975), viii.
5. I. Waddington, "The Development of Medical Ethics—A Sociological Analysis," *Medical History,* 19(1):36–51, January, 1975.
6. J. Berlant, *Profession and Monopoly,* (Unical Press, 1975), pp. 67–68.
7. R. Veatch, *A Theory of Medical Ethics* (NY: Basic Books, 1981), p. 90.
8. L. King, "Medicine in the USA: Historical Vignettes V, The 'Old Code,' Medical Ethics and Some Problems it had to Face," *Journal of the American Medical Association,* Nov. 12, 1982, Vol. 284, No. 18, p. 2330.
9. J. Katz, *The Silent World of Doctor and Patient* (NY: The Free Press, 1984), PP. 17–21.
10. See Vol. I, T. Percival, *The Works,* op. cit., p. 5–337.
11. Ibid., p. 7–8.
12. T. Percival, *The Works,* op. cit., Vol. I, p. 7.
13. L.B. McCullough, "The Legacy of Modern Anglo-American Medical Ethics, Correcting Source Misperceptions," op. cit.
14. E. Percival, "Memoirs," in T. Percival, op. cit., Vol. I, ccviii.
15. Ibid., ccv.
16. Ibid., cccxi.
17. T. Percival, *The Works,* op. cit., Vol. II, 526.
18. T. Gisborne, *Enquiry into the Duties of Men in the Higher and Middle Classes of Society in Great Britain Resulting from Their Respective Stations, Professions, and Employment,* B & J White, London, 1794, 648 pp.
19. T. Percival, *The Works,* op. cit., Vol II, p. 370.
20. Ibid., p. 171.
21. T. Percival, *The Works,* op. cit., Vol. I, ccxxiv.
22. T. Percival, *The Works,* op. cit., Vol. II, p 360.

23. E.D. Pellegrino, "The Virtuous Physician, and the Ethics of Medicine," in E.E. Shelp, Editor, *Virtue and Medicine* (Holland: D. Reidel Publishing Co., 1984).

24. E.D. Pellegrino, "The Virtuous Physician, and the Ethics of Medicine," in E.E. Shelp, Editor, *Virtue and Medicine* (Holland: D. Reidel Publishing Co., 1984).

25. T. Percival, *The Works,* op. cit., V2, p. 367.

26. E.D. Pellegrino, "Foreward: Thomas Percival, the Ethics Beneath the Etiquette," op. cit.

27. T. Percival, *The Works,* Vol. II, Chapter I, Article I, p. 373.

28. Ibid., Chapter I, Article ii, p. 374.

29. Ibid., Chapter I, Article vii, p. 376.

30. Ibid., Vol. II, Chapter I, Section xvi, p. 380.

31. Ibid., Chapter I, Article viii. p. 377.

32. Ibid.

33. Ibid., Chapter I, Article xiv, xv, p. 378–379.

34. Ibid., Chapter I, Article xviii, p. 381.

35. Ibid., Chapter I, Article xxv, p. 385.

36. Ibid., Chapter I, Article xxiii, p. 383.

37. Ibid., Chapter I, Article xxvii–xxxi, p. 385–390.

38. Ibid., Chapter I, Article xxx, p. 389.

39. Ibid., Chapter I, Article xxxi, p. 389.

40. Ibid., Chapter I, Article xxvii, p. 387.

41. Ibid., Chapter I, Article xxvi, p. 387.

42. Ibid., Chapter II, Article iii, p. 391.

43. Ibid., Chapter II, Article iv, p. 392.

44. Ibid., Chapter II, Article vi, p. 393.

45. Ibid., Chapter II, Article xv, p. 398.

46. Ibid., Chapter II, Article xxi, p. 402.

47. Ibid., Chapter II, Article xxii, p. 402.

48. Ibid., Chapter II, Article xxxii, p. 408.

49. John Gregory, "Lectures on the Duties and Qualifications of a Physician" (London: Strahan and T. Cadell, 1772), cited in J. Berlant, op. cit., p. 95.

50. Ibid., p. 90,

51. Quotes from the *Oxford English Dictionary.*

52. Ibid., Vol. II, Note III, Chapter I, Section XVI, p. 487.

53. E.D. Pellegrino, "Moral Choice, The Good of the Patient and the Patient's Good," in Earl Shelp, Editor, *Ethics and Critical Care Medicine"* (Holland: Reidel Pub. Co., 1983).

54. F.L. Pleadwell, "Samuel Sorbiere and His Advice to a Young Physician," C. Burns, ed., *Legacies of Ethics and Medicine* (NY: Science History Publications, 1977), p. 237–269.

55. E.D. Pellegrino, "The Virtuous Physician and the Ethics of Medicine," in E.E. Shelp, editor, *Virtue and Medicine,* (Holland: D. Reidel Publishing, Co., 1984).

Humanism and Ethics in Roman Medicine: Translation and Commentary on a Text of Scribonius Largus

 Edmund D. Pellegrino, M.D. and Alice A. Pellegrino, A.B., M.A., J.D.

> It is only when we, as members of a later society, with the gifts of hindsight and differing ideals, attempt to define Roman medicine in modern terms that it falls short. One should recall the basic humanity of Celsus, Aretaeus, and Galen as one assesses the worth of medicine in the Empire.
>
> —John Scarborough, *Roman Medicine,* p. 148

In the closing words of his last public address—his presidential oration before the British Classical Association in 1919—William Osler summarized his philosophy of medicine and life in two words—*philotechnia* and *philanthropia*—"love of the art" and "love of humanity."[1] He was quoting from a well-known Hippocratic text that many physicians before him, and since, have taken as the inspiration for those humanistic qualities that have characterized the best physicians in all ages.

Osler's view has long been the standard account of the origins of medical humanism and especially its ethical expression. In 1955, however, Ludwig Edelstein, a distinguished humanist and authority on ancient medicine, disagreed. In his Osler oration, he suggested instead that a fuller and perhaps loftier expression might be found in the writing of an obscure Roman of the first century A.D.—one Scribonius Largus.[2] Edelstein expanded upon the opinions of several German classicists whose commentaries on a text of

Read at the annual meeting of the American Osler Society, May 3, 1983.

Reprinted with permission from *Literature and Medicine, 7:* 22, 1988

21

Scribonius—the preface to his *Compositiones*—pointed to a humanistic strain not generally attributed to Roman medicine.[3]

Edelstein's commentary emphasized several distinctive humanistic features of Scribonius's professional ethics–the grounding of the physician's moral obligations in the special nature of his social role, the compassion intrinsic to that role, and its status as a moral imperative. Taken together these created a humanistic ethic in which compassion for the sick person shapes the moral obligations of the physician.

These features of Scribonius's preface merit careful reflection today when both ethics and humanism are foci of public and professional concern. The humanistic strain in medicine is being threatened by some of the same forces that are weakening the ancient edifice of medical ethics—the commercialization and industrialization of medical care, specialization and technology, and moral pluralism. As a result, the physician's technical and professional moral obligations are becoming progressively disengaged from each other. Osler's hope for a fusion of *philotechnia* and *philanthropia* seems less possible now than ever.

Equally sincere and dedicated physicians differ sharply on most of the prescriptions and proscriptions of the Hippocratic ethic.[4] Many recognize only competence and nonmaleficence as moral obligations, denying any obligation to efface self-interest in the interests of the sick. The physician as professional is giving place to the physician as entrepreneur, proletarian, or corporate employee. Compassion is increasingly depreciated as unrealistic and ancillary in the face of medicine's technologic prowess.

Given the likely continuation of these trends, a central question is whether it is still possible to define some set of moral commitments common to the profession that can transcend the deep philosophical differences that divide it. If such commitments are to be found, they will reside in the one medical reality that does not change with time—the need of the sick person for the physician's help and the promise the physician makes when he or she offers to provide that help.

Scribonius Largus illuminates the humane and ethical nature of that relationship in a unique way. In a few pregnant words embedded in a treatise devoted to pharmacotherapeutics, he defines precisely what it is to *be* a physician. He writes squarely in the Hippocratic tradition but adds dimensions drawn from the ethics of the middle Stoa that enlarge that tradition significantly.

J.S. Hamilton recently provided the first English translation of Scribonius's preface.[5] Ours differs in emphasis but not in substance. In this paper we extend Edelstein's commentary on the ethical substance of Scribonius's work, particularly as it relates to the search for a humanistic medical ethic today. Our intent is to focus attention on the origins of the philosophical argument all too briefly presented in Scribonius's text.

Scribonius Largus and His Text

We know very little for certain about Scribonius. He is variously described as physician, freedman, slave, pharmacist, Greek or Roman.[6] His Latin is crude by Augustan standards, suggesting that he was poorly educated or a foreigner who wrote first in Greek and then translated into Latin.

Some authorities make Scribonius the personal physician of Claudius, others of Claudius's wife Messalina, or simply a member of the Claudian household. He is reputed to have accompanied Claudius on his campaign in Britain in 43 A.D., although the evidence is scanty. He did, however, have access to a powerful figure in the Claudian household—G. Julius Callistus—to whom he addressed and dedicated his *Compositiones.*

The body of the *Compositiones* consists of a compilation of some 271 remedies. They must have been of interest to Claudius, whose fascination with drugs and magic potions was well-known. Scribonius's compendium followed the well-established tradition of the Roman encyclopedists, for example, the elder Cato, the elder Pliny, Varro, and Vitruvius, each of whom had drawn up lists of medical recipes.[7] These were commonly used as guides to home- and self-therapy by the practical-minded Romans.

Written between 44 and 48 A.D.—sometime after the return of Claudius's British expedition and before the death of the empress Messalina—Scribonius's *Compositiones Medicamentorum* seems to have been quickly relegated to a secondary position behind the works of his more famous colleagues.[8] From the time of the earliest manuscripts, which date to the ninth and tenth centuries, to the codices of the sixteenth century, Scribonius's book has been published in tandem with the works of a variety of other medical authors, including Celsus, Benevenius, and Marcellus Empiricus. Indeed, the *Compositiones* was published with the work of Marcellus so often that many editors and scholars attributed the book to that author.

The *editio princeps* of Scribonius was compiled by Johannes Ruelle, who incorporated it into the medical writings of Aulus Cornelius Celsus, Scribonius's probable teacher, in his publication of 1528, now in the National Library of Medicine in Bethesda, Maryland. This edition was soon followed by several others, including a 1529 Aldine edition of Andernaco's concerning those ancient doctors who wrote on diseases and their cures in Latin, and Stephanus's 1567 edition of the writings of the leading medical practitioners after Hippocrates and Galen.

In 1887, following two more editions in 1655 and 1786, Georg Helmreich produced what proved to be the definitive edition of Scribonius. Succeeding scholars from Karl Deichgräber to Aldo Marsili used Helmreich's work in producing papers, translations, and new editions of the *Compositiones.* In 1983, however, Sergio Sconocchia, using the newly discovered sixteenth-century Toledo code rather than the edition of Ruelle, which was based on several imperfect and sometimes contaminated manuscripts, published the new Teubner Scribonius. It is this text of Sconocchia on which our translation (and that of Hamilton as well) is based.

Translation
Scribonius Largus: *Compositiones*

Scribonius opens in the usual manner with a salutation to his patron Gaius Julius Callistus.[9]

Herophilus, who was once considered to rank among the greatest physicians, is reported to have said—with good reason, I believe—that drugs are the hands of the gods; the use of drugs that have been perfected through testing, after all, can produce the same kind of results of which divine influence is capable. During my own searches among the works and disputes of the more distinguished physicians for methods of treatment for my patients,

I have often discovered otherwise humble men who have gained importance because of their experience. Unfortunately, I have also come across men who, to their shame, have no ties to the discipline of medicine, yet manage to free their patients from pain and danger simply by administering an effective drug: it seems to be the work of some god! For this reason, those who attempt to diminish medicine by using drugs—calling what they do *medicine* not because they actually heal but because of the imagined power and efficacy of those drugs—ought to be despised. On the other hand, those who are simply eager to help their patients in every possible way should be applauded.[10] Certainly, I myself have sought to win great honor of science by the fruitful use of the drugs I have given, the same honor which many other men have attained by that means. This area of medicine, in fact, is the most important and, therefore, it was the first to be practiced and celebrated—if it is indeed true that the ancients cured their illnesses with herbs and roots. Even from its very beginnings, the human race in its timidity distrusted the iron and fire of cauterization. Nowadays, many men, although still not all, do turn to the latter expedient; yet, unless great necessity and fear for their health impels them, men tend to avoid things that they could barely tolerate even when healthy. I do not know, therefore, why some physicians refuse to use drugs to heal, unless they are thus displaying their ignorance of their craft. If, indeed, they have no experience of this type of remedy, then they are justly condemned for neglecting to learn so vital an area of their art. If, on the other hand, they have experienced the utility of drugs, yet still reject their use, they are all the more culpable because they are subject to bias, an evil that should be despised in every living creature, especially physicians. All gods and men should hate the doctor whose heart lacks compassion and the spirit of human kindness. These very qualities, after all, preclude the physician, bound by the sacred oath of medicine, from giving a harmful drug even to an enemy—yet the physician will attack that same enemy, when occasion demands, in his role as a soldier and good citizen. Medicine, however, does not measure a man's worth according to his wealth or character, but freely offers its help to all who seek it, and never threatens to harm anyone.

Hippocrates, the founder of our calling, transmitted the beginnings of this discipline in the form of our sworn oath, which ordains that no physician should give, or even show, an abortifacient drug to a pregnant woman. In this way, Hippocrates long ago prepared his students' hearts and minds to learn humane feelings. How much more evil would this man, who thought it wrong to destroy even the tenuous possibility of a man, judge the harming of a living human being! In truth, he believed it to be of the utmost importance that each and every physician preserve the name and honor of medicine by working conscientiously, even reverently, in accordance with the maxim which he himself set down: ''Medicine is the science of healing, not of harming.'' If, while aiding the suffering, the doctor does not concentrate his whole being on following this ideal in every way, then he does not truly practice the compassion he promises. Those men who either cannot, or do not, wish to help the afflicted, therefore, should cease to discourage others by denying that powerful drugs can frequently offer the sick much-needed aid. The true doctor uses medicine to succor the sick in a series of specific steps. He should first try to heal his patients by giving them food, in a calculated amount over a suitable period of time. If the sick man does not respond to this treatment, then the physician should turn to the power of drugs, which are more potent and, thus, more effective than food. Only when the disease does not yield to these cures, should the physician perforce turn to surgery or, as a last resort, cauterization.

But surely, Asclepiades,[11] the greatest proponent of medicine, denied that drugs should be given to the ill! Such is the fiction certain men still use to support their argument against drugs. Even if it is true, I could yet say that Asclepiades provided for what he had experienced. Perhaps he did not carefully consider this particular area of medicine. He was, after all, a man and, in this matter at least, did not conduct himself very favorably. No one can deter me when I see something so clearly manifested. What more can I say, therefore, about those men who so shamelessly contrive such claims than that they commit a crime tantamount to patricide and sacrilege. Certainly Asclepiades did state that drugs should not be given to patients suffering from fevers or from that illness that the Greeks call "severe suffering" (ὀξέ α πάθη). He felt that food and wine given at suitable intervals would more safely cure them. In his book *Parasceuasticon,* or "Preparations," however, he contends that the doctor who does not possess two or three tested compounds for each type of illness, which he can prepare at a moment's notice, should be employed only as a last resort. Thus does Asclepiades denigrate the use of drugs: if a doctor does not have various drugs, compounded for each type of illness, at hand, the great physician considers him unworthy of the vocation of medicine! Yet the negligence of certain men, who are doctors in name only, has caused widespread license. For this reason, no man should entrust himself and his family to any doctor whom he has not carefully judged. Certainly, he would never consider allowing any untested artist to paint his portrait. All people, however, have exact weights and measures, so that no mistakes will occur in the less important areas of life. They are not so careful of their health, but value all things at a higher price than they do their lives. Thus, not all aspiring physicians need study seriously or at all; some are not only ignorant of the ancient founders who shaped and perfected their professional abilities. They even dare to devise false teachings about them. When there is no careful selection process, but instead good and bad men are given equal consideration, regard for discipline and principle is lost. Each man pursues with greater vigor that which he can attain without labor, but which yet seems useful and capable of maintaining his dignity.[12] Thus, every man practices medicine in whatever way he wishes, nor can those who choose charlatanry be diverted from their course. The very size of the field of medicine allows everyone free rein. Many men, therefore, although they may have full knowledge of but one area of medicine, yet possess the name and reputation of the true doctor. We judged, nevertheless, that from the beginning we followed the right course—in so far as anyone can—when we chose to believe that nothing is more important than the skill as a whole. For, moved not so much by our desire for glory as by our empathy for the art itself, we trusted that we could obtain true good from it. To be capable of protecting or restoring someone's good health, seemed, for us, a great, almost divine, achievement. And so, as with other aspects of the discipline, we eagerly followed up that whose virtue the use of drugs demonstrates, particularly since we daily observed its successes and, despite the disbelief of the majority, we could display them, from time to time, in practice.

Do I truly need to give you, Callistus, further proof that drugs have a necessary use? You have asked me for certain compounds because you already understand their efficacy. Mindful of the kindness and brilliance that you have shown to all men, particularly to me, I have gathered into this book not only those compounds that you specifically requested, but also any others I had at hand. I am eager to repay somehow those kindnesses that you have so often shown me, both in the past and more recently, kindnesses that you have now compounded. After you yourself had read them and given me your opinion, you handed my writings on Latin medicine, control of which I entrusted to you, to our divine Caesar. I, for the most part, bow to your judgment. With your extraordinary generosity toward me, you sheltered my work's reputation under the aegis of your great name, not simply with words but by the very fact that you approved it. Indeed, when you praised this work, dedicating it with your noble hands, you faced as much risk through that judgment as did I through my pen. I readily acknowledge, therefore, that I owe you unique thanks, not only because you so warmly fulfilled my wishes before you were even asked, but also because your favor won me swift reward for and enjoyment of my labors. Forgive me, however, if you find these compounds few and incomplete: we are, as you know, abroad and the necessary number of books has yet to follow us. Later, if you wish, I will collect more remedies for each disease. It is necessary to have a large number for certain remedies are only suitable for certain people. All remedies are not suitable for all since their bodies differ. I will start from the head, which holds the highest and the most important place when action is needed. I will take care to place the uncompounded remedies first. They are often more effective than those compounded of many ingredients. It is like the number of denarii and Greek drachmae in a Roman pound. For us a pound contains eighty-four denarii but remains a pound no matter how many drachmae it comes to for the Greeks. I have listed first and marked by number those diseases for which remedies were requested and appropriate so that readers can easily find what they want. Then I listed the names and weights of the drugs compounded for each disease to which they apply.

Commentary on the Text

Scribonius's Latin is somewhat awkward and unpolished, prompting the belief that he first wrote the *Compositiones* in Greek and later translated parts of it into Latin. But his use of some very important words was in close accord with the usage of his contemporaries. These few words are particularly significant because they reveal an underlying philosophy of medicine and medical ethics that is singularly humanistic.

Professio originally meant "a declaration of intent," especially a formal declaration before a magistrate. It is so used in writings from Cicero to Tacitus and Quintilian. In Scribonius's meaning of "one's occupation," it is first found in the Tiberian historian Vellius Paterculus and then in writers such as Celsus, Ulpian, and Suetonius, all of whom were Scribonius's contemporaries or successors.[13]

Scribonius's use of *humanitas* and *misericordia*—respectively "humane feeling and kindness" and "compassion"—is common to many authors of the Golden Age (ca. 60 B.C.–14 A.D.). *Humanitas* appears in the anonymous *Rhetorica ad Herennium,* in Cicero, in Caesar, and in the writers of the second and third centuries A.D. For all of them, *humanitas* is "that quality by which man is distinguished from the beasts."

The same classical precedents apply to *misericordia,* for it can be found in Plautus, Terence, Cicero, Seneca, and Tacitus, among others.[14] Thus, despite his lack of style, Scribonius's use of these Latin words is consistent with usage of the best authors of his time. These words carry nuances of meaning of particular significance for his humanistic philosophy of medical ethics.

We should, however, distinguish Scribonius's use of *misericordia* from Seneca's use. Writing a decade after Scribonius, Seneca (5 B.C.–65 A.D.) equates the word with "pity," a "mental defect" that "blunts" the mind, interfering with discernment of facts, good judgment, justice, and prudence.[15] Yet these are the very qualities Scribonius would want in the physician. His usage, therefore, suggests not pity in Seneca's sense but "empathy" and "compassion" combined with "rationality and humaneness."

In the same way, Scribonius's use of *sacramentum* conforms to usage by his literary contemporaries. *Sacramentum* was at first the legalistic term for "an oath made to support a claim in court," and was so used by Cicero, Varro, and Gaius. In Cicero's *De Officiis,* Caesar's *De Bello Gallico,* the *Res Gestae* of Augustus, or Pliny's letters, it was a purely military oath. *Sacramentum* came to refer to a "solemn obligation" in the first century A.D. The *Oxford Latin Dictionary* cites Petronius's *Satyricon* (written during the reign of Nero) as the first literary appearance of *sacramentum* with this meaning. It seems likely that Scribonius was using this word in the same sense as his literary contemporaries.[16]

John Scarborough has warned of the difficulties of any research into Roman medicine—the fragmentary texts, their uncertain provenance, the difficulties of finding contemporary equivalents for Latin words, and the paucity of translations and commentaries on medical texts.[17] Gilbert Murray points out, in addition, that in the Greco-Roman world books were viewed differently than they are in our own. They were intended more as mnemonic aids to conversation rather than as works to be read. Thus, textual criticism and interpretation put ancient books to tests most were not expected to meet.[18]

Any interpretation of Scribonius's text is beset with all of these difficulties and is further complicated by the structure of some of his sentences. Nevertheless, as Edelstein so clearly demonstrated, certain conclusions about Scribonius's moral philosophy can be safely gleaned from the available text.

Although the body of the *Compositiones* is yet to be translated into English, it has an intrinsic interest as evidence of the kind of therapeutic armamentarium available to the Roman physician. The remedies range from the barely rational to the outrageously fanciful. It is filled with fascinating prescriptions, such as electroshock by the torpedo fish to cure headaches or gladiator's liver for hemoptysis. Scribonius was mistaken about the use of tourniquets and perhaps over-enchanted with the use of even legitimate drugs.[19] Yet intermingled with the oddities are some very rational elements: the first description of the preparation of opium extract, a defense of the proper use of effective drugs, denunciations of superstition and magical remedies, and drug usage based on experience and observation of effects. How much of his compendium Scribonius or his contemporaries actually used we do not know. Nevertheless, the bizarre therapeutics must not alienate us from the lofty medical morality of the preface.

Commentary on Ethical Content

In that preface, Scribonius's purpose is to justify the use of drugs against those who eschewed their use. In his time, these were the followers (or misinterpreters) of Asclepiades who preferred diet, baths, and exercise, and had a parsimonious or even nihilistic attitude toward the use of drugs. Against this view, Scribonius contends that drugs should be used when necessary, and that to withhold them is to do an injustice to the patient and to be unfaithful to the physician's primary obligation, which is to help the sick by all legitimate means.

Scribonius argues his case on grounds of professional morality, especially the obligation of beneficence, and its intrinsic connection with the nature of a physician's activities. The key words in his argument are *professio, misericordia, humanitas,* and *sacramentum.* We have noted their philological significance above. They had their origins in Stoic moral philosophy and complement even as they offer a contrast to, Hippocratic conceptions of profession and medical beneficence.

Scribonius pays proper tribute to the founder of medicine, writing that the Hippocratic Oath prepared the profession for *humanitas*—"human kindness," or "compassion." His reference to the Oath, apparently the first in any Latin text, uses the Oath in an interesting way. Scribonius takes the Hippocratic proscription against abortion as evidence for the acute sensitivity to compassion. Indeed, compassion becomes an explicit moral obligation that the physician ought to manifest in every medical act or cease to be a physician at all. Compassion is, in fact, role-specific, since it is required of physicians but not of soldiers. Nor is it required of physicians when they are not serving as physicians but acting as citizens in defense of their countries.[20] This is a very critical point for the Roman citizen who was expected to fulfill his obligations to his state and fellow citizens despite his private beliefs. To say that the obligation to compassion supercedes this civil duty is—for a Roman—high praise indeed.

In fact, the physician's "profession" is a promise of compassionate beneficence, a *sacramentum* that he is morally obliged to respect.[21] This promise is what unites physicians as a special group. This profession is so holy that when he defaults on it, the physician is to be condemned by gods as well as by men. Being a member of the profession is more than a mastery of a *technē,* therefore, in the Greek sense of "an art or craft." It is also a way of life to which one publicly and voluntarily commits himself. Medicine calls for a concentration of one's whole being. It does not discriminate among patients because it "does not measure a man's worth according to his wealth or character, but freely offers its help to all who seek it."

To be faithful to Hippocrates, Scribonius calls for an uncompromising dedication to medicine as an art of healing and not harming. In Scribonius's own words—*scientia enim sanandi non nocendi est medicina*—"the prime end of medicine is healing"; to harm the patient in any way is to violate the physician's reason for being. But Scribonius goes well beyond non-maleficence, which is the lowest level of beneficence. He says the doctor must concentrate his whole being on the relief of suffering. The physician who does not, or will not, offer compassion (*misericordia*) should not practice medicine at all, since compassionate healing is the primary end of medicine. Nor is it defensible for those who deny the utility of drugs to discourage their use by those who are dedicated to healing. Scribonius thus demands a positive view of beneficence—one must do good and even at some risk to his own self-interest.

The profession of medicine demands an effacement of self-interest since the physician must not have money or glory as his primary motivation. Moreover, medicine requires that the physician be a virtuous person since physicians have great freedom and may practice as they wish. Scribonius even alerts patients and their families to scrutinize the character of their physicians since they must entrust themselves to their care and are dependent upon their integrity and competence.

Taken together, these elements of Scribonius's moral code may justifiably be called humanistic. His is a virtue-based, role-specific, deontologic ethic. Scribonius is explicit in his exhortation on behalf of the humanity of the person who is ill. He makes compassionate healing the specific moral aim of medicine. He subordinates the physician's self-interest to the interests of his patients. Scribonius thus enriches and deepens the Hippocratic concept of *philanthropia*. The aim of medicine is always healing. The vulnerability and exploitability of the patient are always part of being sick. Thus, Scribonius's conception of medicine as an enterprise of compassion, joined to competence and a good character, has a significance beyond his own time and place.

Stoic Origins of Scribonius's Medical Humanism

Rome in the first century A.D. and Roman medicine, itself, seem among the most unlikely places to nurture the kind of ethical and humanistic sentiments expressed by Scribonius. The city and the empire had just been relieved of its grosser atrocities by the death of Caligula. It had yet to be assaulted by Nero's special brand of madness.

Roman medicine was in a no less parlous state. It was beset by a multitude of charlatans and incompetent itinerants marketing a mixture of magic and empiricism, combined with remnants of Hippocratic medicine. When they were ill, Romans first turned to superstition and their tradition of homespun medicine. Then they consulted their Greek physicians. Neither the science nor the ethics of Roman medicine would seem to be congenial soil for Scribonius's lofty doctrines.

Yet, one of the paradoxes of this complex period of history is the influence—at least on educated Romans, their thinkers, politicians, and writers—of the demanding moral philosophy of the middle Stoa. The most influential Stoic philosopher for the Romans was Panaetius of Rhodes (185–110/9 B.C.).[22] He introduced Stoicism to Rome in the second century B.C. through his influence on Scipio the Younger, Laelius, and Q. Mucius Scaevola. His greatest disciple was Poseidonius of Apamaea (135–51 B.C.), whose lectures Cicero attended in Rhodes in 78 B.C. Panaetius made significant changes in the moral philosophy of the old Stoa. He gave it a more practical turn, making its duties more specific to everyday life and, indeed, relating them to the several roles each of us plays. Most important for the dominant spirit of Scribonius's work is the fact that Panaetius also placed stronger emphasis than his predecessors on the duties of generosity and humaneness. He is usually credited with softening the harshness of the ancient Stoa and with introducing its humanistic strain.[23]

This turn to the human and the practical was most congenial to the Roman mind. Stoicism became Romanized to some extent by its emphasis on the old virtues of courage, justice, temperance, honesty, and benevolence, and on the solidarity of family ties. This Romanized moral philosophy of the middle Stoa was the basis for Cicero's treatise on morals, *De Officiis*,[24] a work that seems most likely to have provided, through the writings of Seneca, a contemporary of Scribonius, the Stoic substratum for Scribonius's medical moral philosophy.

Cicero's last work, *De Officiis,* was written sometime between 46 and 43 B.C. for the edification of his son, Marcus. By the time Scribonius wrote his *Compositiones* one hundred years later, *De Officiis* had already become a classic in the Roman world. Some have suggested that Cicero's work is nothing more than a paraphrase or translation of Panaetius. Cicero, however, wrote that this is not so but that he has taken from Panaetius what is most reasonable while emphasizing a topic Panaetius did not cover adequately, the conflict of duties and their resolution. This is a particularly important point since so much of ethics is indeed the resolution of conflicts of obligation rather than a choice between absolute good or evil.[25]

Cicero's work touches only tangentially on medicine. On one occasion he recognizes medicine as a useful role worthy of a gentleman.[26] In another place, he labels *inhumanus*—"inhuman," "unfeeling"—a doctor who would hold his patient to a promise not to use a remedy more than once.[27] He thus shows himself sensitive to the special plight of the ill person. It is less what Cicero says about medicine than his general philosophy of duty, promise-keeping, and conflicts of obligation that is most important for Scribonius's medical ethics.

Cicero's treatise speaks of the classical virtues: wisdom, justice, courage, and restraint, decorum, or temperance. These virtues are based in the idea of *humanitas.* Humans differ from animals, because rationality gives humans the capacity to choose and to make those choices known in speech. For the Stoic moralist, these are the most distinctively human qualities. They constitute the common bond that binds all humanity together.[28] They are the source of the obligations we owe to each other. Cicero devotes much attention to the nature of oaths and promises, the sacredness of good faith and trust, the relationship of morality to our roles in life, the superiority of morality over exigency, financial gain, business advantage, and even over law.[29] He uses practical examples from Roman life and history to illustrate these points in a concrete way.

One quotation will illustrate the emphasis Cicero puts on keeping promises—keeping one's profession of faith:

> But in the taking of an oath we ought to bear in mind not so much the consequences of breaking it as the obligations we have brought upon ourselves: for an oath is a sacred declaration. A solemn promise should be considered as being made before a god as witness and is therefore to be kept. Its fulfillment should be considered not in the light of non-existent divine anger, but of justice and good faith.[30]

Accordingly, the physician's profession is a promise to help, to serve the humanity of his patient with compassion (*misericordia*). It is, therefore, a solemn and sacred oath, and this is the way Scribonius interpreted it.

There are many other features of Cicero's Stoic philosophy that are applicable to medical ethics, for example, his emphasis on the virtue that should characterize a good person, no matter what his profession, the repeated assertions of morality over expediency, whether in business, private life or public life, and the concept of duties owed those who are dependent upon us.[31] It is not our purpose to comment on the whole of Cicero's text but only to cite it as evidence of a very likely source of Sribonius's humanistic medical ethics.

The Roman Stoic idea of *humanitas,* according to Bruno Snell, was different from the Greek concept of *philanthropia.*[32] Snell demonstrates that *philanthropia* was, for the Greeks, a feeling of solidarity of all men as shortlived and frail subjects of fate. A helpless person as a fellow human merited consideration by that fact alone. A conqueror like Cyrus does nothing wrong if he takes his foes' property. But if he leaves them something, he shows *philanthropia*. *Philanthropia* is a restraint, and a hospitality beyond legal behavior.

The Ciceronian notion of *humanitas* was exceeded in beneficence only by the Christian notions of *agape* and *caritas*. These virtues were based on the obligation of Christians to follow the example of the Beatitudes and the Sermon on the Mount. The early date of Scribonius's work makes Christian influences improbable, although we know that in later centuries Stoicism and Christianity did influence each other.[33]

Amundsen and Ferngren, in an admirable review of the notion of philanthropy in medicine, take note of the special meaning of the term *humanitas*.[34] They compare and contrast the meanings of *philanthropia* as used in Hippocrates', Galen's, and Scribonius's works. We agree with these authors that Scribonius's use suggests a deeper feeling of compassion than we find in Hippocrates or other authors in earlier Roman medicine. Scribonius sees compassion as intrinsic to what it is to be a physician, as did Galen later. This is crucial to our own conception of the philosophical foundations for medical ethics.[35] We agree with Amundsen and Ferngren that even Scribonius's notion of *humanitas* is different from the Christian notion of *agape* and *caritas*.[36]

The ethical principles we find in Scribonius are based in an evolution of Greek *philanthropia,* as exemplified in the Hippocratic ethic, and Roman *humanitas,* as exemplified in Cicero. These two concepts provide a solid basis for a humanistic ethic—one that sees the essence of the physician-patient relationship in a promise that the physician will serve beyond self-interest. It is a sacred promise that invites trust and, therefore, imposes a sacred obligation of fulfillment. It is, in fact, a covenantal promise—not a contract.

The Stoic philosophy and the medical ethical imperatives derived from it by Scribonius are virtue-based. Virtue-based ethics is the oldest ethical theory. It emphasizes the kind of person the physician should be rather than the resolution of complex medical ethical dilemmas. It is at the foundation of the Hippocratic ethic and the ethic of Thomas Percival (1740–1804), whose own work was used so extensively in drafting the American Medical Association's first code of ethics.

Scribonius's ethic is authentically humanistic in the best sense of that belabored term. It is based in the humanity of both the physician and the patient, and in the special kind of human relationship that binds physician and patient to one another. It places the source of the physician's obligations on the dependent and afflicted humanity of the person who is ill.

To opt for a virtue-based ethic is not to deny the utility or importance of ethical analysis and clarification that dominate Anglo-American medical ethics. But, when all is said and done, the patient is dependent upon the character, the trustworthiness, the moral sensitivity, and the resources of the physician. This is understandably difficult to accept in an egalitarian and democratic age, but is ultimately inescapable.

References and Notes

1. William Osler, *The Old Humanities and the New Science* (Boston: Houghton Mifflin, 1920) 63–64.

2. Ludwig Edelstein, "The Professional Ethics of the Greek Physician," in *Ancient Medicine: Selected Papers of Ludwig Edelstein,* ed. Owsei Temkin and C. Lilian Temkin (Baitimore: Johns Hopkins Press, 1967), 319–48.

3. See Georg Helmreich, ed., *Scribonii Largi Compositiones* (Leipzig: Teubner, 1887); Karl Deichgräber, "Professio medici: Zum Vorwort des Scribonius Largus," *Abhandlungen Akademie der Wissenschaften und der Literatur im Mainz, Geistes und Sozialwissen-schaftliche Klasse* 9 (1950): 856–57; and Julius Hirschberg, *Vorlesungen über Hippokratische Heilkunde* (Leipzig: G. Thieme, 1922), cited by Edelstein, "Professional Ethics."

4. See Edmund D. Pellegrino, "Toward a Reconstruction of Medical Morality: The Primacy of the Act of Profession and the Fact of Illness," *Journal of Medicine and Philosophy* 4 (March 1979): 32–56; and Edmund D. Pellegrino and David C. Thomasma, *A Philosophical Basis of Medical Practice: Toward a Philosophy and Ethic of the Healing Professions* (New York: Oxford University Press, 1981).

5. J.S. Hamilton, "Scribonius Largus on the Medical Profession," *Bulletin of the History of Medicine* 60 (Summer 1986): 209–16.

6. See T. Clifford Allbutt, *Greek Medicine in Rome* (London: Macmillan, 1921), 371–72; Paul Jourdan, "Notes de critique verbale sur Scribonius Largus," *Revue de Philologie* 42 (1918): 170–75; Pauly-Wissowa, *Real Encyclopadie der Classichen,* Alter Wissenschaft, 80 vols., ed. J.B. Metziersche (Stuttgart, 1893); and Sergio Sconocchia, ed., *Scribonii Largi Compositiones* (Leipzig: Teubner, 1983).

7. John Scarborough, *Roman Medicine* (Ithaca, N.Y.: Cornell University Press, 1969, 55–65.

8. Our account of the provenance of the text is taken from Sconocchia's "Praefatio," viii–x.

9. G. Julius Callistus was one of the four influential freedmen whom the emperor Claudius appointed to run the increasingly complex bureaucracy of the Roman state. Along with his colleagues Pallas, Narcissus, and Polybius, Callistus controlled all access to the emperor. As secretary, *a libellis,* he oversaw the emperor's private correspondence and all petitions. It was in this capacity that he approached Scribonius and commissioned the *Compositiones.*

10. There is some dispute over the meaning of this sentence. J.S. Hamilton, in his recent translation of Scribonius, prefers to take *probandi* as meaning "tested" or "proved," referring to the same subject as *spernendi.* We believe, however, that the following *autem* and the parallel passive periphrastics *spernendi* and *probandi,* as well as the general context, create a contrast between two separate subjects. We have thus translated *probandi* as "approved" to counterbalance "scorned" (*spernendi*).

11. Asclepiades was the scion of an old and distinguished Pergamese family long connected with medicine. Inscriptions indicate that this family had held a hereditary priesthood of the healer god Asklepios, from as early as the fourth century B.C. He was born circa 130–124 B.C. and came to Rome in 91 B.C.—see Allbutt, 177–91.

12. *Dignitas,* the most important possession a Roman could have, contained all the ideas of worth, honor, glory, and reputation. To maintain it, most Romans would make any sacrifice. It was in defense of his *dignitas* that Caesar crossed the Rubicon in 49 B.C. and began the civil war with Pompeius Magnus. Here, Scribonius seems to suggest that for the physician, at least when practicing medicine, even *dignitas* must take second place to *humanitas.*

13. *Oxford Latin Dictionary*, s.v. *"professio."*

14. Ibid., s.v. *"misericordia."*

15. Seneca, *De Clementia*, bk. 2, sec. 4, in *Moral Essays*, trans. John W. Basore, 3 vols., Loeb Classical Library (Cambridge: Harvard University Press, 1958), 1:437–39.

16. *Oxford Latin Dictionary*, s.v. *"sacramentum."*

17. Scarborough, 162–67.

18. G.G.A. Murray, "Prolegomena to the Study of Greek Literature," in *Greek Studies* (Oxford, 1946), cited in Arnold J. Toynbee, *Civilization on Trial* (New York: Oxford University Press, 1948), 42.

19. Guido Majno, *The Healing Hand: Man and Wound in the Ancient World* (Cambridge: Harvard University Press, 1975), 404.

20. See Teo Forcht Dagi, "Medical Ethics and the Problem of Role Ambiguity in Mikhail Bulgakov's 'The Murderer' and Pearl S. Buck's 'The Enemy,' " which addresses this very conflict, in original publication, pages 107–22.-ED.

21. We still recognize the special nature of the *professio*—the public declaration of commitment to a certain way of life—when we administer an oath (Hippocratic or some other version) at medical commencements. Conferral of the degree is, therefore, not the authentic entry into the "profession." Rather, it is the taking of a voluntary Oath of Commitment, the promise to use professional competence for the benefit of the sick. Some who take and administer the Oath may take it as merely symbolic, but the audience and the public take it as a serious promise of service.

22. See J.M. Rist, *Stoic Philosophy* (Cambridge: Cambridge University Press, 1969), especially chap. 10, "The Innovations of Panaetius," 173–200, and chap. 11, "The Imprint of Poseidonius," 201–18; Émile Bréhier, *The Hellenistic and Roman Age*, trans. Wade Baskin (Chicago: University of Chicago Press, 1965), 127–35; Ludwig Edelstein, *The Meaning of Stoicism* (Cambridge: Harvard University Press, 1966); and Peter Green, *Essays in Antiquity* (Cleveland and New York: World Publishing, 1960), especially chap. 4, "The Garden and the Porch: Stoics and Epicureans," 74–95.

23. See Rist, 173–200; and Giovanni Reale, *A History of Ancient Philosophy: 3. The Systems of the Hellenistic Age*, ed. and trans. John R. Catan (Albany: State University of New York Press, 1985), 296.

24. *Cicero on Moral Obligation: A New Translation of Cicero's "De Officiis,"* with introduction and notes by John Higginbotham (Berkeley: University of California Press, 1967).

25. Ibid., bk. 2, sec. 60; and bk. 3, sec. 7–9.

26. Ibid., bk. 1, sec. 151.

27. Ibid., bk. 3, sec. 92.

28. Ibid., bk. 1, sec. 50.

29. Ibid., bk. 3, sec. 46–72.

30. Ibid., bk. 3, sec. 104.

31. An example of the last point is Cicero's approving citation of Hecato of Rhodes, who stated that a ship did not belong to its owners but to the passengers until they arrived at their destination. Ibid., bk. 3, sec. 89.

32. Bruno Snell, *The Discovery of the Mind: The Greek Origins of European Thought*, trans. T.G. Rosenmeyer (Cambridge: Harvard University Press, 1953), 246–63.

33. G. Verbecke, *The Presence of Stoicism in Medieval Thought* (Washington, D.C.: Catholic University of America Press, 1983).

34. Darrell W. Amundsen and Gary B. Ferngren, "Evolution of the Physician-Patient Relationship, Antiquity through the Renaissance," in *The Clinical Encounter*, ed. Earl Shelp (Dordrecht, Holland: Reidel, 1983), 26–29.
35. See Pellegrino and Thomasma.
36. E.D. Pellegrino, "*Agape* and Ethics: Some Reflections on Medical Morals from a Catholic Christian Perspective," in *Catholic Perspectives on Medical Morals: Foundational Issues,* Philosophy and Medicine Series (Dordrecht, Holland: Reidel), in press.

Rx: Hope

 E.A. Vastyan, B.A., B.D., L.H.D.

"In the gloom gold gathers the light about it."

—Ezra Pound[1]

Let me open not only with a word of gratitude for the privilege of your invitation, but with a warning as well. In his famous—or as some termed it, infamous—valedictory address at this great institution, which Osler titled "The Fixed Period," he remarked on the "absolute uselessness of men more than 60 years old." That makes the task of my lecture quite carefree, for the men who invited me were fully aware that they had a sexagenarian—well past 60—in hand. So you must be content with listening to uselessness.

One further warning as well. Oslerians like you all know that not only was he born to a father who was a missionary Anglican priest, but that young Osler himself intended to enter Holy Orders. My warning is this: I, too, am an Anglican priest. My primary vocation, despite the fact that I've been a medical educator for a quarter-century, has been that of ministry. And so, although religion is still often a taboo topic in polite company, my perspective today will be that of religion and of pastoral ministry—and specifically, of the only ministry I know—the Christian ministry.

Although one could make generalizations about hope and spirituality that could be applicable to religion in general, I shall speak admittedly from within the Christian context alone, and hope that the necessary connections to other religious traditions which you may wish to make, can be drawn by inference. I like what Carlyle once said: that he could learn religion only from someone who knew God other than by hearsay. My only experience and knowledge of God—and of hope—are related to my practice of my Christian vocation. I will try rigorously to limit my remarks to what I know from that experience, and hope you will freely draw whatever connections are necessary to connect it with your own spiritual experience, and with your own knowledge and practice of medicine.

One further introductory clarification needs to be made. Let me suggest

The John P McGovern Award Lecture. Read at the annual meeting of the American Osler Society, May 8, 1990.

35

it with a story. One of my favorite physician-mentors, with whom I frequently made teaching rounds, was not only an excellent clinician, but an excellent teacher. Pithy aphorisms ("pearls" to the students) would fall from him like seed following the sower. Three basic principles, he would tell all medical students, would see them safely through Emergency Room duty: "First, air goes in and out. Second, blood goes round and round. Third, oxygen is good." One day an even wiser colleague corrected him: "Ah, but one more is needed: 'bleeding always stops.' "

So I ask your indulgence for a paper also based on certain very simple presuppositions that I hold, and that I believe apply not only in an emergency room—but in the emergency situation we know as the human condition. My remarks will be those of one who stands frankly and forthrightly on one side of that great, perhaps most basic, divide in humankind: I am a supernaturalist, a theist. I suspect many of you, perhaps even most of you, are naturalists. Further, I believe hope can be understood only by a supernaturalist; certainly hoping behavior is appropriate only for a supernaturalist—one who believes there is meaning and purpose in a spiritual world that is beyond reason, beyond our finite world.

My presuppositions are also simple, also three:

1. God is God, and is in control of every aspect of life—temporal life, and eternal life.
2. We know God as He reveals Himself to us in his Holy Word and Sacraments; and we know him not by inquisitiveness or imagination or inventiveness—but only by obedience.
3. The basic, most fundamental principle of the cosmos is redemptive, not rational. This may be another way of stating the fourth emergency principle above: bleeding always stops.

Another clinical friend has confided to me that when he speaks of a single case in any paper or lecture, he speaks from "my experience." Two patient histories, for him, constitute "a series of cases." Let me now get to the substance of my remarks with the first of "a series of cases" I want to use to frame our consideration of hope.

For some 20 years, one of my standard courses at the College of Medicine at Hershey has been one titled "Dying, Death and Grief." Since most of my students had not yet begun clinical rotations, I assign them to clinical preceptors, with the request that they be assigned to specific patients. Their duties were clearly spelled out: they were to pretend to absolutely no professional expertise, but were to seek the patients' permission to interview them simply as person to person, seeking to understand more deeply what it was like to be seriously ill.

One of our senior faculty members refused to act as preceptor; finally, over a serendipitous lunch one day, told me why. "I'd cooperate," she said, "if you taught it to seniors; but I want those students to learn some real medicine before they see any patients." My counter was that, if such were the case, I would be even more eager to have my turn at bat with the students first. Yet that very afternoon she telephoned me, and asked if I would, in a pastoral capacity, see one of her patients. I'll call him "Brownie."

"I was just with him," she said, "to confide to him that I had exhausted all therapeutic possibilities. That there was no way I knew to delay further the progress of his disease. And," she continued, "he met that with effusive gratitude, almost with joy. I was pretty wiped out by that. Would you visit him?"

I did, and a series of daily visits followed. We not only prayed together; we talked together at length. This was the first time in my experience that I fully realized how important reminiscence can be to a dying patient—a recovering and remembering of the times of life that had been replete with meaning and purpose, as a rich way to launch off into the unknown. Many of his stories were of living through danger during his duty as a bombardier in American Flying Fortresses during World War II.

After about a week, his physician called me again. She had made rather carefully conceived provisions to have Brownie go home, to be with his wife and daughters for his final days. To her surprise, he refused. He wanted to remain in the hospital, and his physician couldn't understand why. Could I shed any light on that, she wondered.

I asked him that afternoon. Instead of responding directly, he began a story: "Our bombing missions would go deep into Germany long before our fighter escorts had the range to go with us. They'd go to the limit of their range, turn back, refuel, and meet us again at their limit on our homeward course. After one particularly rough mission over Berlin, where we had lost many planes, we were limping back to England—badly damaged, with a gunner dead in the tail. Over France, one of our engines had begun to smoke. As I was hunched up there in the bombardier's bubble, an American fighter plane came buzzing past. When he saw how badly we were hurt, he throttled back, pulled almost alongside me in the bubble, and raised his arm in a sign: 'Thumbs up!' I could almost hear him say it. Just as he did it, pow!, an anti-aircraft shell exploded, and his plane disintegrated before my eyes." He paused for a long moment. "That's what I want to do for my family. That's why I want to die here, not at home."

He died a few days later. I wasn't present, but I was later told it had the air of a celebration—with wife, daughters, nurses, residents—singing hymns, and exchanging hugs and kisses and tears.

Experiences like this may be relatively infrequent; they are not unique. Something like it will even be described in medical literature on occasion. Many of you probably saw the moving paper in *The New England Journal of Medicine*—a few years ago—by a self-described "successful, hard-driving and competitive" surgeon.[2] Robert M. Mack published a very personal account of what he called the "lessons" he had learned from living with cancer, an adenocarcinoma of the lung. After a successful surgical resection he experienced two years of symptom-free life, until a new growth was discovered in the lung, with metastases to at least three sites of bone. Following a time in which he was "devastated, bewildered and very frightened," he wrote, "I am happier than I have ever been. These are truly among the best days of my life."

He continued: "It became poignantly clear to me . . . that this was a time of real choice. I could sit back and let my disease and my treatment take their course, or I could pause, and look at my life and ask, "What are my priorities? . . . One of the really ironic things about the human experience is that many of us have to face pain or injury or even the possibility of death in order to learn the real purpose of being and how best to live a rewarding life."

Dr. Mack's experience was even more eloquently expressed by Senator Paul Tsongas, who titled the memoir of his life with cancer, *Heading Home.*[3] In that book, he wrote: "The illness made me face up to the fact that I will die someday. It made me think about wanting to look back without regret whenever that happened . . . My illness has forced me to understand that I have true spiritual needs whether I am healthy or unhealthy . . . Now the entire matter of belief is central to me and gives me a truer sense of direction . . . . These changes, or more accurately reinforcements, are a precious gift. The cancer gave them to me. I treasure them.''

Such reactions, however, while not rare, are probably not the norm among cancer patients—or among patients with ominous diseases generally. Patients and families, within experience I suspect is common to most of us, are much more often torn by anguish, often tragically crushed by the burden of lethal illness and suffering. Perhaps even more frequently, such patients avoid any outward expression of the effects of their illness, bearing in silence and solitude—and so often in depression and despair—their inner agony.

Yet experiences like those of Brownie, Dr. Mack, Senator Tsongas—are not simply anomalies. I have repeatedly encountered that same affirming joyfulness in patients—and so, too, I suspect, have most nurses and physicians who have been willing to let such patients share their inner lives.[4]

Experiences like these are what I refer to as hoping behavior. What happens in the lives of such people? How shall we understand such reactions to life-threatening illness? How should we respond? Suggestive questions abound:

1. What is it that lies at the root of such behavior?
2. What is the nature of such hope?
3. Can religious concepts—specifically, can Christian concepts—help us understand as well as recognize such hope?
4. What implications would such understanding have for medical care of such patients, when we encounter such behavior?
5. Can we foster such behavior amid the dire circumstances of grief, and suffering, and dying? Should we?

Within the category of medical literature, I've been able to find very little that deals with hope, either explicitly or implicitly. *Index Medicus* has no category for hope. There are, of course, categories that index the psychological and behavioral ramifications of illness, but still very little of hope or hoping. But a few papers can be found. I have long known, and used, one by Brody, published in *JAMA* in 1981[5] and I was surprised last week by a physician-friend who sent me a clipping from the most recent issue of *JAMA* (May 2, 1990)—entitled, as was Brody's paper, simply, "Hope."[6]

Both are interesting papers. And both assume that hope can be a prescription—an "Rx"—something which can be ordered by the physician and can even be dispensed, to order, by ancillary medical personnel.

Indeed, Buchholz, in that most recent paper, writes with tongue-in-cheek of hope as a generic product of the pharmacopeia of wise physicians— as "a naturally occurring substance created by an individual's ability to project himself or herself into the future and imagine something better than what exists in the present." He writes further: "The only limit on maximum dosage is the patient's ability to receive and the professional's ability to administer HOPE at an appropriate rate."

Both papers have valuable suggestions for fostering hope, but I wish to suggest another perspective: that hope is fundamentally a gift to be received— not a behavior or a concept or an emotion that can be prescribed.

Further, I want to suggest it is a gift which is received by physician as well, a gift from the patient, a gift which can be fostered, encouraged, wondered at—but which is, paradoxically, one of the truly great gifts that cannot be given, but must be humbly received, by the "care-giver."

I believe it is a myth that we can either "give" or "take away" hope.

Moreover, it's a myth that goes with the arrogance of believing the "caregiver" is a spiritually superior person, or in a spiritually superior position. There exists a vast religious experience and literature, ancient as well as modern, which suggest the opposite is almost always the case.

Hope has, however, been relatively neglected, both as a philosophical and theological concept, until relatively recently. Within classical theology, it seems to be the poor third sister among the great theological virtues of faith, love, and hope—often being subsumed in discussions about faith.

Within the past three decades, there has appeared a "Theology of Hope"—usually associated with two German theologians, Jurgen Moltmann and Wolfhart Pannenberg. This has emerged in a strident Marxist form of politics called "Liberation Theology;" what I know of it has not seemed of much use for our purposes in discussing hope in a medical context.

Much more useful to me have been three other Europeans. Two were French philosophers of the World War II era, Gabriel Marcel and Simone Weil, and the third was a transplanted Dutchman, Paul Pruyser, who spent most of his life at the Menninger Clinic as a psychologist of religion.

Marcel produced an important work under the oppression of the Nazi occupation of France, which he called a "Sketch of a Phenomenology and a Metaphysic of Hope."[7] Simone Weil, during the same period, produced much more modest but, I believe, even more profound, observations in a series of letters and brief essays—the most useful for me being her study of "Affliction and the Love of God."[9] Pruyser both influenced and was influenced by Karl Menninger's own contributions to the study of hope—and is, to the best of my knowledge, the only medically related person to explore the ramifications of Marcel's work.[9–10]

Out of their work, there emerges a strong consensus about some of the basic characteristics of hope. Marcel emphasized a key point: that it is most helpful and useful to talk about the phenomenon as hoping, rather than as hope; to view it always as a verb, rather than a noun. For hoping, he insists, is much more a matter of being than of having, of a process rather than a static entity, of behavior rather than concept.

Hoping, moreover, he sees as a global condition. It affects the whole person, and is directed at what we might term basic purpose or meaning. In this way, it can be clearly differentiated from wishing or desiring—which are usually directed at very specific objects. And to separate hoping from wishing or desiring, understanding its fundamental differences, is key to recognizing it.

The self's involvement in hoping is very different from one's involvement in wishing or desiring. With a wish or desire, I am usually deeply and strongly involved. I develop strong emotional attachment or longing; I engage in obsessive behavior to attain a wish. With hoping, the process is much more quiescent. Hoping always has the nature of humility—of responsiveness, of waiting, really of awaiting.

Another basic, differentiating characteristic of hoping is its communal character. It is different, for instance, from either optimism or pessimism—both of which have an assertive, aggressive element. Both optimist and pessimist tend to say, "If only you could see things as I do." In both there persists a zeal to convert the hearer to my point of view. So, too, to doubt something, or conversely, to assert something, is rooted in the nature of self–assertiveness: *my* point of view should prevail.

Not so with hope. Rooted as it is within calamity, or catastrophe, hoping knows deeply a tragic sense of life. And within that knowledge of suffering and anguish, hoping remains always modest. Hoping knows no assertiveness. While it is intimate and private, it is usually shared quietly, without argument, without aggressiveness. It unites rather than divides, even when the auditor (perhaps physician or nurse) doesn't truly share the hope offered by the hoping person.

It's at this point, Simone Weil observes, that the most significantly spiritual act occurs when hoping appears. She writes, "We possess nothing in this world other than the power to say I. This is what we should yield up to God, and this is what we should destroy." Hoping, for Weil, involves giving up the right to oneself, offering the self as at once a gift-received from God, as a gift-given to God, in an act she terms "de-creation."

These are fundamental characteristics noted by Marcel, Weil and Pruyser. Let me suggest several more.

I have always found hoping behavior rooted in expectancy; desiring or wishing, on the contrary, seems almost always rooted in expectation. And the difference between expectancy and expectation is the difference between freedom and bondage.

A strong wish or desire enslaves me very specifically to the object of my longing, my expectation—whether this be romantic love, sexual obsession, or material gratification. Nothing satisfies Mercedes lust but a Mercedes; that poor person can never again drive either happily or safely in a Cadillac. Expectation is always concrete, always pressing, always urgent.

Expectancy is fundamentally different. It is freeing, for it is openness to an open future—a trusting, even eager, waiting for whatever is about to happen. One patient with an ominous cancer once put it this way to me: "I'm watching—really eager—to see how God is going to handle this thing." And there's usually an element of joy to the waiting, even to the waiting that is immersed in danger.

For danger is a frequent companion of hope. Hoping appears most characteristically—and some would say, only—under conditions of suffering, of catastrophe, of calamity. C.H. Spurgeon, the great 19th century London preacher, put this point succinctly: "Hope is like a star—not to be seen in the sunshine of prosperity, and only to be discovered in the night of adversity."[11] Even more stark is Simone Weil: "The dereliction in which God leaves us is his own way of caressing us."

Another element must be strongly emphasized. Hoping never emerges as some decorative aspect of confident living; it is no part of the power of positive thinking, or living. Hoping appears if, and only if, the tragic human condition—of vulnerability, of mortality, of helplessness is forthrightly faced, accepted—and, finally, both affirmed and celebrated. "Life is the destiny you are bound to refuse," W.H. Auden warns, "until you have consented to die."[12] Symbolically manifested in the sacrament of Holy Baptism, that dying—giving up one's right to oneself—Auden sees (in common with traditional Christian theology) as the key to hoping behavior, the key to life.

Explore this a bit further with me in our own context in contemporary medicine. Medicine has provided us such awesome relief from suffering, pain, anguish—that we can be easily sidetracked from facing our own personal vulnerability. Indeed, we tend to think it morbid to face either disease or death as an inevitable condition of humankind. And yet, though anesthesia, analgesics and medical technology have all been remarkable achievements of the past century, the fourth rule of Emergency Room medicine still holds immutable: bleeding always stops. Death comes.[13–14]

Hoping suggests that this basic vulnerability must be recognized, faced, even cherished—in the midst of, in spite of, our technological prowess and human ingenuity. Otherwise our lives are lives of denial, self-deception, and illusion. The prophet Jeremiah expressed this long ago—

> "They have healed the wound of my people lightly,
>> saying 'Peace, peace,'
>>> when there is no peace.

(Jeremiah 7:14, NIV)

The Biblical attitude is "always robust . . . .there's not the tiniest whine about it . . . .there is always a sting and a kick all through the Bible."[15]

The most basic Christian understanding goes even further, suggesting that *living vulnerably* is the only true sharing of the broken human condition, the only true living of hopeful lives, free lives, in this world.[16] Look for instance at the most hallowed teaching of Jesus of Nazareth, in the Beatitudes:

> Blessed are the poor in spirit,
>> for theirs is the kingdom of heaven.
> Blessed are those who mourn,
>> for they will be comforted.
> Blessed are the meek,
>> for they will inherit the earth . . . . .
> Blessed are those who are persecuted because of righteousness,
>> for theirs is the kingdom of heaven.

(Matthew 5:3ff, NIV)

This is an insistence that losing is finding, that sharing is possessing, that vulnerability—accepted, affirmed, cherished, lived—is the very key to fulfilled, purposeful life. This was put simply and starkly in a fragment of verse by Puritan divine, Richard Baxter:[17]

> I preached as never sure to preach again,
> And as a dying man, to dying men

Living hopefully, living vulnerably, in this fashion means one is willing to celebrate the temporary—to accept with a sense of joy all of that which finite, mortal, limited, conditioned, suffering, tragic, broken human life has to offer—as today's life, temporary life, abundant life, all of life. It is this affirmation which lies behind the provision of daily manna to the Israelites wandering in the desert: it was food for today. If you picked enough for tomorrow, it would spoil. If you didn't pick enough, your neighbor had enough to share. So, too, it undergirds the petition in the prayer Jesus taught: Give us this day our daily bread. John Donne emphasized the point eloquently: "We ask *panem quotidianum*, our daily bread, and God never says you should have come yesterday, he never says, you must come again tomorrow, but *today if you will hear his voice,* today he will hear you."[18]

My final point is perhaps but a repeat of all the others—hoping is basically intense concentration on God's point of view. Hoping behavior is a living, daring confidence in God that is so sure, so certain, the hoper would stake his life on it a thousand times. Paul of Tarsus, who lived through shipwrecks, floggings, imprisonments, stonings, could write from his final prison in Rome, before his execution, a letter to the Philippians that is the New Testament's paean to joy—and to hope. To vulnerable, joyful hoping. He concludes: "I have learned to be content whatever the circumstances. I know what it is to be in need, and I know what it is to have plenty . . . I can do everything through him who gives me strength . . . And my God will meet all your needs according to his glorious riches in Christ Jesus." (Philippians 4:10ff, NIV)

Let me conclude with a simple story from personal experience. The wife of a close friend, (I'll call her Hannah) had been rushed to our Emergency Room, and then to intensive care, with severe internal hemorrhaging. Physicians had told her husband that the situation looked bleak. Following a Sunday church service, he asked if I would go with him to visit his wife, and share with them prayers for healing. We went to her bedside in the ICU—where tubes and wires, as usual, stretched everywhere. He greeted her, and began what I thought was superbly understated encouragement: "You are brave, you are superb, you are my love. You're doing well. Hang in there, hang tough." It was a good sermon.

She rasped a response neither of us could understand. He asked her to repeat. She did so in the same words, apparently. Again we couldn't understand. Once more he asked her to repeat; once more with the same result. At the fourth time, she finally opened her eyes and virtually yelled, with feeble strength and failing breath, distinct, individual words, spaced out and clear: "My . . . . hand . . . . is . . . . in . . . . the . . . . hand . . . . of . . . . Jesus."

And it clearly was, for whatever outcome was impending—neither of us could any longer have doubt about that. Hannah survived.

Are there clinical ramifications to these observations? I suggested that I'd explore some, but most, I suspect, have already been readily apparent. Yet my major points perhaps should have stark, simple emphasis: There is no technology of hope. There is no technique of hope-giving. There are no professional hope-givers. "RX: Hope?" No, that's not a prescription a single one of us can write for any human being.

Hope is a gift, a gift of grace to the sufferer, in the midst of suffering, whenever it appears.

It can be a gift from the sufferer, when hope appears, to us—to anyone privileged to be a "care-giver" in the midst of suffering, if we can expectantly accept it.

We can find the gift, and recognize it, accept it—only when we are willing to admit our own vulnerability, our own final helplessness.

And my strong conviction is that we'll find it much more often than we have—if we look for it, if we're willing to find it, if we're willing to accept it, from those who suffer in our presence and under our care. We'll find that hope, and see it in our patients, if we're willing, from time to time, to put aside our expertise and our professionalism—and let heart speak to heart. If we're willing to be free, as one writer put it, "free to be merely man." And, I'll add, free to let God be God—the God of hope.

REFERENCES

1. Pound, Ezra. *The Cantos.* New York: New Directions, 1948.
2. Mack, Robert M. "Lessons from Living with Cancer," *New England Journal of Medicine* 311:1640–1644, 1984.
3. Tsongas, Paul. *Heading Home.* New York: Alfred A. Knopf, 1984.
4. Vastyan, E. A. "Spiritual Aspects of the Care of Cancer Patients," *CA-A Cancer Journal for Clinicians* 36:111–114 1986.
5. Brody, Howard. "Hope," *JAMA* 246:1411–1412 1981.

6. Buchholz, William M. "Hope," *JAMA* 263:2357–2358 1990.
7. Marcel, Gabriel. *Homo Viator.* Gloucester, MA:Peter Smith, 1978.
8. Paniches, George A. (ed.), *The Simone Weil Reader.* New York:David McKay Company, Inc., 1977.
9. Pruyser, Paul W. "Phenomenology and Dynamics of Hoping," *Journal for the Scientific Study of Religion,* Fall, 1963, pp. 86–96.
10. Pruyser, Paul W. "Maintaining Hope in Adversity," *Bulletin of the Menninger Clinics,* 463–474, 1987.
11. Spurgeon, C.H. *Morning by Morning,* Springdale, PA: Whitaker House, 1984.
12. Auden, W.H. "For The Time Being — A Christmas Oratorio", *The Collected Poetry of W.H. Auden,* New York:Random House, 1945, pp. 407–466.
13. McGill, Arthur C. "Human Suffering and the Passion of Christ," in Flavian Dougherty, C.P. (ed.), *The Meaning of Human Suffering,* New York:Human Sciences Press, 1982.
14. McGill, Arthur C. *Suffering: A Test of Theological Method,* Philadelphia: The Westminister Press, 1982.
15. Chambers, Oswald. *My Utmost for His Highest,* New York: Dodd, Mead & Company, 1935.
16. Weil, Simone. *Waiting on God,* Glasgow: William Collins Sons & Co. Ltd., 1951
17. Baxter, Richard. *Poetical Fragments,* quoted in Roger Pooley and Philip Seddon (eds.), *The Lord of the Journey,* London: Collins, 1986.
18. Donne, John. "Sermon preached at Pauls upon Christmas Day, in the evening, 1624," *The Sermons of John Donne, Vol. VI,* George R. Potter and Evelyn M. Simpson (eds.), Berkeley: University of California Press, 1953.

SECTION II

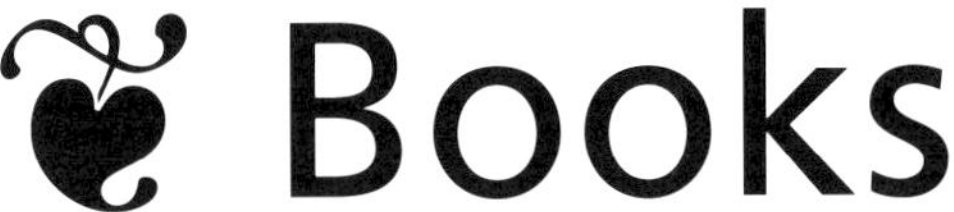 **Books**

Osler's Legacy: The Principles and Practice of Medicine

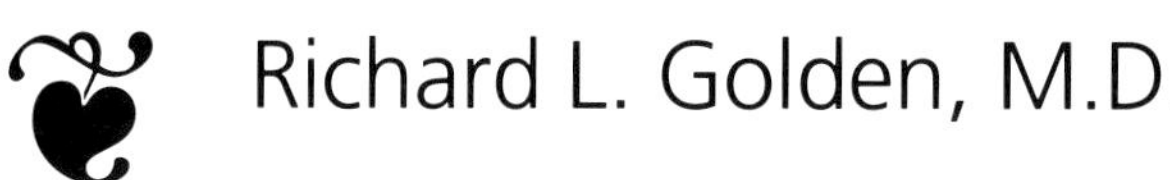 Richard L. Golden, M.D.

It was in 1890, some twenty years after beginning what he called his "inkpot career",[1] that Osler began work on the Textbook. Although there then existed no lack of competitive works, Osler in 1881 had commented on the "paucity of American text-books of medicine, and upon the modesty of the sixty-five professors of 'Theory and Practice' who for nearly twenty years had left the field in the possession of foreign authors, with whom Wood and Flint alone competed."[2] In Britain, Sir Thomas Watson's *Practice of Physic* had held sway for over four decades; and the textbook of John S. Bristowe had gone through five editions. In America there were works by Alfred L. Loomis, Nathan S. Davis, Alonzo B. Palmer, and Roberts Bartholow, which had appeared in the early 1880s. Notable among others were Pepper's *System of Practical Medicine* and Keating's *Cyclopaedia for the Diseases of Children,* to both of which Osler had contributed chapters. Watson's book was seriously out of date, and some of the others did not achieve great success, nor receive Osler's approval in review. The time was ripe for a new textbook of general medicine, and the profession looked to Osler, who, with his extraordinary background in pathology and clinical medicine, was eminently suited to the task. Moreover, his relentless pursuit of the current literature, his familiarity with the history of medicine, and his experience and facility with the written word were additional factors that promised success. His appointment as Professor of Medicine at Johns Hopkins in 1889 gave him the additional leisure time that he needed for the task. The Hospital was functioning efficiently and his subordinates were competent and able to relieve him of much of his clinical responsibilities. Fortuitously, the financial problems of the Baltimore and Ohio Railroad, whose shares endowed the University, led to a delay in the opening of the Medical School. Frustrating as this was for Osler, it reduced the level of his teaching responsibilities and gave him greater freedom for the task at hand.[2-6]

Presidential Address. Read at the annual meeting of the American Osler Society, May 8, 1990.

Reprinted with permission from *Annals of Internal Medicine, 116:*255, 1992

Osler has written graphically of the events leading to his decision:

> On several occasions, in Philadelphia, I was asked by Lea Bros. to prepare a work on Diagnosis and had half promised one; indeed I had prepared a couple of chapters, but continually procrastinated on the plea that up to the 40th year a man was fit for better things than text-books. Time went on and as I crossed this date I began to feel that the energy and persistence necessary for the task were lacking. In Sept. 1890 I returned from a four-months trip in Europe, shook myself, and towards the end of the month began a work on Practice. I had nearly finished the chapter on Typhoid Fever when Dr. Granger, Messrs. Appleton's agent, came from N.Y. to ask me to prepare a Text-book on Medicine. We haggled for a few weeks about terms and finally, selling my brains to the Devil, I signed the contract. My intention had been to publish the work myself and have Lippincott or Blakiston (both of whom offered) handle the book, but the bait of a guaranteed circulation of 10,000 copies in two years and fifteen hundred dollars on the date of publication was too glittering and I was hooked.

He goes on to describe how he accomplished the actual task of writing:

> October, November, and December were not very satisfactory months and Jan 1st 1891, saw the infectious diseases scarcely completed. I then got well into harness. Three mornings of each week I stayed at home and dictated from 8 a.m. till 1 p.m. On the alternate days I dictated after the morning hospital visit, beginning about 11.30. The spare hours of the afternoon were devoted to correction and reference work. Early in May I gave up the house, 209 Monument St., and went to my rooms at the Hospital. The routine there was: 8 a.m. to 1 p.m. dictation, 2 p.m. visit to the private patients and special cases in the wards, after which revision, and so forth. After 5 p.m. I saw any outside cases; dined at the club about 6.30, loafed until 9.30, bed at 10, and up at 7 a.m. I had arranged to send a MS. by July 1st, and on that date I forwarded five sections, but the publishers did not begin to print until the middle of August.

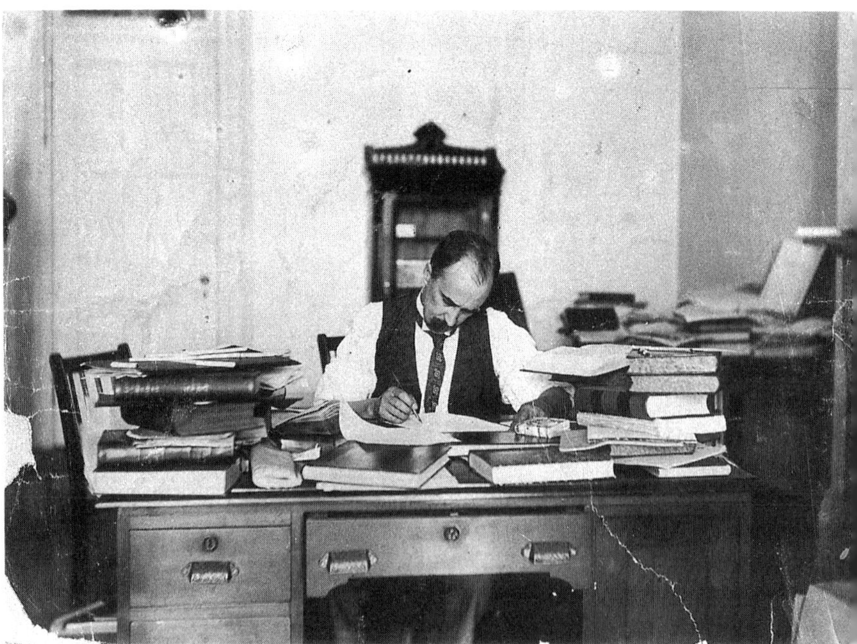

FIGURE 1.   Sir William Osler at work on *The Principles and Practice of Medicine* at The Johns Hopkins University in July 1891.

> The first two weeks of August I spent in Toronto, and then with the
> same routine I practically finished the MS. by about October 15th. During the
> summer the entire MS. was carefully revised for the press by Mr. Powell of the
> English Department of the University. The last three months of '91 were
> devoted to proof reading. In January I made out the index, and in the entire
> work nothing so wearied me as the verifying of every reference. Without the
> help of Lafleur and Thayer who took the wards off my hands I never could
> have finished in so short a time; my other assistants rendered much aid in
> looking up references and special points.
>
> During the writing of the work I lost only one afternoon through a
> transient indisposition and never a night's rest. Between September 1890 and
> January 1892 I gained nearly 8 lbs in weight.[7]

Osler did much of his writing in the suite of Hunter Robb, commandeered for its size and favorable location. Robb, the senior resident in gynecology at Johns Hopkins Hospital humorously describes the scene from a rather different viewpoint:

> He asked me if I would loan him the use of my library for an hour or so
> in the mornings. I of course said, 'Yes, with great pleasure'. The first morning,
> he appeared with one book under his arm accompanied by his stenographer,
> Miss Humpton. When the morning's work was over, he left the book on my
> library desk, wide open with a marker in it. The next morning he brought two
> books with him, and so on for the next two weeks, so that the table and all the
> chairs and the sofa and the piano and even the floor was covered with open
> books. As a consequence I was never able to use the room for fully six months.
> Oftentimes right in the middle of his dictating he would rush into my other
> room, and ask me to match quarters with him, or we would engage in an
> exchange of yarns. It was a great treat for me, and except when he would court
> inspiration by kicking my waste-paper basket about the room, I thoroughly
> enjoyed his visits.[8]

Although Robb makes no mention of it, he apparently cured Osler of his waste basket indiscretion by filling it one day with a quantity of concealed bricks![9]

The book was a great success in more ways than one. He received the first copy on February 24, 1892 and the next day, according to the time honored story, presented it to Grace Revere Gross, tossing the large red book into her lap saying, "There, take the darn thing; now what are you going to do with the man?"[10,11] This apparently referred to a previous proposal when he had threatened to let the book "go hang." The "widow Gross", as he sometimes facetiously referred to her, had sagely advised the shoemaker to stick to his last.[12] While perhaps not the most romantic of proposals, it served as the successful forerunner to their marriage on May 7th, 1892. The book that he gave to Grace was the first state of the first edition distinguished by the superfluous *'e'* in *G(e)orgias* in the Platonic inscription on the verso of the third leaf. Three thousand copies were quickly distributed before the appearance of the second state in April 1892 in which the *Gorgias* error was corrected.[7,11,13] It is a curious and little known fact that this same error reappeared in the first printing of the tenth edition in 1925.[14] Osler did not retain a copy of the first state other than the one given to Grace. His working copy of the second state was a specially bound two volume interleaved set in which he inscribed, *"Private copy.* May all the curses of the good Bishop Ernulphus light on the borrower-and-not-returner or upon the stealer of this book."[7] The curse, recorded by, but unjustly attributed to the good Bishop, no doubt came from Laurence Sterne's, *Tristram Shandy,* a favorite of Osler.[15,16] On a prospectus

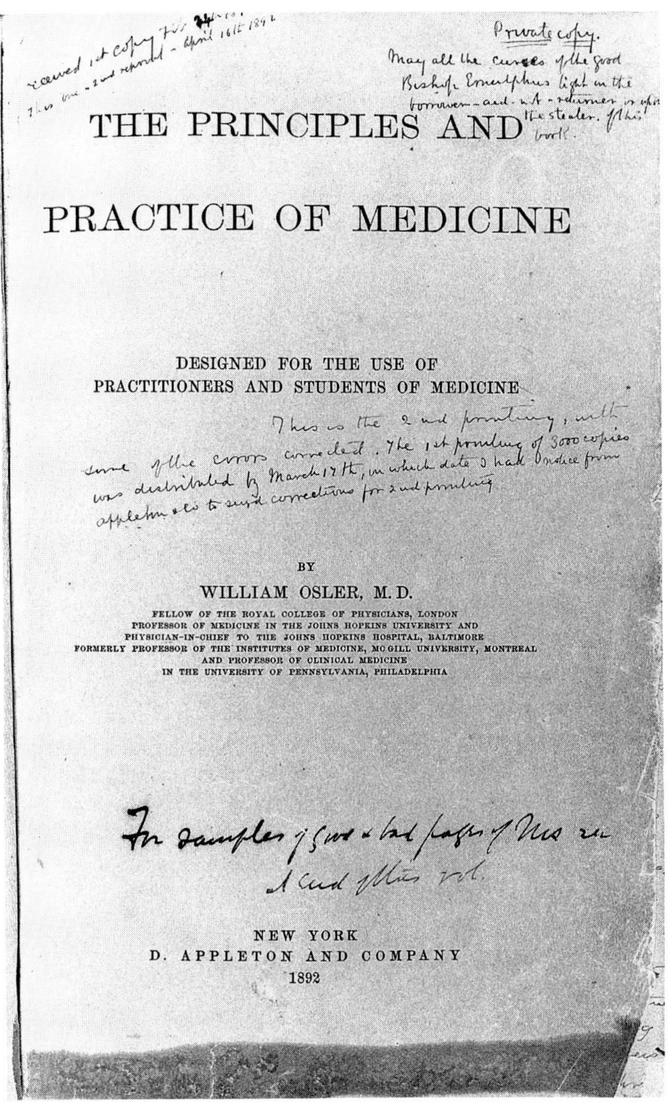

FIGURE 2.   The title page of Sir William Osler's copy of the first edition (second state) of the textbook with his annotations.

inserted into the volume he wrote, "This, thank the Lord, I did not write."[7] An astounding 23,500 copies of the first edition were sold before the appearance of the second edition in 1895, more than fulfilling the Appelton guarantee, and providing him with a new found measure of financial independence.[17]

Osler's textbook was a marvel of precision, clarity, and up–to–date information based on a solid foundation of pathology. It was filled with literary and classical allusions and written with such style as to make it eminently readable and enjoyable. Falconer Madan, the Bodleian Librarian, eloquently expressed these feelings when he said that Osler "succeeded in making a scientific treatise literature."[3] The book, sometimes irreverently referred to by the students as "the given word," was based on morbid anatomy and oriented to specific diseases. Each disease was generally defined, its historical background given when possible, and followed by an analysis divided into etiology, transmission, morbid anatomy, symptoms, diagnosis, prognosis, prophylaxis and treatment. Osler leaned heavily on his experience as a pathologist, using the material in the volumes containing his autopsy notes, which he borrowed from the Montreal General Hospital. This is reflected in the textbook in the emphasis on morbid anatomy.[3,6,18,19] The one major criticism leveled against *The Principles and Practice* was the paucity of therapeutic information. Labelled a "therapeutic nihilist" by some, and more euphemistically a "therapeutic conservative" or "sceptic" by others, Osler forthrightly acknowledged the lack of effective therapy for most diseases.[3,20] By way of example, in the discussion on pneumonia he states that, "Pneumonia is a self-limited disease, and runs its course uninfluenced in any way by medicine. It can neither be aborted nor cut short by any means at our command. Even under the most unfavorable circumstances it will terminate abruptly and naturally, without a dose of medicine having been administered."[21] His conservative attitude on the value of most contemporary drugs was characterized uncharitably, as "paranoia antitherapeuticum Baltimorensis."[22] Osler did not subscribe to the polypharmacy and homeopathy of his day and had pronounced upon the problem in his famous aphorism: "The desire to take medicine is one feature which distinguishes man, the animal, from his fellow creatures."[23] In describing Osler's trip to France in 1909, Cushing whimsically relates a local practitioner's observation that medical practice in Cannes was divided into two parts—practice for the English ladies and practice for the American ladies. For the latter group, great caution was necessary in prescribing "since every American lady travelled with Osler's *Practice of Medicine* in her trunk."[24] Humor aside, it should not be construed that Osler's conservatism precluded the use of all drugs.[25] He advocated, among others, the use of iron in anemia, quinine in malaria, nitroglycerine and amyl nitrite in angina pectoris, and 'G.O.M.', ("God's own medicine") as he called morphine, for pain. Nevertheless, one of his favorite prescriptions was "Time, in divided doses."[26]

The Principles and Practice of Medicine was an immediate 'best seller' and was received with acclaim in America and Britain.[11] It quickly superceded all other competing textbooks including William Pepper's, *An American Textbook of the Theory and Practice of Medicine,* to which Osler had contributed several chapters.[27] In addition to some 23,500 copies of the first edition, an additional 17,500 of the second were sold, for a total of 41,000 copies of the first two editions.[17] By the time of the sixth edition in 1905, some 105,000 copies had been printed, with the 100,000th copy presented to Osler's son, Revere.[28,29] His royalties on the textbook at this time amounted to $54,512, equivalent to just over $1,000,000 in 1992 terms.[25] Ultimately almost five hundred thousand copies were sold.[30] This was truly a remarkable achievement for a medical textbook and stood in solid support of Cushing's characterization as the "most used and useful book in medicine."[31]

The multiplicity of literary and historical allusions that embellish the textbook bear testimony to Osler's firm grounding in the classics and his knowledge and passion for the history of medicine. Fielding H. Garrison commented on this as a stimulus to the reader's ignorance, and as a means of catching his attention.[32] Where else but in Osler is chlorosis described by Maudlin's song from Issak Walton's *The Compleat Angler,* telling of the "green sickness" which spares country bred girls?[33] Obesity becomes an "oily dropsy" in the words of Lord Byron.[34] In a remarkable correlation of literature and medicine he relates that, "An extraordinary phenomenon in excessively fat young persons is an uncontrollable tendency to sleep—like the fat boy in Pickwick."[35] This Dickensian description has come to be known as the Pickwickian syndrome.[36] In the discussion on syphilitic aortic valvular disease,

Osler writes, "I was in the habit of enforcing upon my students the etiological lesson by a mythological reference to Bacchus and Vulcan, at whose shrine a majority of those cases of aortic insufficiency has worshipped, and not a few at that of Venus."[37] We are told that the *pesta magna* described by Galen is believed to have been small pox and that Marcus Aurelius died of it.[38] Lobar pneumonia is graphically described in John Bunyan's phrase as the "Captain of the Men of Death."[39]

Osler called the book his "quiz compend" and it was the subject of much affectionate humor.[40] In 1902 an amusing mock examination paper, based on the fourth edition, was published in *St. Thomas's Hospital Gazette* on the many erudite and obscure literary allusions in the text. It began with "Who was Mephibosheth?" and included such arcana as "Who had a translucent head?"[41,42] The examination was expanded in 1907 according to Osler by the "boys" at the Johns Hopkins Hospital, although the suggestion is said to have come from Osler himself.[42–45] The test was reprinted in different versions over the years, the last in 1973 by Tigertt, with a complete set of answers.[46] In 1907, Tales from Osler, a game of "Consequences," appeared in *St. Thomas's Hospital Gazette* which again put the well–read student of Osler to the test.[47]

1909 saw the appearance of a poem entitled "The Student's Guide to Osler" in *Guy's Hospital Gazette*.[44,48,49] With a cadence somewhat reminiscent of Gilbert and Sullivan it was another spoof of Osler's erudition and use of esoteric references and names in the sixth edition. The poem gently chides Osler as follows:

> For why should it matter to usward,
> > If Osborn has sent you a screed,
> Or why have you sought a brief mention of Porter,
> > Or Barker, or Caton or Reed?
> I sometimes am seized with a yearning,
> > In Appelton's ledger to look,
> What fun it would be if only we could see
> > Whether each of them purchased the book!

Humor was but one minor aspect of the book. A dramatic and far reaching event took place in July 1897 when a member of John D. Rockefeller's philanthropic staff, Frederick T. Gates, read the second edition of the Textbook from cover to cover during his summer vacation. Gates, a Baptist minister, was deeply impressed with the book. His account of this event deserves retelling:

> In the early summer of 1897 my interest in medicine was awakened by a . . . Minneapolis boy who in his loneliness in New York often spent his week-ends with us in Montclair. . . . . I determined as a result of my talks with the enthusiastic young student to make myself more intelligent on the whole subject of medicine, and at his suggestion I bought a copy of Dr. Osler's *Principles and Practice of Medicine* . . . I read the whole book without skipping any of it. I speak of this not to commemorate my industry or intelligence but to testify to Osler's charm, for it is one of the very few scientific books that are possessed of a high literary quality. There was a fascination about the style itself that led me on, and having once started I found a hook in my nose that pulled me from page to page, and chapter to chapter, until the whole of about a thousand large and closely printed pages brought me to the end.
>
> But there were other things besides its style that attracted and intensified my interest . . .To the layman student, like me, demanding cures, and specifics, he had no word of comfort whatever. In fact, I saw clearly from the work of this thoroughly enlightened, able and honest man, perhaps the

> foremost practitioner in the world, that medicine had—with the few exceptions . . . noted—no cures, and that about all medicine up to 1897 could do was to suggest some measure of relief, how to nurse the sick, and to alleviate in some way the suffering. Beyond this, medicine as a cure had not progressed. . . .
>
> When I laid down this book I began to realize how woefully neglected in all civilized countries and perhaps most of all in this country, had been the scientific study of medicine. . . . It became clear to me that medicine could hardly hope to become a science until it should be endowed, and qualified men could give themselves to uninterrupted study and investigation, on ample salary, entirely independent of practice. . . . Here was an opportunity for Mr. Rockefeller to become a pioneer. . . .

Gates goes on to tell of how he brought these ideas to Rockefeller's attention:

> Filled with these thoughts and enthusiasms, I returned from my vacation . . . and . . . dictated for Mr. Rockefeller's eye a memorandum in which I aimed to show to him the actual condition of medicine in the United States and the world as disclosed by Dr. Osler's book. . . . I remember insisting that even if the proposed institute should fail to discover anything, the fact that he, Mr. Rockefeller, had established such an institute of research, would result in other institutes of a similar kind, or at least other funds for research being established, until research in this country would be established on a grand scale; and that out of the multitudes of workers we might be sure in the end of abundant rewards, even though those rewards might not come directly from the institute which he might found.

Gates then relates the outcome of these proposals:

> These considerations took root in the mind of Mr. Rockefeller and, later, of his son. Eminent physicians were consulted as to the feasibility of the project, a competent agency was employed to secure the counsel of specialists on research, and out of wide consultation the Rockefeller Institute of Medical Research came into being. It had its origin in Dr. Osler's perfectly frank disclosure of the very narrow limitations of ascertained truth in medicine as it existed in 1897.[50]

Gates's fascination with Osler's scientific candor and literary style in *The Principles and Practice* began a chain of events that influenced the establishment of the Rockefeller Institute in 1901, and the Rockefeller Foundation in 1913.[51] The Harvard Medical School received $1,000,000 from the Institute in 1902, a gift described by Gates as growing directly out of Osler's book.[52] In 1904, following a devastating Baltimore fire, the Johns Hopkins Hospital received $500,000 in Rockefeller aid after Osler had appealed to Gates for help.[53] In 1913 the General Education Board of the Rockefeller Foundation under the chairmanship of Frederick Gates gave $1,500,000 towards the establishment of the full-time system at Johns Hopkins.[54] Rockefeller funds were also instrumental in the establishment of the Johns Hopkins School of Hygiene and Public Health in 1918, and the Institute of the History of Medicine and the Wilmer Institute in 1929.[55] The China Medical Board, a division of the Rockefeller Foundation, was established in 1914, and financed numerous health and education projects in China, including the Peking Union Medical College.[56] In a full cycle it helped to finance the translation of Osler's textbook into Chinese.[57,58]

Although the book had a profound effect on medical philanthropy and its derivatives, its major impact was from its influence on the education and practice of generations of students of medicine, both in the English-speaking world and beyond through its translations.[17] Recognized as a "medical masterpiece'' it quickly became the standard textbook of medicine and went through sixteen editions from 1892 to 1947, encompassing almost five hundred thousand copies.[30,59] The pursuit of the more than 100 editions, states, printings, variants, and translations would be an almost impossible task today even for the most dedicated bibliophile. Cushing wrote that, ''Someone, some day, could well write a volume devoted to a study of the successive editions of this famous work, which continues to exert an enormous influence on students of medicine. . . . ''[17]

Each edition with the exception of the 14th, 15th and 16th editions carried a dedication to Osler's revered teachers, William Arthur Johnson, priest of the parish of Weston; James Bovell of the Toronto School of Medicine; and Robert Palmer Howard, professor of medicine at McGill. The new editions generally appeared at three to five year intervals, major exceptions being the fifth and ninth editions. The fifth edition appeared in 1902 only one year after the publication of the previous edition. This was necessitated by an oversight in which the copyright had not been taken in Great Britain. An unauthorized fourth edition was promptly printed in Edinburgh by Young J. Pentland at a substantially reduced price—the so called pirated edition.[14,60] In London, Henry Kimpton published a fourth British edition made from American sheets. Thus in 1901, there were three distinct American and British fourth editions on the market.[61] Osler wrote, ''I regret the mistake which has disturbed the normal process of triennial parturition, but the circumstances justify what Rabelais called 'the pretty perquisite of a super-foetation'.''[62] The seventh edition, sometimes considered the zenith of the series, reflected the considerable scientific advances that had taken place since 1892, and was the last that Osler did alone. The eighth edition of 1912 and the

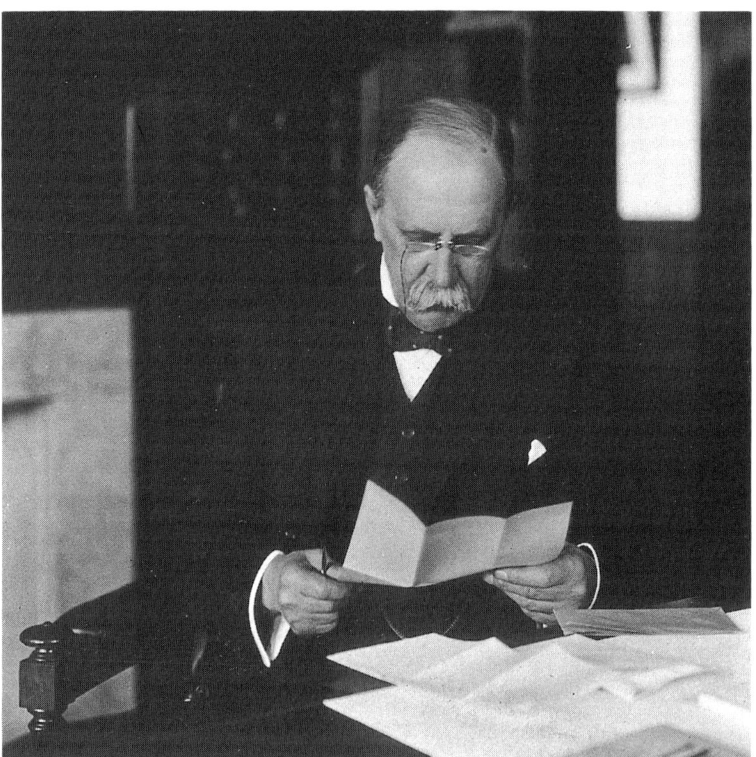

FIGURE 3. Sir William Osler as Regius Professor of Medicine at Oxford.

posthumous ninth edition of 1920 were done with the assistance of Thomas McCrae, marking an unusual hiatus of eight years between them. This no doubt resulted from the burdens of the war, the death of Revere, and Osler's deteriorating health. McCrae continued the revisions through the twelfth edition, after which the mantle passed to Henry A. Christian of Harvard University. Christian, maintaining the one-man book tradition, carried it through the sixteenth and final edition.[63] Thus, after an extraordinary run of fifty-five years, publication ceased in 1947. This can be attributed to diminished sales, the decline in popularity of single author textbooks, the advent of newer books such as Cecil's, and the gradual loss of Osler's imprint. Perhaps he was prophetic when he once said that "even great textbooks die like their authors."[64]

Among the overseas publications there was a series of British editions which was for the most part Appleton volumes with cancel titles and appropriate bindings.[63] This, together with the many translations of *The Principles and Practice,* gave the book and Osler's teachings a truly global impact. Osler's bibliographers show the first translation into French in 1908, followed by German, Chinese, Spanish and Portuguese editions.[63,65,66] Newer research, however, reveals that the first translation was a hitherto unknown Russian edition in 1905, preceeding the French work by almost three years. The Russian translation entitled *Handbook of Internal and Neurological Diseases. For Doctors and Students,* was published in two volumes, the first in 1905 and the second in 1906. These were translated from the fifth edition by Dr. S. Z. Serebrennikov, and published in St. Petersburg by *Contemporary Medicine and Hygiene.*[67] In 1928 still another Russian translation appeared which also remained unknown in the West. Entitled *Handbook on Internal Medicine,* it was translated from the tenth edition by T. and V. Ravinskii and edited by Professor M. Breitman. It contained a portrait and biography of Osler and was published by the *Practical Medicine Company* of Leningrad.[67]

The German edition, a translation of the sixth American edition, was published in Berlin in 1909.[63] There were three Chinese editions, based on the fifth through the ninth editions. These were printed initially in Yokohama and later in Shanghai. They were translated through the efforts of Dr. Philip B. Cousland, a Scottish medical missionary. The Chinese books spanned the years 1909 to 1934 including reprints and appendices.[58,63] Cousland in a letter to Osler said of the book that, "It is the first complete textbook in medicine to be translated into Chinese and should be the means of relieving and preventing untold suffering among the teeming population."[68] A Spanish translation based on the eighth edition was published in Barcelona in 1915 and reprinted by Appleton in New York the following year. A Portuguese translation of the fourteenth edition was brought out in Rio de Janeiro in 1945. A further Spanish translation of the fifteenth edition appeared in Buenos Aires in 1949, the last of the foreign editions.[63] These translations, together with the discovery of the Russian editions, attest strongly to Osler's truly world-wide influence.

The burden of the frequent revisions of his textbook was quickly felt by Osler. In the words of Cushing, "The birth of a successful text-book, like that of a child, may hold its authors in unexpected bondage. . . . "[20] This sentiment was expressed by Osler in a letter to Francis J. Shepherd in 1898, in which he lamented: "I am over head & ears in my 3rd Edition—infernal nuisance."[69] In 1907 while in the midst of the revision of the seventh edition he began to have thoughts and concerns about the future evolution of the textbook, and the transfer of responsibility. He wrote of this to Lewellys S. Barker, who had taken his place at Johns Hopkins.

> I want an hour's chat with you about the Text-book. This new edition, due October 1908, will not be a very serious revision, as they will not break up the plates, but in the next edition we can do as we like. It would be very nice if you and Thayer came in with me as joint authors. It would be possible, I think, to arrange to have the work kept up as a Johns Hopkins Hospital Text-book of Medicine. I think some arrangements could be made with the publishers and some plan devised by which the head of the Medical Department would have *ex-officio* rights in it. In the IXth edition I would probably go out altogether and the book would appear from you and Thayer—perhaps I retaining a small financial interest.[70]

Barker was apparently unreceptive, and the issue remained dormant until January 1910 when Osler again suggested that Barker take over the forthcoming 1912 edition. He wrote,

> Naturally, I have a strong sentiment about the book, but I know quite well that the life and success of a work depends upon the life of a man, and it is quite to the interests of the publishers as well as my own, to make provision for a gradual or immediate transfer of editorial control.[71]

The proposal was withdrawn several months later and it was Thomas McCrae, his former resident and now professor of medicine at the Jefferson Medical College, who became co-author of the eighth edition.[72] With the passing of Osler in 1919, McCrae assumed full control of the ninth through the twelfth editions, retaining the single author concept.[63]

It was not until 1968, after a publication hiatus of twenty-one years, that Osler's dream of a Johns Hopkins textbook of medicine achieved reality. Using the same name and numeration, the seventeenth edition of *The Principles and Practice of Medicine* was published by Appleton-Century-Crofts under the editorship of Dr. A. McGehee Harvey and his co-workers from Johns Hopkins.[73] This was not a revision of Osler's book, nor the work of a single man; but rather a multi-authored work by the Johns Hopkins faculty, employing a patient- rather than a disease-oriented approach. Successive quadrennial editions have appeared, the last being the twenty-second edition of 1988.[63,74] The book is the product of a medical school maintaining the tradition of Osler and continuing the name and numeration of the original series, thus preserving the spirit of Osler and his magnum opus, and bringing to fruition his vision of a Johns Hopkins textbook of medicine.

References

1. Osler W. *Bibliotheca Osleriana*. Montreal and London: McGill-Queen's University Press, 1969:xxiii.
2. Osler W. *Review of recent works on practice*. Am J Med Sc 1885; n. s., 89:175-181.
3. Cushing H. *The Life of Sir Wiliam Osler*. Oxford: Clarendon Press, 1925:i, 339–340.
4. Pepper W, ed., (assisted by Starr L). *A System of Practical Medicine by American Authors*. Philadelphia: Lea Bros. & Co., 1885.
5. Keating JM, ed. *Cyclopaedia of the Diseases of Children: Medical and Surgical*. Philadelphia: J. B. Lippincott, 1889.

6. Harvey AM, McKusick V. *Osler's Textbook Revisited*. New York: Appleton-Century-Crofts, 1967:1–7.

7. Osler W. *Bibliotheca Osleriana*. Montreal and London: McGill-Queen's University Press, 1969:# 3544.

8. Cushing H. *The Life of Sir William Osler*. Oxford: Clarendon Press, 1925:i, 349.

9. Cushing H. *The Life of Sir William Osler*. Oxford: Clarendon Press, 1925:i, 350

10. Osler, W. *Bibliotheca Osleriana*. Montreal and London: McGill-Queen's University Press, 1969:# 3543.

11. Cushing H. *The Life of Sir William Osler*. Oxford: Clarendon Press, 1925:i, 357–358.

12. Cushing H. *The Life of Sir William Osler*. Oxford: Clarendon Press, 1915:i, 351.

13. Golden RL, Roland CG. *Sir William Osler. An Annotated Bibliography with Illustrations*. San Francisco: Norman Publishing, 1988:1375

14. MacDermot HE. *Notes on the early editions of Osler's Textbook of Medicine*. Ann Med Hist 1934; n. s., 6:224–240.

15. Francis WW. *At Osler's shrine*. Bull Med Library Assoc 1937; 26:1–8.

16. Sterne L. *The Life & Opinions of Tristram Shandy, Gentleman*. New York: The Heritage Press, 1935:Book III, Chapt. XII.

17. Cushing H. *The Life of Sir William Osler*. Oxford: Clarendon Press, 1925:422, 473.

18. Abbott ME. *"More about Osler."* Bull Hist Med; 1937; 5:765–796.

19. Rodin AE. Oslerian Pathology. *An Assessment and Annotated Atlas of Museum Specimens*. Lawrence, KS: Coronado Press, 1981:5–19.

20. Cushing H. *The Life of Sir William Osler*. Oxford: Clarendon Press, 1925:i, 359, 391.

21. Osler W. *The Principles and Practice of Medicine*. Ed. 1, New York: D. Appleton and Company, 1892:529.

22. Golden RL, Roland CG. *Sir William Osler. An Annotated Bibliography with Illustrations*. San Francisco: Norman Publishing, 1988:152.

23. Bean RB, Bean WB. *Sir William Osler. Aphorisms from his Bedside Teachings and Writings*. Springfield: Charles C Thomas, 1961:# 210.

24. Cushing H. *The Life of Sir William Osler*. Oxford: Clarendon Press, 1925:ii, 158.

25. Harrell GT. *Osler's Practice*. Bull Hist Med 1973; 47:545–567.

26. Toulmin H. *Recollections of Sir William Osler*. Int Assoc Med Mus Bull (Special Osler Memorial No.) 1926:9, 229–231.

27. Cushing H. *The Life of Sir William Osler*. Oxford: Clarendon Press. 1925:i, 360.

28. Cushing H. *The Life of Sir William Osler*. Oxford: Clarendon Press, 1925:ii, 21.

29. Golden RL, Roland CG. *Sir William Osler. An Annotated Bibliography with Illustrations*. San Francisco: Norman Publishing, 1988, # 1399.

30. Robb-Smith AHT. *The story behind the Osler plaque*. Ox Med Sch Gaz (amended reprint). 1988; xxviii (3):18–20; 1989; xxix (1):17–19; (2):18–20.

31. Cushing H. *William Osler, the man*. Ann Med Hist 1920; 2:157–167.

32. Garrison FH. *Sir William Osler's contribution to medical literature*. Ann Med Hist 1919; 2:184–187, 1919.

33. Osler W. *The Principles and Practice of Medicine*. Ed. 2, New York: D. Appleton and Company, 1895:1077.

34. Osler W. *The Principles and Practice of Medicine.* Ed. 6, New York: D. Appleton and Company, 1905:721.

35. Burwell CS et al. *Extreme obesity associated with alveolvar hypoventilation—A Pickwickian Syndrome.* Am J. Med 1956; 21:811–818.

36. Osler W. *The Principles and Practice of Medicine.* Ed.6, New York: D. Appleton and Company, 1905:431.

37. Osler W. *The Principles and Practice of Medicine.* Ed. 1, New York: D. Appleton and Company, 1892:603.

38. Osler W. *The Principles and Practice of Medicine.* Ed. 1, New York: D. Appleton and Company, 1892:46.

39. Osler W. *The Principles and Practice of Medicine.* Ed. 4, New York: D. Appleton and Company, 1901:108.

40. Cushing H. *The Life of Sir William Osler.* Oxford: Clarendon Press, 1925:i, 356, 413.

41. D.M.S. (Dudgeon LS, Mavrogordato A, Scott SG) *An examination paper on Osler (fourth edition).* St. Thomas's Hosp Gaz 1902; 12:59–60.

42. Osler W. *Bibliotheca Osleriana.* Montreal and London: McGill-Queen's University Press, 1969:# 3586.

43. D.M.S. (Dudgeon LS, Mavrogordato A, Scott SG) *"Hospital Notes."* St. Thomas's Hosp Gaz 1907; 17:196–197.

44. Osler W. *Bibliotheca Osleriana.* Montreal and London: McGill-Queen's University Press, 1969:# 3587.

45. MacDermot HE. *The lighter aspects of Osler's textbook.* Can Med Assoc J 1949; 61:76–78.

46. Tigertt WD. *Annotated answers to the 1902 examination on Osler's Principles and Practice of Medicine.* Ann Int Med 1973; 79:460–472.

47. *Tales from Osler.* St. Thomas's Hosp. Gaz 1907: 17:195–197.

48. "S. S." (Brookhouse HO). *The student's guide to Osler.* Guys Hosp Gaz 1909: 23:420.

49. LeRoy EC, Wallis F, Sawyer WA. *A student's ode to Osler's text republished with notes.* Can Bull Med Hist 1989: 6:57–66.

50. Cushing H. *The Life of Sir William Osler.* Oxford: Clarendon Press, 1925:i, 454–456.

51. Cushing H. *The Life of Sir William Osler.* Oxford: Clarendon Press, 1925:i, 550–551; ii, 245.

52. Cushing H. *The Life of Sir William Osler.* Oxford: Clarendon Press, 1925:i, 573–574.

53. Cushing H. *The Life of Sir William Osler.* Oxford: Clarendon Press, 1925:i, 633–635.

54. Cushing H. *The Life of Sir William Osler.* Oxford: Clarendon Press, 1925:ii, 383.

55. Bernheim BM. *The Story of Johns Hopkins.* New York, Toronto, Whittlesey House, 1948:118, 170–176,

56. Wong KC, Wu L. *History of Chinese Medicine.* Ed. 2, Shanghai: National Quarantine Service, 1936:633–635, 686.

57. Cousland PB. Preface. In: Osler W. *The Principles and Practice of Medicine.* 2nd Chinese ed., Shanghai: China Medical Missionary Association, 1921.

58. Golden RL, Summers GV. *The history of the Chinese translations of Sir William Osler's textbook.* Hong Kong Library Assoc J 1984; no. 8:27–37.

59. Cushing H. *The Life of Sir William Osler.* Oxford: Clarendon Press, 1925:i, 242.

60. Osler, W. *Bibliotheca Osleriana.* Montreal and London: McGill-Queen's University Press, 1969:# 3548, 3549.

61. Golden RL, Roland CG. *Sir William Osler. An Annotated Bibliography with Illustrations*. San Francisco: Norman Publishing, 1988:# 1394, 1447, 1448.
62. Osler W. *An Explanation*. Lancet 1903;i, 1058.
63. Golden RL, Roland CG. *Sir William Osler. An Annotated Bibliography with Illustrations*. San Francisco: Norman Publishing, 1988:136–148.
64. Gilcreest EL. *Sir William Osler—physician and philanthropist—Glimpses during the World War*. Int Assoc Med Mus Bull (Special Osler Memorial No.) 1926:9, 409–418.
65. Blogg MW. *Bibliography of the Writings of Sir William Osler*. Baltimore: Lord Baltimore Press, 1921.
66. Abbott ME. *Classified and Annotated Bibliography of Sir William Osler's Writings*. Montreal: The Medical Museum, McGill University, 1939.
67. Golden RL. *A note on the Russian translations of Sir William Osler's textbook*. J Hist Med & Allied Sci 1990:45, 490–493.
68. Golden RL. *Osler and Oriental Medicine*. Princeton: Science Press Associates, Inc., 1982:5–6.
69. Cushing H. *Life of Sir William Osler*. Oxford: Clarendon Press, 1925:i, 470.
70. Cushing H. *Life of Sir William Osler*. Oxford: Clarendon Press, 1925:ii, 86–87.
71. Cushing H. *Life of Sir William Osler*. Oxford: Clarendon Press, 1925:ii, 209.
72. Cushing H. *Life of Sir William Osler*. Oxford: Clarendon Press, 1925:ii, 293, 303, 308.
73. Harvey AM, Johns RJ, Owens Jr. AH, Ross RS. *The Principles and Practice of Medicine*. New York: Appleton-Century-Crofts, 1968.
74. Lambert RH. *Osler and his publishers*. Tran & Studies of the Coll of Phys of Philadelphia; 1983; ser. 5, vol. 5, no. 3:177–190.

A Student's Ode to Osler's Text Republished with Notes

 E. Carwile LeRoy, M.D., Faith Wallis, Ph.D., and Warren A. Sawyer

Sir William Osler's *The Principles and Practice of Medicine,* first published in 1892, was the standard textbook of internal medicine for more than 50 years.[1] The text was exemplary in its systematic organization and original observations and, as one reviewer of the first edition stated: "everywhere throughout the work one feels the delightful personality of the man."[2] Tucked between the leaves of William Osler's own copies of *The Principles and Practice of Medicine,* or mounted into his private scrapbook, are dozens of letters from readers in praise of his textbook. Most of these correspondents were prominent physicians, and being Victorian professional gentlemen, they concentrated their admiration on the book's learned, lucid, and practical qualities. A few of them stepped outside this conventional mode—Alfred Stillé, for instance, appeared to think that the best thing about *The Principles and Practice* was the degree with which Osler's views coincided with his own—but the great majority echoed the judgment of William White, the Philadelphia surgeon: "I have thus far found the information I sought conveyed in a clear and satisfactory manner and embodying the latest clinical and pathological views in a condensed, but sufficiently comprehensive form."[3]

Yet not one of these stately letters bends from the nineteenth-century proprieties to admit that *The Principles and Practice* is not only useful, but vastly entertaining and even occasionally funny. The locus of this humor is the literary allusions, historical anecdotes, and curiosities of medicine that Osler slipped between the lines of his didactic prose, often with devastating dead-pan wit. Medical students, troubled by no scruples of seriousness, took many opportunities to celebrate the amusing side of Osler's textbook.

Because *The Principles and Practice* is a textbook, the obvious vehicle for a

Read at the annual meeting of the American Osler Society, May 4, 1988.

Reprinted with permission from *Canadian Bulletin of Medical History, 6*:57, 1989 student "roast" is a bogus examination paper. Such was "An Examination Paper on Osler (4th Edition)," printed in the *St Thomas's Hospital Gazette* in 1902.[4] When Osler visited St Thomas's in 1907, the president of the Medical and Physical Society presented him with a bound copy of the examination paper, now no. 3586 in the *Bibliotheca Osleriana*. On the flyleaf Osler noted that "at the J[ohns] H[opkins] H[ospital] the boys added to the examination paper," and in its expanded form, "with the interpretations of American scholiasts," it was reprinted in the *St Thomas's Hospital Gazette* in 1907.[5] The "boys" at JHH were none other than Osler himself, abetted by his pseudonymous *alter ego*, E.Y. Davis.[6]

With the St Thomas's students in the van, even their sober-sided elders joined the fun. The same White of Philadelphia who had measured out much cool and businesslike praise of the textbook sent Osler a complete set of answers to the "Examination Paper" a month after it was published.[7] The "Examination Paper" was reprinted in the 1930s and 1940s[8] and answers to the questions were still being tracked down in 1973.[9] An updated version was presented before the Osler Club of London by G. F. Abercrombie in 1959.[10] But the St Thomas's joke was not the only shaft of student wit aimed at *The Principles and Practice of Medicine*. The poem presented here was first published in *Guy's Hospital Gazette* on 2 October 1909.[11] Entitled, "The Student's Guide to Osler," it is a humorous piece, gently poking fun at Osler's use of obscure persons, places, and things in the text.

We publish the poem again, with notes, to provide the reader not familiar with Osler's text a glimpse from a student's perspective of writing that is excellent, alive, and memorable. Has any student of *The Principles and Practice of Medicine* forgotten Conoquenessing?

The poem is as follows:

The Student's Guide to Osler

Some people are keen upon Taylor[12]
  When studying medicine's wiles,
While others will steal a few moments with Wheeler[13]
  —Both excellent books in their styles—
But give me the text-book of Osler
  (Or don't, for I've bought it by now!)
And set *con amore* the laurel of glory
  On William of Baltimore's brow.

It isn't so much that it's brainy,
  Although it's undoubtedly that,
I'm not eulogistic because each statistic
  Comes out so impressively pat.
It's all for the sake of the stories
  He tells with a vigour so rare;
No poisonous bloater has dogged Minnesota,
  But goes to posterity there.

Micawber, Tom Brown, Colonel Newcome,[14]
  And other most excellent men,
My late predilections in popular fictions
  Have passed from my ultimate ken.
For now I would dream of new heroes,
  Physicians from every clime,
And Surgeons of valour in Osler's Valhalla
  Who tell of the deeds of their time.

Hippocrates gaily discourses
    Of Erysipelatous lore,[15]
And tells what the sight is of peritonitis[16]
    For those who've not seen it before.
Pneumonia spurred Aretaeus[17]
    To study its devious laws,
Which object titanic was followed by Laennec,[18]
    Till Fraenkel[19] discovered the cause.

And doubtless our myriad Guy's men
    May well be turgescent with pride,
As they scan with delight the remarks of Hale White[20]
    On a case of cirrhosis that died!
There's a whole paragraph about Pitt's[21] work
    On effects of arterial flaw,
Which makes me repine at the solit'ry line
    That's allotted to Perry and Shaw.[22]

But dearest are those to you, William
    Who shed in impetuous pars
Their knowledge like manna beneath the bright banner
    That glows with the Stripes and the Stars.
Gerhard,[23] Cushing,[24] Fitz,[25] and Weir Mitchell,[26]
    We honour, but what of each name
That you print till they're more than the sands
    of the shore,
And equally worthy of fame?

For why should it matter to usward,
If Osborn[27] has sent you a screed,
    Or why have you sought a brief mention of Porter,[28]
Or Barker,[29] or Caton,[30] or Reed?[31]
    I sometimes am seized with a yearning,
In Appleton's[32] ledger to look,
    What fun it would be if we only could see
Whether each of them purchased the book!

But when of the names we are weary
    (Directories muddle the brain),
We're provided by you with philosophy too
    In the trite Aphorisms of Cheyne.[33]
Geography also you teach us.
    Until I came under your thrall,
I don't mind confessing that Conoquenessing[34]
    I never had heard of at all.

And those who would seek for emotions
    No longer are destined to grope
In the desolate train of Corelli or Caine,
    Or the pseudo-heroics of Hope.[35]
Sir Walter's historic romances[36]
    Appear by comparison vague,
To the terrible tale from the "Pioneer Mail,"
    On the ramifications of plague.[37]

What fun when the "Western Physician,"
    With colic and devious doubt
His judgement upsetting, insisted on getting
    His blameless appendix cut out![38]
What pathos and woe when the extern

Came down the proud father to tell
That bouncing young Barney, the fifteenth Morgagni,
   Was born with the jaundice as well![39]

When night had enshrouded the College,
   Unhindered by pallid moon beams,
The bleeding remains of the Appleton-Swains[40]
   Came galloping into my dreams.
And Dr. R.P. Cooke[41] of Cuba
   (While Oliver drearily bled),[42]
Stood draining his bumpers to Frenchmen[43] with jumpers,
   And gazing thro' Cardinal's head.[44]

How useful it is in the Conjoint,[45]
   To be able urbanely to talk
Of the folk at Ellezelles,[46] who were really unwell
   After eating a portion of pork!
(Thus, we, by the way, should be thankful
   We never fell under the ban
Of a greater disease than extreme D & Vs[47]
   When we've dined at the Café Farnan.)

But no European can honour,
   E'en were he with genius rife,
With adequate Bravo, Your *multum in parvo,*
   That glorified Bradshaw of Life![48]
It hails from the beautiful country
   Where Modesty's flower never dwells,
And from goosb'ries and pears up to Trust Millionaires
   Things are bigger than everywhere else.

And now you are with us at Oxford
   You've plenty of Leisure, no doubt,
So make, I petition, another edition,
   And leave the Pathology out;
Cut symptoms and treatment, and give us
   More tales, repartees, epigrams,
It would leave the whole screed more amusing to read,
   And quite as much use for exams!
1909
                       S.S.

Discussion

We attribute the poem to Herbert Orpe Brookhouse. W. W. Francis in the *Bibliotheca Osleriana* refers to the poem (item 3587) as follows: "... extracts from another skit, in verse, 'the student's guide to Osler', with references to the 6th edition. Signed S.S., but by H.O. Brockhouse."[49] We have found no evidence to support Francis' contention that the poem was ever part of a skit. MacDermot[50] published a portion of the poem in 1949 giving the author as S. Brockhouse. The misspelling of Brookhouse as Brockhouse first appeared in the *Bibliotheca Osleriana.* Cushing,[51] who cited this work while it was in press, adopted the misspelling as did MacDermot more than 20 years later.

    While we have not been able to follow Francis' path to Brockhouse or Brookhouse as the purported author of the poem, circumstantial evidence supports this attribution. Herbert Orpe Brookhouse of Bromley, Kent, matriculated at the University of London in October of 1900 and entered Guy's Hospital Medical School in October of 1902. He received his MB, BS with honors in 1908 and his MD in 1910 from the University of London. While at Guy's his marks, according to the present Sub Dean for Admissions, were very good indeed:[52] he was awarded the Michael Harris Prize, the Woodridge Prize in physics, and the Junior Professors' Prize; he also received a Special Certificate in Anaesthetics for House "Appt." in December, 1908. He became a member of the Royal College of Surgeons and a licentiate of the Royal College of Physicians in 1908. Brookhouse established a private practice in Bromley in 1910; his name disappears from all calendars, registers, and lists, including *Guy's Men,* during the Great War. Cushing lists 1917 as the year of Brookhouse's death,[53] and a manuscript copy of the poem, believed to be in the hand of Sir Arthur Salusbury MacNalty, bears the notation "killed in the War." Neither Cushing nor the MacNalty manuscript are correct as to the year and manner, respectively, of Brookhouse's death. The death certificate of Herbert Orpe Brookhouse gives the cause of death as a suicide "whilst of unsound mind by placing himself in front of a train."[54] The date of death is given as 3 December 1916. Brookhouse had been a patient at Dr. C.F. Fothergill's hospital at Chorley-Wood. Arrangements had been made to transfer Brookhouse to Moorecroft, Hillingdon. While awaiting this transfer, Brookhouse slipped away from the hospital and placed himself on the tracks of the Metropolitan and Great Central Railway. A note found on the body stated: "My name is H.O. Brookhouse. I am a patient at Dr. Fothergill's, Hemsol, Chorleywood. If there were the least chance of my ever being useful to any one again I would not have done it."[55]

Poems signed "S.S." appear in *Guy's Hospital Gazette* throughout Brookhouse's Guy's years; no poems use this *nom de plume* prior to his matriculation or after his graduation.

The Residents' Theatricals at Guy's, the first of which was produced in 1901, were an institution by Brookhouse's time. He co-authored plays for the Theatricals in 1906 and 1908. In 1907, however, Brookhouse was sole author of "Ortocure," a play in two acts. The reviewer for the *Gazette* stated: "Throughout Messrs Brookhouse and Chapple (Brookhouse's assistant) have given their characters many good things to say. Perhaps too many good things, for quite a number are lost owing to the laughter which has greeted the preceding quip."[56] Brookhouse himself delivered the Prologue to the play, the first stanza of which is as follows:

We have had a sly instruction
   That a play—to be a play—
Ought to have an introduction,
   Or a Prologue, so to say.
With unanimous contrition
   We have raised some tags of rhyme,
And, obeying old tradition,
   We have come to waste your time.

While the rhyme scheme and meter differ from the Osler poem, the wit and humor of "S.S." are present. It is difficult to imagine that a person afflicted with the urge to raise some tags of rhyme would suffer from such an urge only upon the annual occasion of the Theatricals. A more frequent outlet for these cruel urges would be necessary and, we believe, was found in the authorship of the "S.S." poems.

References and Notes

1. A. M. Harvey and V. A. McKusick, *Osler's Textbook Revisited* (New York: Appleton Century Crofts, 1967).
2. Review of *The Principles and Practice of Medicine* by William Osler, *Medical News,* 60 (1892): 422.
3. White's letter of 21 April 1892 forms folio 13 of Osler's scrapbook of reviews of and correspondence about *The Principles and Practice of Medicine.* This volume, now accession 9432 in the Osler Library, was recovered in Oxford too late to be included in the *Bibliotheca Osleriana,* the catalogue of Osler's library (Oxford: Clarendon Press, 1929; reprinted Montreal, McGill-Queen's University Press, 1969), although Cushing had consulted it for his biography of Osler. Stillé's letter, also dated 21 April 1892, is on the verso of folio 18.
4. "D.M.S.," (initials of L.S. Dudgeon, A. Mavrogordato and S.G. Scott), "An Examination Paper on Osler (4th Edition)," *St Thomas's Hospital Gazette,* 12 (1902): 59–60.
5. "D.M.S.," "Hospital Notes," *St Thomas's Hospital Gazette,* 17 (1907): 196–97.
6. See manuscript note by W.W. Francis on p. 4 of *Bibl. Osl.* 3587, a miscellany containing the 1907 "Examination Paper" and related items, including the "Student's Guide to Osler" which is the subject of this paper.

    Cushing refers to Egerton Yorrick Davis, M.D. as Osler's "fanciful half." Osler created a fictional background for E.Y. Davis of Caughnawauga, PQ, and used this pseudonym freely. See Harvey Cushing, *The Life of Sir William Osler* (Oxford: The Clarendon Press, 1925), vol. 1, p. 239–42.
7. Osler's note in *Bibliotheca Osleriana,* item 3586, transcribed in *Bibliotheca Osleriana.*
8. Henry R. Veits, "An Amusing Examination Paper," *New England Journal of Medicine,* 212 (1935): 531–32; H.E. MacDermot, "The Lighter Side of Osler's Textbook," *Canadian Medical Association Journal,* 61 (1949): 76–78.
9. W.D. Tiggert, "Annotated Answers to the 1902 Examination on Osler's *Principles and Practice of Medicine,*" *Annals of Internal Medicine,* 79 (1973): 460–72.
10. Inserted in *Bibliotheca Osleriana,* item 3587.
11. "The Student's Guide to Osler," *Guy's Hospital Gazette,* 2 October 1909. The original poem contained numerical footnotes as above. These gave only page references to the sixth edition of the text. We have added topical subject headings and (within quotation marks) the passages from *The Principles and Practices of Medicine* to which these footnotes refer.
12. Sir Frederich Taylor (1847–1920), author of *Taylor's Practice of Medicine.*
13. Alexander Wheeler (?–1903), author of *Student's Handbook of Medicine and Therapeutics.*
14. Wilkins Micawber, a character in Charles Dickens' *David Copperfield;* Tom Brown, protagonist of Thomas Hughes' novel, *Tom Brown's School Days;* Thomas, Clive, or Ethel Newcome, characters in Thackeray's *The Newcomes.*
15. p. 213 (Erysipelas, treatment of)

"Perhaps as good an application as any is cold water, which was highly recommended by Hippocrates."

16. p. 582 (Acute general peritonitis, symptoms of)
"The appearance of the patient when these symptoms have fully developed is very characteristic. The face is pinched, the eyes are sunken, and the expression is very anxious. The constant vomiting of fluids causes a wasted appearance, and the hands sometimes present the washer-woman's skin. Except in cholera, we see the Hippocratic facies more frequently in this than in any other disease—'a sharp nose, hollow eyes, collapsed temples; the ears cold, contracted, and their lobes turned out; the skin about the forehead being rough, distended, and parched; the color of the whole face being brown, black, livid, or lead-colored.' "

17. p. 165 (Lobar pneumonia, history of)
"Among the ancients, Aretaeus gave a remarkable description. 'Ruddy in countenance, but especially the cheeks; the white of the eyes very bright and fatty; the point of the nose flat; the veins in the temples and neck distended; loss of appetite; pulse, at first, large, empty, very frequent, as if forcibly accelerated; heat indeed, externally, feeble, and more humid than natural, but, internally, dry and very hot, by means of which the breath is hot; there is thirst, dryness of the tongue, desire of cold air, aberration of mind; cough mostly dry, but if anything be brought up it is a frothy phlegm, or slightly tinged with bile, or with a very florid tinge of blood. The blood-stained is of all others the worst.' "

18. p. 170 (Lobar pneumonia, morbid anatomy of)
"Since the time of Laennec, pathologists have recognized three stages in the inflamed lung: engorgement, red hepatization, and gray hepatization."

19. p. 167 (Lobar pneumonia, bacteriology of)
There was, however, no suspicion that this organism was concerned in the etiology of lobar pneumonia, and it was not really until April, 1884, that A. Fraenkel determined that the organism found by Sternberg and Pasteur in the saliva, and known as the coccus of sputum septicaemia, was the most frequent organism in acute pneumonia. At first there was a good deal of confusion between this and the organism described by Friedlander, November, 1883, which is now known as the pneumo-bacillus. Fraenkel and Weichselbaum, in 1886, demonstrated the diplo-coccus in most cases of croupous pneumonia, and later studies have made it probable that this organism is the sole cause of genuine acute lobar pneumonia."

20. p. 563 (Capsular cirrhosis, surgical treatment of)
"As Hale White remarks, a case of cirrhosis of the liver which is tapped rarely recovers, but there are instances in which early and repeated paracentesis is followed by cure."

21. p. 982 (Aneurism of the cerebral arteries, etiology of)
"Males are more frequently affected than females. Of my 12 cases 7 were males. The disease is most common at the middle period of life. One of my cases was a lad of six. Pitt describes one at the same age. The chief causes are (a) endarteritis, either simple or syphilitic, which leads to weakness of the wall and dilation; and (b) embolism. As pointed out by Church, these aneurisms are often found with endocarditis. Pitt, in his recent study of the subject, concludes that it is exceptional to find cerebral aneurism unassociated with fungating endocarditis. The embo-

lus disappears, and dilatation follows the secondary inflammatory changes in the coats of the vessel.''

22. p. 471 (Etiology of gastric ulcer, evidence of)
"Perry and Shaw found it five times in 149 autopsies in cases of burns."

23. p. 57 (Typhoid fever, historical note on)
"Among these were certain young American physicians, to one of whom, Gerhard, of Philadelphia, is due the great honor of having first clearly laid down the differences between the two diseases (typhoid and typhus)."

24. p. 110—no reference to Cushing found on 110; however, the following is found on pp. 99–100 (Typhoid fever, treatment by diet):
"Water is given at fixed intervals. A good plan is to have a jug beside the patient and a tubing with a glass mouth-piece, so that he can drink as much as he wishes. A washing-out plan of treatment is advised by E.W. Cushing and T.W. Clark, of the Lake-side Hospital, Cleveland. A gallon or more may be taken in the day. The water causes polyuria, and is a sort of internal hydrotherapy by which the toxins may be washed out."

25. p. 519 (Intestinal obstruction, etiology and pathology of)
"Of the 101 cases of strangulation in Fitz's table, which has the special value of having been carefully selected from the literature since 1880, the following were the causes: Adhesions, 63; vitelline remains, 21; adherent appendix, 6; mesenteric and omental slits, 6; peritoneal pouches and openings, 3; adherent tube, 1; peduncular tumor, 1."

26. p. 388 (Sunstroke, treatment of)
"In the cases in which the symptoms are those of intense asphyxia, and in which death may take place in a few minutes, free bleeding should be practised, a procedure which saved Weir Mitchell when a young man."

27. p. 1055. Chronic chorea (Huntington's chorea)
"Osborn, of East Hampton, L.I., writes (Jan. 28th, 1898) that the disease still continues to recur in certain families described by Huntington, as it has done, so it is said, for fully two centuries."

28. p. 533 (Embolism and thrombosis, infarction of bowel)
"Jackson, Porter, and Quimby have made an exhaustive study of 30 Boston cases, and have collected 214 cases. They recognize two groups—acute and chronic. In the former the onset is sudden, with colic, nausea, vomiting, and a bloody diarrhoea, so that the picture is one of acute obstruction. The abdomen becomes distended and death occurs in collapse within a few days. In the chronic cases the onset is insidious, and there may be no symptoms referable to the abdomen."

29. p. 11 (Footnote referring to work on malaria in Osler's clinic including a publication by Barker)
"Barker, on Fatal Cases of Malaria, Johns Hopkins Hospital Reports, 1899.

30. p. 431 (Obesity)
"An extraordinary phenomenon in excessively fat young persons is an uncontrollable tendency to sleep—like the fat boy in Pickwick. I have seen one instance of it. Caton has reported a case."

31. p. 470—no reference found to Reed on 470; however, the following is found on p. 740 (Hodgkin's disease, histology of)
"The study of D.M. Reed, from the laboratory of my colleague, Dr. Welch, suggests that there is a specific histological picture in Hodgkin's disease characterized by (1) proliferation of the endothelial and reticular cells; (2) the formation of lymphoid cells (uniform in size and shape)

from the mother cells of the lymph-nodes and from the endothelial cells of the reticulum; (3) characteristic giant cells, formed from proliferating endothelial cells, which differ from the giant cells of tuberculosis; (4) great proliferation of the connective-tissue stroma leading to fibrosis; and, lastly, eosinophile cells, which form a marked feature in a large proportion of the cases. The metastatic nodules present the same structure as the glandular growths.''

32. p. title page (reference to publisher of text).

33. p. 463 (Chronic gastritis, dietetic treatment of)
"George Cheyne's thirteenth aphorism contains a volume of dietetic wisdom: 'Every wise man, after Fifty, ought to begin to lessen at least the quantity of his ailment, and if he would continue free of great and dangerous Distempers and preserve his Senses and Faculties clear to the last he ought every seven years go on abateing gradually and sensibly, and at last descend out of Life as he ascended into it, even into the Child's diet.' ''

34. p. 62 (Typhoid fever, infection of water in outbreak of)
"Quite as instructive an instance is afforded by the recent outbreak at Butler, Pa., a town of about 18,000 people, situated in the mountainous region of western Pennsylvania. The major portion of the water-supply was drawn from the Conoquenessing Creek, the minor portion from a small tributary called Thorn Creek. In the neighborhood of the latter was erected by the water company a filtration plant and reservoir, giving the town a presumably pure supply. On August 28th, 1903, a dam on Conoquenessing Creek broke interfering with the company's supply, and necessitating the sinking of wells near the creek and filtering the water. In the middle of September the filter broke down, and water was pumped for about a week from the creek directly into the reservoir. On August 18th, a case of typhoid fever occurred in a house near Thorn Creek reservoir, and following it four more. The excreta, carelessly disposed of, were washed by the rains into the reservoir. This resulted in an alarming outbreak, the total number of cases reaching 1,364, with 115 deaths. That not a few cases arose by contact may be judged from the fact that 10 per cent of the nurses contracted the disease. A most interesting feature of the outbreak, and one offering indirect proof of the water-supply being the cause, if evidence were otherwise lacking, was the relatively small number of cases arising in a quarter of the town supplied by artesian wells (Anderson).''

35. Marie Corelli, Sir Thomas Henry Hall Caine, and Anthony Hope Hawkins, who wrote as Anthony Hope, were popular English novelists of the time.

36. Sir Walter Scott, English novelist and master of the historical romance.

37. p. 239 (Plague, historical and geographical distribution of)
"The revival of the plague within the past eleven years has aroused universal interest. Since the outbreak at Hong-Kong, in 1894, the disease has appeared in many parts of the world. In India it has proved a terrible scourge since 1896. In the Punjab during the three years 1901–1903 a million of people have died of it. For the year ending May, 1904, there were 913,784 deaths from this cause in India, an increase of more than 25,000 over 1903. (240) Setting all canons of sanitary science at defiance, 'it will ravage healthy districts and leave notoriously unhealthy tracts alone; it will suddenly die out for a year or even more, and then reappear in more virulent form than before. It will spread to the north and not to

the west, as instanced by the immunity enjoyed by the Frontier Provinces; it will depopulate irrigated lands, and equally villages in the midst of sandy wastes; it will spare a busy city like Delhi, and yet take heavy toll of other towns' (*Pioneer Mail*)."

38. p. 517–518 (Appendicitis, diagnosis of)
"A well-known physician in a Western city having one night a bellyache, and feeling convinced that his appendix had perforated, summoned a surgeon, who quickly removed the supposed offender!"

39. p. 537 (Hereditary icterus)
"Glaister states that the children of Morgagni, fifteen in number, all had icterus neonatorum."

40. p. 748 (Haemophilia, etiology of)
"In a majority of cases the disposition is hereditary. In the Appleton-Swain family, of Reading, Mass., there have been cases for nearly two centuries; and F.F. Brown, of that town, tells me that instances have already occurred in the seventh generation."

41. p. 235 (Yellow fever, mode of transmission)
"Dr. R.P. Cooke and two privates of the hospital corps, all non-immunes, entered this building and unpacked the boxes, and for a period of twenty days occupied the room, each morning packing the infected articles in the boxes, and at night unpacking them. In their experiments with the fomites, in all seven non-immune subjects during the period of sixty-three days lived in contact with the fomites and remained perfectly well."

42. p. 749 (Haemophilia, prognosis)
"The longer the bleeder survives the greater the chance of his outliving the tendency; but it may persist to old age, as shown in the case of Oliver Appleton, the first reported American bleeder, who died at an advanced age of haemorrhage from a bed-sore and from the urethra."

43. p. 1055 (Saltatory spasm)
"One of the most striking of these occurs among the 'jumping Frenchmen' of Maine and Canada. As described by Beard and Thornton, the subjects are liable on any sudden emotion to jump violently and utter a loud cry or sound, and will obey any command or imitate any action without regard to its nature. The condition of echolalia is present in a marked degree. The 'jumping' prevails in certain families."

44. p. 997 (Congenital hydrocephalus)
"Even when extreme, the mental faculties may be retained, as in Bright's celebrated patient, Cardinal, who lived to age of twenty-nine, and whose head was translucent when the sun was shining behind him."

45. The Conjoint was a qualifying exam jointly offered by the Royal College of Surgeons and the Royal College of Physicians of London.

46. p. 381 (B. botulinus)
"Van Ermengena isolated an organism, to which he gave the name *B. botulinus*, from a diseased ham, which poisoned thirty-four persons, all members of a musical society, at Ellezelles, in Germany."

47. D & V is medical shorthand for diarrhea and vomiting.

48. Bradshaw was the common name of an annual timetable for all United Kingdom trains.

49. *Bibliotheca Osleriana*, p. 393.

50. H.E. MacDermot, "The Lighter Aspects of Osler's Textbook," *Canadian Medical Association Journal*, 61 (1949): 76–78.

51. Harvey Cushing, *The Life of Sir William Osler* (Oxford: The Clarendon Press, 1925), vol. 1, p. 685, n. 2.

52. R.G. Spector, personal communication. Sub-Dean for Admissions, Guy's Hospital Medical School, London Bridge SE1 9RT.
53. Cushing, *Life,* p. 685, n. 2.
54. London. General Register Office. Register of Deaths (Watford District). DX 369314.
55. *The West Hartfordshire and Watford Observer,* 9 December 1916, courtesy of Professor H. P. Lambert and P. Swain, St. George's Hospital Medical School, London.
56. Review of "Ortocure" by H.O. Brookhouse, assisted by Harold Chappel, *Guy's Hospital Gazette,* December 28, 1907.

On the Need for a New Biography of Sir William Osler

 Charles G. Roland, M.D.

Any essay demands a point of view, and I state mine at the outset: I believe that there is most definitely a need for a new biography of the namesake of our Society. My intent is to try to convince you of that need and to suggest some of the material such a work might contain and some of the directions that it might go. At the end of the evening, on the basis of a completely random draw conducted by an internationally renowned firm of chartered accountants, one of you will be selected to carry out this task!

Although the mere passage of time does not itself prove the need for additional biographic examination of any subject, the fact remains that it is 62 years since Harvey Cushing's justly celebrated, much read, and constantly referred-to *Life of Sir William Osler* was published by the Oxford University Press. The book is still in print, incidentally. It is not simply the passage of time that makes a new biography appropriate, but rather what has happened during that time. My thesis is that two changes of enormous importance mandate such a work. One of these is essentially worldwide. The second relates to Osler alone.

The first change is obvious and ubiquitous. We look at things differently than we did 60 and 70 years ago. It may be the arrogance of the present to imagine that there have been more profound changes in these two generations than in any previous similar period, but in fact this competitive aspect doesn't matter. What does matter is that we perceive and interpret events differently. This change is not the result of any single revolution. Rather, it bespeaks an amalgam of innumerable events such as the theory of relativity, the Freudianization of the western world, the Holocaust, the atomic bomb, television, space travel, the so-called sexual revolution, and the apparently ubiquitous erosion of privacy.

The second major factor that, in my opinion, makes desirable another examination of the life of William Osler, relates specifically to Osler. I refer

Presidential Address. Read at the annual meeting of the American Osler Society, April 29, 1987.

here to the cumulating mass of literature—a word I use here in its scientific rather than its esthetic sense—about our patron. The awful implications of the exclamation, "Of the making of books there is no end!" confront us most dauntingly when we survey the scientific literature, but even in assessing Osleriana the dimensions are remarkable.

Let me hasten to say that I do not believe nor propose that everything that has been written about Osler since Cushing's book has advanced our knowledge of the man. I can disprove that notion easily, looking no further than at some items from my personal bibliography. But I believe that I can show very substantial changes in our knowledge that need to be taken into general account.

Here I need to declare a caveat and request your indulgence. A major portion of the Oslerian scholarship published in recent decades has been written by members of the American Osler Society—including many of those here in this room. If I misinterpret your work, I accept full responsibility and make advance apologies; if I do not mention something you have written that you know is pertinent to my theme, I beg you not to take this failure on my part as an affront. The literature is voluminous and this, after all, is a presidential address, not an attempt at a comprehensive analytical *catalog raisonée.*

In considering whether or not there is a need for a new biography of anyone, several possible reasons suggest themselves, either individually or in combination. These include (1) substantial error in previous biographies; (2) an accretion of new facts, previously unknown or unused; (3) significant alterations in interpretation, either of the individual's life, or of society in general, or both; (4) an altered readership.

I do not approach this question as a revisionist historian suggesting that Cushing GOT IT ALL WRONG. That is not my position at all. I believe that Cushing's *The Life of Sir William Osler*[1] will remain a standard source for the indefinite future—certainly as a reference. If Cushing's work fails to be completely satisfactory today, 62 years after it was published, it is because of some subtle and some not so subtle changes that have occurred since its publication, not because of any inherent substantive weakness.

Nevertheless, there is one faulty area in Cushing that needs to be redressed by our new biographer. Welch pointed out the flaw (though he did not refer to it as such) in a review he wrote of the *Life* for the *Saturday Review of Literature* in 1925:

> With much ingenuity [Cushing] has carefully obliterated all direct personal reference to himself, his name with one trifling exception not appearing in the book after the title page, although many of the published letters are to him and the initiated may readily penetrate such disguises as 'one of the latchkeyers,' 'a quondam Baltimore neighbor,' 'his young friend,' 'an overseas American,' etc.[2]

Cushing's reasons for effacing himself in this way may have seemed compelling to him, but it makes for bad biography in at least this one area. I am reminded of Homer Smith, in that splendid book, *Circulation of the Blood: Men and Ideas,* writing a detailed chapter on the history of the kidney and never mentioning Homer Smith![3] Misplaced modesty to the nth degree.

But all the other three categories that I just mentioned—new facts, new interpretations, and new readership—are operative and provide substantial reasons for recommending that some appropriate scholar undertake what would inevitably be a major task. Let me consider each, briefly.

New Data

The accumulation of additional factual knowledge about the life, career, and thought of Sir William Osler, his family, his close friends and associates, and other relevant individuals, has been enormous. A bibliography prepared more than a decade ago contained information about 1367 items published about Osler up to the 1970's.[4] The flood of Osleriana has only increased since that time, and a contemplated second edition of the bibliography will certainly contain more than 2000 items. No one would suggest that every one of these publications makes a substantive contribution to Osleriana, either with respect to fact or interpretation, but the data that can be considered "new" are enormous. It seems a feckless task to attempt to suggest which of this mass represent genuine contributions to our knowledge of Osler and which are simply reworkings of an old theme. No one, surely, would question my suggestion that the second rubric is by far the largest. But it is the new that compels our attention.

Think of the information we lacked 60 years ago. Major collections of letters to Osler and by him have been published. One of the earliest of these was Gwyn's publication of the letters of "Father" Johnson to his son James.[5] These appeared in 1939 and were iconoclastic in revealing the doubts the senior Johnson had about the wisdom of James associating too much with Osler.

Amongst other cumulations there has been Palmer Howard's book of correspondence between the Wrights and the Oslers, which not only contains dozens of letters, but also about 40 previously unpublished photographs, certainly the largest such trove that has become available in many decades and including such candid gems as scenes during an Easter egg hunt at The Open Arms in 1916.[6] The Osler-Camac correspondence, published by two of our founders, Earl Nation and Jack McGovern, makes available another 100 or so letters, the correspondence between Osler and Camac, the originator of *Counsels and Ideals from the Writings of William Osler.*[7] Howard Holley's series of letters between Ned Milburn and W.O.[8] demonstrate the lifelong continuity of a youthful friendship. There is also the recently published *Life and Letters of Dr. Henry Vining Ogden*—Ogden was a young contemporary of W.O.'s who moved to Milwaukee in 1882, and with whom Osler corresponded for years—the book contains about 100 letters from W.O. to Vining, plus 50 from Cushing to Vining, providing some new insights both into Osler and into Cushing's work on the *Life.*[9]

In addition to the hundreds of letters that have come to light over the years, there is much more writing by Osler available now than there was 60 years ago, though it is true that Cushing had access to most or all of the unpublished corpus in the Osler papers. Even so, his use of the material must have been constrained by Osler's interdiction of their publication for a half century. Moreover, the scope of Osler's own publications has been enlarged by the recently published, amended and enlarged, annotated bibliography of W.O.[10]

The late Garth Huston, a former president of this society, produced a handsome little book in 1972, thus bringing to public view an unfinished essay of Osler on Sir Kenelm Digby's Powder of Sympathy, work that W.O. presented in 1900. Osler's interest in Digby represents, of course, an extension of his great affection for Sir Thomas Browne; the essay begins with an attention-getting generality that seems typically Oslerian: "The history of the progress of the human mind is a history of a struggle with its delusions. A fine piece of work indeed, noble in reason, infinite in faculty, man may be in action like an angel, in apprehension like a god; but there is another side to this flattering picture, which makes us feel that even at his best he is a poor, feeble creature, as little fitted, in the words of Johnson, for thinking as for flying."[11] How typical indeed: the high thought, the recognition of human weaknesses, the allusion in a single sentence both to Shakespeare and to Johnson, and so on.

In this same rubric of Osleriana, and of even more fundamental importance, has been the appearance in print of Osler's autobiographical notes, his "Inner History" of Johns Hopkins medical school, and his observations of his own dreams and nightmares.

Of these, the Inner History appeared first, in 1969, the first year that such material might legally be published. Edited by Don Bates and Edward Bensley, it was found to contain useful observations on various of the early faculty and staff at Hopkins. There is little that would seem truly intimate to a jaded audience of the 1980s, but many interesting notes on such items as the fees—*very* high—charged by William Halsted, the strong and weak points of Kelly and Welch, and this note on Miss Caroline Hampton, first Head Nurse in one of the wards:

> . . . Miss Caroline H. a niece of Gen. Wade Hampton, fell victim [to romance] much more quickly. She was very soon transferred [to] the surgical operating room. Dr. Halsted the surgeon had very advanced ideas of teaching the nurses bacteriology and it was soon evident that he was becoming very interested in his pupil.[12]

In 1976, Bensley and Bates also produced W.O.'s autobiographical notes, containing entries from 1896 till 1916.[13] These cover a wide ground, including details of his practice, information about his selection to the Regius Professorship, and so on. The dreams and nightmares I shall refer to again later. There is no time to say more here, other than that these sources will be fundamental to our still unidentified new biographer.

On a smaller scale, the archives and the literature abound with new stories, of which the following is representative. Anne Wilkinson (1910–1961), whose name I shall mention again, writes about her first visit to meet her great-uncle, William Osler, in 1914:

> We were taken to the dining room to pay our respects during the elders' Sunday breakfast—six of us, counting cousins. How could I forget? for he gave the whole of his radiant attention. I have an idea, he said, but first you must go to your aunt's bathroom and bring me everything you find in the medicine cupboard—then we shall see what we shall see. Our joy was in no way diminished by our aunt's disapproval. The joke was mainly to please the children but a little to tease his niece because she believed in dosing and he didn't. When pills and syrups and gargles and creams and tonics and shaving soap, toothpaste and unguents and laxatives were set before him, he mixed together a small quantity of each ingredient in a saucer. This, he said, is a cure for every pain, a prescription for immortality. And while he stirred he repeated incantations. We were spellbound, joyous and mildly fearful too, for the moment came when every child must take from the tip of his outstretched spoon a portion of this supernatural formula. Then, filled with the elixir of life, we retired to the nursery.[14]

We have learned much about some aspects of Osler's physical being that could be relevant to a modern biographer. Palmer Futcher has reproduced his father's clinical notes on an attack of renal colic suffered by W.O. on 31 December 1904, one that came on while "reading at the Medical and Chirurgical Library [in Baltimore] an article on "Strangulation of the Bile Ducts by Round Worms"! No renal calculi were found in the urinary specimens, but one of them did contain several quartz stones slipped in by the patient, or perhaps by Dr. Egerton Yorrick Davis, from the gravel walk at 1 West Franklin Street.[15]

On a quite different scale, Jerry Barondess,[16] Harold Segall,[17] and AHT Robb-Smith[18] have studied Osler's last illness, death, and postmortem. And thanks to the scientific labours of Henry H. Donaldson we know a great deal about the gross and microscopic appearance of Osler's remarkable brain—though I think it is not unfair to suggest that these investigations do nothing to help us to understand *why* his brain was remarkable. In 1928, Donaldson published his analysis of the brains of three scholars: Granville Stanley Hall, Edward Sylvester Morse, and Sir William Osler.[19] He concludes that ". . . variations in the convolutions can hardly be used to explain mental traits and abilities as between persons of ordinary and of superior intelligence."[20] He does, however, suggest that better nutrition may be significant in producing better brains. For those interested in likenesses of our hero, the brain photographs are an unusual addition for the family photograph album.

We know much more about Osler's professional activities than did Cushing, too. Of numerous instances to which I might refer, let me select one, prepared by a guest of this Society who is on the programme here in Philadelphia. Dr. Leon Saunders has studied the history of his profession, veterinary medicine, and has shown that William Osler's contributions have been even more important than we previously guessed. Indeed, Osler should be identified as the first teacher of veterinary pathology in North America, his seminal labours at the Montreal veterinary school from 1876 on being followed only some years later in the schools of the United States.[21]

Sometimes, serendipity plays a role in opening up the vistas. I have a very particular instance in mind. The Classics of Medicine Library, two years ago, produced three large volumes reproducing Osler's non-scientific essays. Our intent had been simple enough, in undertaking the task: we wished simply to make life easier for the student (of any age) who wanted to investigate Osler's thought systematically. Nothing remarkable there. But a quite unlooked for benefit occurred. The president of the company put one of his staff to work on a name index and a subject index, and Miss Linda Beam laboured for weeks to produce what is perhaps the chief contribution of the entire project—53 pages of index that make everything in this large corpus far more accessible than it has been in the past. This is not, of course, *new* knowledge, but I believe that for many it will have the same effect, leading them to Osleriana not known, otherwise, to be pertinent to a given task at hand.

New Interpretations

The question of interpretation is an especially interesting one, in my view. There have been quite marked alterations in the way the 1980's interprets heroes generally, and there seems quite evidently a change in the way we look at Osler. But far beyond that, and perhaps of even greater importance in justifying the preparation of an additional biography, are new ways that we look at the world in general.

Perhaps this change can be demonstrated most obviously in the question of privacy, and the change in what was considered to be private in the 1920's versus what seems to be private today. *Nothing* seems to be private any more. Thus it would be natural for a biographer today to at least inquire into Osler's sex life. I should add quickly—to both allay the worries of the traditionists and to dampen the excitement of the prurient—that I know nothing whatever about Osler's sex life that is not already in public print. But certainly, as one reads Cushing's biography, it is obvious that he skirts this area carefully—if indeed there was anything unreported that he thought needed to be skirted. For example, he does not address the question of Osler's somewhat advanced age at the time of his marriage—42—nor the related and more impertinent question of what his sexual activities may have been in the years between puberty and marriage; this occupied, after all, the substantial period of more than 25 years, of which we seem to know nothing of a sexual nature. There is no reason to suppose that Osler lacked the customary male sex drive, but his consummation of it remains a mystery. There is some evidence in Osler's own accounts of his dreams that sexuality was very much a part of his life; how else could one interpret this dream, for example—a Freudian delight:

> . . . . Again I woke in an agony, feeling the snake crawling up my left sleeve and squirming about to make itself comfortable. It was a bigger one and in the dim light I could see the tail crossing the back of my hand obliquely. . . . It seemed hours and the beast had evidently coiled in my armpit and his head was on my breast. Then it uncoiled and slipped away. . . . I fell back in a sort of faint and when I came to [Rissien] Russell was there again . . . . He said 'I had better reexamine you and see if the snake has bitten you.' I saw a disturbed look on his face as he said 'Have you always had these large breasts Osler?' 'No,' I said, 'I felt there was something curious.' 'My God,' he said, 'there's milk in them. He has given you the wrong injection.' He put his hand on my abdomen, which for the first time I noticed to be very big, and said 'We are ruined. You are in the family way. . . .[22]

Would a modern biographer uncover more material in this area? Should he, or she?

Incidentally, Osler himself seems to have made a private joke about his age when he became a father. This has to do with the nickname "Ike" for Revere. Most of us have assumed that this referred to Isaak Walton and thus to Revere's love of fishing. But the nickname, it turns out, was in use before Revere was two years old, and thus presumably before he evidenced much enthusiasm for angling. It now seems that the name refers to the birth of Isaac when Abraham was 100 and Sarah 91. Though hardly a fundamental advance in our knowledge, it does emphasize Osler's Biblical knowledge, his sense of humour, and his ability not to take himself too seriously.[23]

On the narrower question of how we interpret Osler, there are far too many examples to do more than merely allude to them here. Many members of this audience have been prominent in this endeavour. One has only to think of George Harrell's several important papers, perhaps especially the provocative investigation of Osler's income, when we first learned that he had earned the modern equivalent of many millions.[24] Macht has studied Osler's prescribing habits, basing his work on surviving prescriptions in a Baltimore pharmacy—a study of particular interest given Osler's reputation as a therapeutic nihilist, yet one I have never seen cited.[25]

Phil Teigen has elucidated Osler's historical craftsmanship from a historiographic point of view.[26] Several of us have had a go at explaining Osler's continued popularity, though that seems one of the more ineffable aspects of Osleriana. Rarely referred to, but important nonetheless, is the thesis and a resulting string of papers on various aspects of his literary and historical writings that came from the busy pen of William White.[27] The list goes on, at considerable length.

It is both fair and important to note, too, that not all commentary and interpretation has been favorable. In my own writings about Osler I have tried to present a balanced view of the man, laying some stress, for example, on what I termed, in one paper,[28] Osler's rough edge—his ability to be critical and, at times, harsh—and there and elsewhere I have tried to make the point that Osler's sense of humour could be and often was hurtful, despite it being overall a splendid asset. Taking this approach carries some risk in itself; I published an analysis of the Fixed Period episode, 20 years ago, entitled "The Infamous William Osler,"[29] and received a testy letter from an Oslerolator claiming that I had no right to combine the words "infamous" and "Osler" in the same phrase!

But some of the criticism of Osler is more pointed and seems intended to be destructive. Perhaps the best known recent example of this genre is Weissmann's essay, "Against *Aequanimitas*," which appeared both separately and as a chapter in the author's much-lauded book, *The Woods Hole Cantata*.[30] I am not one of those who think Osler should be—or needs to be—protected from dissection and analysis. Indeed, I strongly favour such analysis. But the work must be done according to accepted rules of argument; Weissmann fails to do so, in my opinion. Instead, he resorts to special pleading, presentism, and *argumentem ad hominem*, among other devices. There is no time here for a lengthy dissection, but consider the implications to logic of this segment of Weissmanniana:

> ... I'm afraid that formal instruction in ethics, aesthetics, or the 'larger issues' of the humanities will not assure the goodness—in the general sense—of our students or teachers. Remember Alexis Carrell? A far more distinguished scientist than Osler (Carrell won the Nobel Prize in 1912 for his work in vascular surgery), he was also a prolific essayist and rabid 'humanist.' His social Darwinism, so much a product of the Oslerian school, extended to such examples, taken from 'Man the Unknown':
>
>> Indeed, human beings are equal. But individuals are not, The equality of their rights is an illusion. The feeble-minded and the man of genius should not be equal before the law. The stupid, the unintelligent, those who are dispersed, incapable of attention, of effort have no right to a higher education. It is absurd to give them the same electoral power as the fully developed individuals. Sexes are not equal.
>>
>> Carrell, at the end of his life, voluntarily returned to work for the Vichy regime. . . .[31]

So according to Weissmann there is an Oslerian "school" of which Carrell is a member and, by implication, thus his views represent Osler's. Moreover, membership in this club connotes the kind of person who collaborated with the Nazis in World War 2 and therefore, possibly, had some responsibility for the Holocaust. This is careless and pernicious nonsense.

That Cushing's view, his interpretation, is dated is no criticism of him but simply reflects the inevitable flow of time and the change in society. The biographer invariably, whether he wills it or not, alters his subject by the mere action of examining him or her. With regard to that chimera, objectivity, I refer you to the words of Geoffrey Wolff (biographer of Harry Crosby and of his own father, Thomas Wolff). He said: "I'm not certain that any telling can leave material unaltered; point of view alters data, dogma deforms it, and putative objectivity (the absence of a point of view) confuses it."[32] And the point of view of a biographer of the 1980s must differ profoundly from that of Cushing, in the 1920s.

How does one incorporate someone like Anne Wilkinson into this scenario? I mentioned her earlier as a great-neice of our hero. Wilkinson was also a remarkably gifted poet, one of Canada's best, perhaps, until her early death from cancer more than 20 years ago. She is also the author of a book that must be taken into account by any biographer of her great-uncle, a moving and effective family history of the Oslers entitled *Lions in the Way: A Discursive History of the Oslers.*[33] The book is a significant contribution not only to those interested in William or some other member of the Osler family—for example, most of what we know about Frank, the intriguing black sheep, comes from *Lions in the Way:*—but also to anyone concerned with the social history of late 19th- and early 20th-century Canada.

In addition, though perhaps much less obviously pertinent, is Anne Wilkinson's poetry. She wrote, "I was the child of old men heavy with honour"[34] and her family relationships show up in many subtle ways. Writing of the family summer cottage she observes:

My ears are tied to the tattle of water
That echoes the vows of ancestral lovers,
My skin is washed by a lather of waves
That bathed the blond bodies of uncles and aunts
And curled on the long flaxen hair of my mother[35]

These may not be definitive statements, anecdotes that portray any solid picture, but I think they do illuminate something of the atmosphere. We may be able to learn something about what it was to be brought up an Osler, from these poems. Certainly we can learn something about life in Ontario at the time, and that is, I think, relevant and important to a biographer of Osler.

I cannot go on at any greater length about Anne Wilkinson, except to mention another intriguing fact. Much of her poetry is medically oriented. She created poems entitled "When wound is fresh," and "Poem of anxiety," and "To a psycho-neurotic." The poem "Dissection" shows deep feelings for the human body, ones that she certainly shared with Osler, even if we can't prove that she received them from him (her husband was a surgeon, too). Here it is in its entirety:

We crawl through craniums, stare
Beneath the bones at spasms, redden
At the grey twitched ultimatum when
We touch the guilty puddle where the nerve roots
Launch their tippy boats to shoot the heart.
The towering head observes which curled inch
Controls the meadow of the hand, which pipe
Dictates the course of sewers in our city;
It clocks the ragged pulse
That hammers out our imagery, unravels
Every sleeping snake
And travels to the threshold of its sting.
And while we squint to focus microscopes,
Dissect each bleeding head,
Sun bursts in splendour from the attic skull,
An angel shedding glory, come to free
The puppet dangling from a mildewed coil.[36]

Finally, the observation that intrigues me most of all. In 1962 Wilkinson published a long poem entitled "Notes on Robert Burton's 'The Anatomy of Melancholy',"[37] which I recommend to your attention.

New Readership

The fourth factor, the change in readership, I believe also to be significant. There are many reasons why medical students, physicians, librarians, and others, are unlikely to read Cushing today. It is, first of all, too long a book by contemporary standards. One might make a comparison here between earlier biographies of Churchill and the recent one by Piers Brendon (1984). This is short enough to fit, without a word deleted, on six audiocassettes; it is much shorter than the standard multivolume tomes, and much more readable.

What of the ultimate purpose of biography? There is, of course, the desire to entertain, and the urge to educate or inform. These goals are fundamental to all kinds of writing. For a group such as the American Osler Society, there is also the question of projecting and perpetuating a role model. Those of us in this room tonight would display a wide spectrum of opinion about Osler the man, perhaps ranging from indifference (at least on the part of a few of the long-suffering spouses present) to unalloyed admiration. But regardless of our personal feelings, we might all agree that some readable account of Osler's life should be available for the benefit of those who might gain from reading it. And this sentiment implies a belief that there such a transfer occurs: that reading the life of a good person may convey some of the goodness to the reader. On this point I am unsure. Theodore Rosengarten disagrees. Rosengarten wrote the life of Nate Shaw, in 1974. He concludes that "In the end, we do not find a single life that can be imitated, or one that we would imitate if we could. This letdown is one of the chief pleasures of reading biography, the satisfaction that you are not the other person."[38] But are we all satisfied not to be Osler?

Missing Information

Of course, there are still areas of *terra incognita* on Osler's map. One hopes that scholars will hasten to fill in these areas. For example, there is the question of Osler's attitude towards women. I keep hearing that Osler was a terrible chauvinist, though such evidence as I have found personally suggests that he was at least no worse than the generality of men of his time. Weissmann takes delight in pointing out that Osler moved, in a faculty meeting, that Gertrude Stein not be permitted to proceed in medicine. How this can be seen as prejudice or misogyny, we are not enlightened; Edward Bensley seems to suggest that she had not done well and should have been plucked, having failed four of nine examinations.[39] But there is much scattered information on Osler's feelings about women; why does not someone undertake the work, in a careful, scholarly, unexcited manner, so that we might all have a better view of his attitudes?

Similarly, we need to know what the man felt about Jews. In many places he refers to "Hebrews" in ways that would not be used today. Are these evidence of hidden anti-semitism, or merely a convention from his day that no longer is followed? His personal relationship with Jews seems to have been excellent—Abraham Jacobi was a friend, and there were many others. This aspect of his life surely could be illuminated. And so on.

Conclusion

Let me conclude, then, by reaffirming my conviction that there is a job to be done here. We know a different Osler than could have been known in 1925: not necessarily a better Osler, nor a worse Osler, but I believe we have a better balanced view of a complex individual. If I am correct, then there is a gauntlet to be thrown down, and I do so here and now.

Nor is this gesture merely a rhetorical flourish. I do not offer myself up as the new Cushing. I have absolutely no intention of writing this book. But someone must. I would hope that it might be someone listening to me tonight. What better reward could I have, a crown to an otherwise unremarkable presidency, than to be able to think, ten or twenty years from now, that these words may have played some small role in persuading one of you to take up your pen—or, rather, your keyboard—and to settle in to the task. Many of you will be thinking at this moment that this would be a congenial task indeed, were there but time. Let me end by reminding you of the words of William Osler:

> While medicine is to be your vocation, or calling, see to it that you have also an avocation—some intellectual pastime which may serve to keep you in touch with the world of art, of science, or of letters. Begin at once the cultivation of some interest other than the purely professional. . . . No matter what it is—but have an outside hobby.[40]

What better hobby could a member of the American Osler Society have than preparing an honest, judicious, spirited, and sympathetic Life of our namesake?

References

1. Harvey Cushing, *The Life of Sir William Osler* (1925)
2. William H. Welch, "A great physician and medical humanist: a review of Harvey Cushing's Life of Sir William Osler," *Saturday Review of Literature* November 1925.
3. Alfred P. Fishman and Dickinson W. Richards (eds.), *Circulation of the Blood: Men and Ideas* (New York: Oxford University Press, 1964), pp. 859.
4. Earl F. Nation, Charles G. Roland, & John P. McGovern, *An Annotated Checklist of Osleriana* (Kent State University Press, 1976), pp. xii+289. An additional 211 items are cited in a supplement, Earl F. Nation, *An Up-Dated Checklist of Osleriana* (Pasadena: Earl F. Nation, [1986]), pp. 60+11.
5. Norman B. Gwyn, "The letters of a devoted father to an unresponsive son, student of medicine at McGill and London: being the letters of Osler's great inspiration, W.A. Johnson to his son James . . . ," *Bulletin of the History of Medicine* 7: 335–51, 1939.

6. R. Palmer Howard, *The Chief: Doctor William Osler* (USA: Science History Publications, 1983).

7. Earl F. Nation & John P. McGovern (eds.), *Student and Chief: The Osler-Camac Correspondence* (Pasadena: The Castle Press, 1980).

8. Howard Holley, *A Continual Remembrance: Letters from Sir William Osler to his Friend Ned Milburn, 1865–1919* (Springfield, IL: Charles C Thomas, 1968), pp. 132.

9. Leonard Weistrop, *HVO: The Life and Letters of Dr. Henry Vining Ogden, 1857–1931* (Milwaukee: The Milwaukee Academy of Medicine, 1987).

10. Richard L. Golden and Charles G. Roland (eds.), *Sir William Osler: An Annotated Bibliography with Illustrations* San Fransisco: Norman Publishing, 1988), pp. xv+214, illust.

11. K. Garth Huston (ed.), *Sir Kenelm Digby's Powder of Sympathy: An Unfinished Essay by Sir William Osler* (Los Angeles: The Plantin Press, 1972), p. 1.

12. Donald G. Bates & Edward H. Bensley (eds.), "The inner history of the Johns Hopkins Hospital," *The Johns Hopkins Medical Journal* 125: 184–194, 1969; see p. 188.

13. Edward H. Bensley & Donald G. Bates (eds.), "Sir William Osler's autobiographical notes," *Bulletin of the History of Medicine* 50: 596–618, 1976.

14. Toronto, University of Toronto Archives, Anne Wilkinson Papers. This excerpt is from her essay "Curate's Egg."

15. Thomas B. Futcher, "Dr. Osler's renal stones," *Journal of Urology* 135 (1966): 1272.

16. Jeremiah Barondess, "A case of empyema: notes on the last illness of Sir William Osler," *Transactions of the American Clinical & Climatological Association* 86 (1974): 59–71.

17. Harold N. Segall, *Osler Library Newsletter* 50 (Oct.): 1–3, 1985.

18. AHT Robb-Smith, "Did Sir William Osler have carcinoma of the lung? Sir William Osler and the Tonypandy phenomenon," *Chest* 66: 712–16, 1974, and 67: 82–87, 1975.

19. Henry H. Donaldson, "A study of the brains of three scholars," *Journal of Comparative Neurology* 46 (1928): 1–84.

20. Donaldson, "Brains," 83.

21. Leon Z. Saunders, "From Osler to Olafson: the evolution of veterinary pathology in North America," *Canadian Journal of Veterinary Research* 51 (1987): 1–26.

22. Charles G. Roland, "Sir William Osler's dreams and nightmares," *Bulletin of the History of Medicine* 54: 418–446, 1980; see pp. 433–434,

23. Personal communication, Alistair Robb-Smith to George Harrell, 3 July 1985 (copy supplied by G. Harrell).

24. George T. Harrell, "Osler's practice," *Bulletin of the History of Medicine* 47 (1973): 545–567.

25. David I. Macht, "Osler's prescriptions and materia medica," *Transactions of the American Therapeutic Society* 35: 69–85, 1936.

26. Philip M. Teigen, "William Osler's historiography: a rhetorical analysis," *Canadian Bulletin of Medical History* 3: 31–49, 1986.

27. Some of White's papers include, "The biographical essays of Sir William Osler and their relation to medical history," *Bulletin History of Medicine* 7: 28–48, 1939; "Walt Whitman and Sir William Osler," *American Literature* 11; 73–7, 1939; "Re-Echoes of Sir William Osler's 'The Fixed Period,' " *Bulletin of the Institute of the History of Medicine* 5: 937–40, 1937; *Aequanimitas:* Osler's inspirational essays," *Bulletin History of Medicine* 6: 820–33,

1938; and "Osler on Shakespeare, Bacon, and Burton: With a reprint of his Creators, Transmuters, and Transmitters, as illustrated by Shakespeare, Bacon, and Burton," *Bulletin History of Medicine* 7: 392–408, 1939.

28. Charles G. Roland, "Osler's rough edge," *Annals of Internal Medicine* 81: 690–692, 1974.

29. Charles G. Roland, "The infamous William Osler," *JAMA* 193: 436–38, 1965.

30. Gerald Weissmann, *The Woods Hole Cantata: Essays on Science and Society* (New York: Dodd, Mead, 1985), pp. 211–230.

31. Weissmann, *Cantata*, p. 219.

32. Geoffrey Wolff, "Minor lives," in *Telling Lives: The Biographer's Art*, edited by Marc Pachter (Washington, New Republic Books/National Portrait Gallery, 1979), p. 65.

33. Anne Wilkinson, *Lions in the Way: A Discursive History of the Oslers* (Toronto: Macmillan Company of Canada Ltd., 1956), pp. 274.

34. Anne Wilkinson, "Summer acres," in *Counterpoint to Sleep* (1951).

35. *Idem.*

36. A.J.M. Smith (ed.), "Dissection," in *The Collected Poems of Anne Wilkinson, and a Prose Memoir* (Toronto: The Macmillan Company of Canada Ltd., 1968), p. 34.

37. Smith, *Collected Poems*, pp. 119–124.

38. Theodore Rosengarten, "Stepping over cockleburs: conversations with Ned Cobb," in *Telling Lives: The Biographer's Art*, edited by Marc Pachter (Washington, New Republic Books/National Portrait Gallery, 1979), p. 109.

39. Edward H. Bensley "Gertrude Stein as a medical student," *Pharos of Alpha Omega Altha* 47 (2): 36–7, 1984.

40. William Osler, "After twenty-five years," in *Aequanimitas, With Other Addresses to Medical Students, Nurses and Practitioners of Medicine* (Philadelphia, P. Blakiston's Son & Co., 1928), p. 213.

Modern Version of Osler's Bedside Library

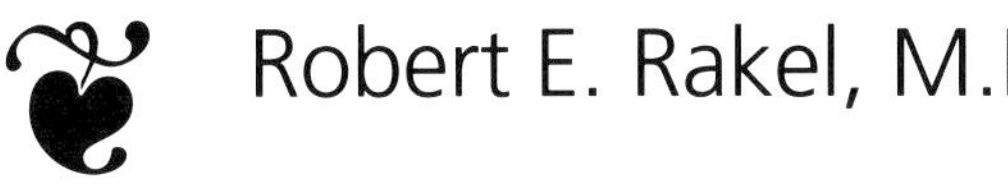 Robert E. Rakel, M.D.

Reading is a personal adventure; our individual preferences in books are influenced and directed by the variety and variability of past influences. Sir William Osler, whom many consider the ideal physician, believed that regular reading provided an "inner education" that was necessary beyond professional training. It is apparent that his own reading habits were influenced by the religious atmosphere in which he spent his early years and in which he received a liberal exposure to the classics. The books and authors he recommended to medical students for their bedside libraries clearly reflect those biases as well as his preferences for evening reading.

Osler proposed that:

A liberal education may be had at a very slight cost of time and money. Well-filled though the day may be with appointed tasks, to make the best possible use of your one or of your ten talents, rest not satisfied with this professional training, but try to get the education, if not of a scholar, at least of a gentleman. Before going to sleep read for half an hour, and in the morning have a book open on your dressing table. You will be surprised to find how much can be accomplished in the course of a year.

Osler recommended 10 books or authors for medical students to read in this manner [1]:

Old and New Testaments
Shakespeare
Montaigne
Plutarch's *Lives*
Marcus Aurelius
Epictetus
Religio Medici

Read at the annual meeting of the American Osler Society, May 15, 1985.

Reprinted with permission from *Perspectives in Biology and Medicine, 31*:577, 1988

Don Quixote
Emerson
Oliver Wendell Holmes—*Breakfast Table* series

The list includes authors who flourished during Osler's young manhood (Emerson and Holmes) but primarily reflects his love of the classics and the attitudes of the last century. I was curious to know which books would be chosen by physicians who share a similar philosophy today. My interest was piqued by Reynolds [2], who conducted a similar but smaller survey. Responses were solicited from the American Osler Society, a group of 95 physician-scholars who share a respect for Osler and an appreciation for the high value he placed on humanism in medicine and the pursuit of excellence.

If what we see in Osler's list is a demonstration of one man's particularly discriminating and scholarly nineteenth-century view of the world, my hope in taking this survey was to see what, if any, patterns or trends might surface if we, as twentieth-century physicians, examined our own reading tastes and habits.

Members of this society were asked to list their favorite books, paying particular attention to those that would be of greatest interest and value to developing physicians. Eighty percent of the members responded (76 of 95).

The survey yielded many interesting results. Although 428 different books and authors were recommended, 300 of the 869 total were mentioned only once. Of the remaining 569 that were mentioned two or more times, 30 books or authors were recommended five times or more. It is evident that variety in reading taste is a prominent feature of this group.

In one day's mail I received a response listing Lewis Thomas as one of the respondent's favorite authors, and then opened a response from Lewis Thomas, who is a member of the American Osler Society. Accompanying Thomas's list of favorite books was the note, ''Herewith the list, written down without much premeditation and while, as always these days, double parked.''

The styles of individual responses to the survey displayed nearly as much variety as the choices of favorite books and authors. Some included a list of books without comment; some commented but felt uncomfortable providing a list, as such; others included brief comments with each book mentioned. The number of recommendations in a single return ranged from zero (those who did not want to impose their preferences on others) to 109. The prize for the most recommendations goes to William Bean, who submitted 16 lists published by himself or others containing a total of over 250 titles.

Although many were of the opinion that Osler's first list would put most modern medical students to sleep and were old-fashioned and stuffy even for that day, seven of Osler's selections were among the 14 books most often cited in the survey, each being mentioned at least nine times. Epictetus was the only one not mentioned two or more times.

It would seem that our group's top 10 books and authors exhibit a willing appreciation of fine quality in modern writing but at the same time preserve a strong tie to a rich and established literary past. Not surprisingly, Sir William Osler topped the list of favorite authors, and Cushing's biography of Osler ranked second. Perhaps a little unexpected for this ''modern'' list was the emergence of the Bible and the works of William Shakespeare in spots 3 and 4; Sir Arthur Conan Doyle at number 5 may either be indicative of the more modern appreciation for clever deductive reasoning or for the opportunity he offers to escape into the refuge of a good mystery. Lewis Thomas was deservedly recognized as one of today's most talented medical writers by appearing at number 6. *Don Quixote* and Oliver Wendell Holmes, both on

Osler's list, seemed to have withstood the test of time and rank seventh and eighth in our poll. And finally, the list is rounded out with a return once again to the more contemporary efforts of James Michener and Sir Winston Churchill, although Charles Dickens tied with Churchill for tenth place.

Preferred Time to Read

Osler made it clear that he considered the pre-bedtime to be optimum for adventuring into outside reading. He once said that, by making a steady practice of a half-hour's reading in bed, "the busiest man can get a fair education before the plasma sets in the periganglionic spaces of his grey cortex."

The majority of those surveyed subscribe to Osler's recommendation to read for 30 minutes at bedtime. This does not mean they read in bed. One specifically notes that he never reads in bed unless he is sick. Those who do not read at bedtime because they fall asleep easily read in the early morning, usually between 4:30 and 7:00 A.M. One physician admits to having "insomnia which I cultivate"; most of his reading is done between 2:00 and 6:00 A.M. Another respondent, although he complains that "one has to have an off-beat circadian rhythm" to indulge in recreational reading early in the morning, says that since student days he often reads in the early morning. Among other reasons, it is the time, particularly when one is in active practice, that one is least likely to be disturbed. He goes on to state that the time and place of reading are irrelevant. What is important is that there be a balance between reading purely for pleasure and reading to increase one's knowledge of a subject. Whatever the purpose, "it should be directed towards helping physicians (mature or embryonic) become well-rounded, educated persons." It is quite clear, however, that these physicians read constantly and compulsively, as if addicted. One physician, commenting upon his own form of the addiction, says "If there is literally nothing that can be read (not even the back of an airplane ticket or a cereal box) I behave a lot like a chain smoker who is out of cigarettes." Another member always carries a lightweight book to read in the barber shop, on the bus, or while his auto is being repaired. At one time he was able to read one French play a month "while waiting for elevators in the hospital."

One member describes his personal reading philosophy as reading "anything I can get my hands on. I will even read junk rather than not read." He admits that his reading is totally undisciplined, and that he reads whenever there is a spare moment, whether it be in the bathroom or while waiting in a line.

Another member shares my penchant for reading two or three books concurrently, switching "from one to another, depending on mood or current interest."

Vacations seem to be another time when people look forward to relaxing with a good book. One member prefers to read in these holiday-type contexts and regards the matter of choosing which books he will read during 1 week at the beach as a decision of major importance each year. He reminds us that these times are precious and "not to be squandered on something trivial." Another regrets that we no longer have the luxury of those lengthy sea voyages taken by Osler and his contemporaries two or three times a year. The physician who reads while waiting for the elevator also enjoys reading on vacation—but says his wife threatens not to go if he takes a book. He admits to sneaking one anyway.

In an effort to pack more reading into shorter available time, speed reading has been tried by some, including myself, and found wanting. One physician said that in trying the rapid reading techniques he felt he was robbed of too much of the opportunity to "savor the writing and the ideas." He prefers to "only use this approach for orientation or to get through something very dull that one feels an obligation to finish." Another comments that:

> Time to read and think are precious commodities in today's society. I believe one hour a day is essential for these activities. A quiet time around lunch and again later in the evening should be set aside to study carefully the day and one's place in the universe. Reading, thinking, and perhaps exercise can be excellent methods of contemplation.

Reading Philosophies

This last comment reflects an attitude shared by other members. Ed Pellegrino describes himself as an omnivorous reader and prefers books that

> deal with the meanings of human life, the relationships that should obtain between individuals, the attempt to understand something of the relationship of man to the world, to his fellows, and to society. . . . I enjoy the opportunity reading gives me for an intense dialogue, conversation and dialectic with great minds. I find in each serious author some insight, some perception, of the meaning of human existence. It is this illumination that helps me understand myself. But most of all, [I read] to stimulate reflection of my own life and the lives of those around me.

Another member specifically chooses books because they "open the mind to aspects of the behavior of human beings and to principles of living which have permanent worth." A Japanese member urges "if you encounter an impressive book, search for the source of the author's thoughts and read his biography."

One physician likes biographies and autobiographies of men who were achievers and in general thinks of reading as nearly the greatest pleasure in life. He paraphrases A. Conan Doyle (in *Behind the Magic Door*), "I face my fate with a braver heart for all the rest and quiet comradeship I find in reading."

One member comments "I am struck by the importance of the iconoclasts in my development. Medical students need an augmented skepticism, a less ready reliance on authority." In a similar vein, another describes the essence of a good doctor and academician. He finds that he frequently encounters a subject that he wants to investigate. All of his reading is in pursuit of these new and fresh ideas. He would prefer to "instill [in students] intellectual curiosity and a feeling of excitement about exploration of a new idea rather than develop a specific recommended reading list."

Touching on another aspect of reading practice, many respondents referred to their fondness for reading and rereading favorite books or chapters, while others never read a book twice. The only book I remember reading a second time was Cushing's biography of Osler.

Histories, biographies, autobiographies, and mysteries emerged as popular categories of reading, although one member points to the more hedonistic tendencies in his list. He receives "pleasure from fishing and sailing books and belly laughs from Saki. He refers to the *Short Stories of Saki* by H.H. Munro, one of the books that, because of this survey, has piqued my interest and has been added to my already lengthy list of books to read "as soon as I have time, but preferably sooner."

Although the works of Shakespeare were frequently recommended, one member is not a proponent of reading Shakespeare since we are exposed to the plays at school and in televised performances. Another feels, however, that it is difficult to develop a rich association with our culture and even with our language if one has not read some Shakespeare.

Stuart Wolf's advice for those planning to become physicians reflects the attitudes expressed by many of the respondents.

> Good reading teaches you to use the language, to write, to become articulate and to organize your thoughts—all very important to physicians. Reading enlarges your frame of reference, teaches you about places, people, emotions and behavior, information that is often seriously deficient among present day young physicians.

Another member comments that "Ambition and poverty are strong motives to work hard, but the power lies in books. They provide the finesse to speak and write effectively."

Reading and the Medical Profession

The survey also produced some provocative individual thoughts about the importance of reading to the well-being of the medical profession—particularly to the personal growth and development of the medical student and the young physician. Osler once said "It is astonishing with how little reading a doctor can practice medicine, but it is not astonishing how badly he may do it."

One physician submits the unqualified but sound advice that the nonmedical reading of students and physicians be "eclectic and voracious." Another refers to the tendency that sometimes develops in students for thinking that there is nothing in the world but medicine and says "One needs to have a bedside library in order to counterbalance this problem."

One physician finds that reading opens up a vast world of human behavior that, in turn, is a tremendous aid to the humanistic aspects of his own practice. He says: "Think of the benefit to the suburban raised medical student who reads *Black Like Me* or *The Autobiography of Malcolm X* before his clinic rotation."

Conclusion

This survey has encouraged me to inspect my own reading habits more closely, but, more than that, it has testified to the very tangible significance of books and reading to professionals throughout the world, many of whose lives are spent in a rush, under pressure, trying to stretch one moment just to reach the next—who seem so often to be figuratively and perpetually—if not literally, double parked.

Osler commented that "it is easier to buy books than to read them, and easier to read them than to absorb them." It is entirely possible that the element of time these days is the primary determinant of how much buying, reading, and absorbing we accomplish. One response contained an appropriate statement by Steven Lock, editor of the *British Medical Journal:* "You have time left for possibly five hundred more books—make the most of it." Perhaps this list of favorites will help us take stock of our lifetime remaining, identifying how many books we want to read per year, and then develop a realistic schedule.

Favorite Books and Authors Selected by American Osler Society Members
Number of times recommended by the 76 respondents
42. Osler, Sir William (1849–1919):
    Aequanimitas
    A Way of Life
    The Principles and Practice of Medicine
    An Alabama Student
    William Osler: The Continuing Education (ed. McGovern and Roland)
    Counsels and Ideals from the Writings of William Osler, C.N.B. compiled by
        Camac (1868–1940)
    The Evolution of Modern Medicine
    Old Humanities and the New Science
    Sir William Osler, 1849–1919: A Selection for Medical Students (ed. Roland)
27. Cushing, Harvey (1869–1939):
    The Life of Sir William Osler
    Consecratio Medici and Other Papers
26. Bible
18. Shakespeare, William (1564–1616):
    Works of . . .
17. Doyle, A. Conan (1859–1930):
    Sherlock Holmes stories
    Round the Red Lamp; Being Facts and Fancies of Medical Life
    Stark-Munro Letters
    The Annotated Sherlock Holmes (ed. William Baring-Gould)
    Through the Magic Door
    The Hound of the Baskervilles
    Micah Clark
    Medical Casebook of Dr. Arthur Conan Doyle (by Rodin and Key, 1984)
14. Thomas, Lewis (1913–):
    Late Night Thoughts on Listening to Mahler's Ninth Symphony
    The Lives of a Cell: Notes of a Biology Watcher
    The Medusa and the Snail: More Notes of a Biology Watcher
    The Youngest Science: Notes of a Medicine-Watcher
11. Cervantes Saavedra, Miguel de (1547–1616):
    Don Quixote
11. Holmes, Oliver Wendell (1809–1894):
    Breakfast-Table series
    Medical Essays
11. Michener, James (1907–):
    Hawaii
    Chesapeake
    The Source
    Centennial
    Tales of the South Pacific
10. Churchill, Sir Winston (1874–1965):
    A History of the English-Speaking Peoples
    The Second World War

Collected Speeches
Lord Randolph Churchill (biography of his father)
10. Dickens, Charles (1812–1870):
    David Copperfield
    Martin Chuzzlewit
    Nicholas Nickleby
    Oliver Twist
    Our Mutual Friend
    Pickwick Papers
    A Tale of Two Cities
9. Browne, Sir Thomas (1605–1682):
    Religio Medici
    Pseudodoxia Epidemica: or, Enquiries . . .
    A Letter to a Friend
    Hydriotaphia
    Clergy in a Country Churchyard ([sic] Gray, Thomas (1716–71), *Elegy*
        Written in a Country Churchyard)
    Christian Morals
9. Emerson, Ralph Waldo (1803–1882):
    Essays
9. Montaigne, Michel de (1533–1592):
    Essays
7. Hemingway, Ernest (1899–1961):
    A Farewell to Arms
    Green Hills of Africa
    For Whom the Bell Tolls
    The Old Ma Finn ([sic] Twain, Mark (1835–1910))
    The Mysterious Stranger ([sic] Twain, Mark (1835–1910))
    Tom Sawyer ([sic] Twain, Mark (1835–1910))
6. Maugham, Somerset (1874–1965):
    Of Human Bondage
6. Stevenson, Robert Louis (1850–1894):
    Treasure Island
    A Child's Garden of Verses
    Virginibus Puerisque
    Travels with a Donkey
6. Wolfe, Thomas (1900–1938):
    Look Homeward, Angel
    You Can't Go Home Again
5. Boswell, James (1740–1795):
    Life of Johnson
5. Carroll, Lewis (1832–1898):
    Alice books
5. Dostoyevski, Fyodor (1821–1881):
    The Brothers Karamazov
    Crime and Punishment
5. Kipling, Rudyard (1865–1936):
    Kim
    Jungle Book
    Short stories
5. Lewis, Sinclair (1885–1951):
    Arrowsmith
5. Mann, Thomas (1875–1955):
    The Magic Mountain
    Confessions of Felix Krull, Confidence Man
5. Marcus Aurelius, emperor of Rome (121–180)
5. Plutarch (46?–120?):
    Plutarch's Lives of Illustrious Men

5. Vallery-Radot, René (1853–1933):
   The Life of Pasteur
4. Watson, James (1928–):
   The Double Helix
   Molecular Biology of the Gene
4. Zinsser, Hans (1878–1940):
   As I Remember Him
   Rats, Lice, and History

References

1. Osler, W. Bed-side library for medical students. In *Aequanimitas and Other Addresses*. Philadelphia: Blakiston's, 1904.
2. Reynolds, R.C. Osler's bed-side library revisited. *Pharos,* pp. 34–36, Spring 1985.

SECTION III

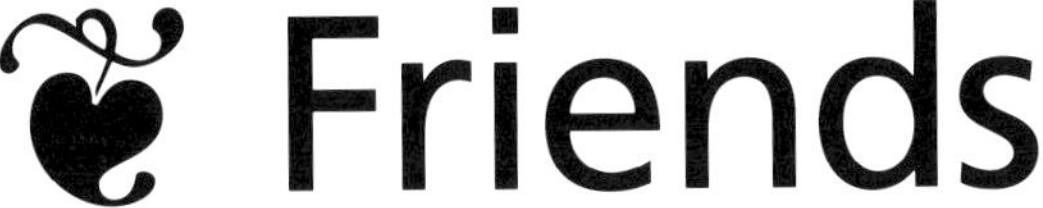

Friends

Cushing and Osler: The Evolution of a Friendship

 Jeremiah A. Barondess, M.D.

WILLIAM OSLER died on December 29, 1919. A month later, Harvey Cushing wrote a touching obituary-memoir, warm, reminiscent and thoughtful, touching on some of the facets of their twenty-three-year friendship that, for him, defined much of its flavor and richness, and the particular intensity it held for him. He wrote:

> Beginning with the kindly admonition (i.e. not to neglect to mention juniors connected with recorded cases) when I was a young surgical house officer at the J.H.H. first trying my feeble literary wings, through letters to a few days before his death—these I find among my papers . . . It was Revere's death unquestionably that so undermined his health he was an easy prey to his terminal pneumonia. The note from Jersey on the 2nd anniversary of the boy's death addressed to 'Dr. Harvey' shows how great was his concealed emotion even then. There are other letters . … . but the extent to which the man influenced my own life as he did that of all others with whom he came in contact is shown by the notes and clippings and pictures which occur in all my books and papers. I had entirely forgotten the Baltimore scrap book until I began to look over the accumulation. In it we found data concerning the Ship of Fools book club—The John Locke dinner—our presentation to him of the Dictionary of National Biography—the slip recalling Revere's annual

Presidential Address. Read at the annual meeting of the American Osler Society, April 27, 1984.

Reprinted with permission from *Transactions and Studies of the College of Physicians of Philadelphia,* 7:79, 1985 celebration of Guy Fawkes' day—the notes from his textbook describing the writing thereof—The Fixed Period address and something of the extraordinary reaction to it in the press which gave us so much anxiety and distress and which sent him to Oxford with a sorry heart I am sure.

. . . . Meanwhile K.C. unearthed many old Kodak pictures among her things which were pasted in her "Willie book" and my journalettes—all contained much about him and 13 Norham Gardens and Lady Osler. When they left Baltimore many of the household possessions were scattered among the "latch keyers" as we were called for a lot of us were given keys and came and went at 1 West Franklin Street as though it were our house—and it was . . . The last thing taken from the house was the door plate which Lady Osler told me to unscrew and keep the morning she departed and which I have had mounted on a block of the Virginia Sandstone from which the house was built. . . There are innumerable things on Dr. Osler's trail that will continue to crop up for many years to come. One thing that I have seen no reference to in the many recent notices is the secret early history of the J.H.H. which is under lock and key to be opened in 100 years. It is probably an amusing skit on the early days. I once saw the book and he read a note from it about Halsted's courting of Miss Hampton."[1]

One should perhaps not find it surprising that these two men developed a friendship of such complexity and warmth, despite the differences in age and status when they first came to know one another, for, in fact, they held common values and interests of immense importance that bound them to each other, quite possibly each as the best friend the other ever had. Their friendship, like most that are strong and lasting, was one in which each found in the other powerful echoes of his own background and interests; echoes, that is, of himself. Each came from a large family and had numerous older siblings. Each was raised in an atmosphere that emphasized traditional virtues, especially hard work, the clear need to make one's own way, and thrift, virtues

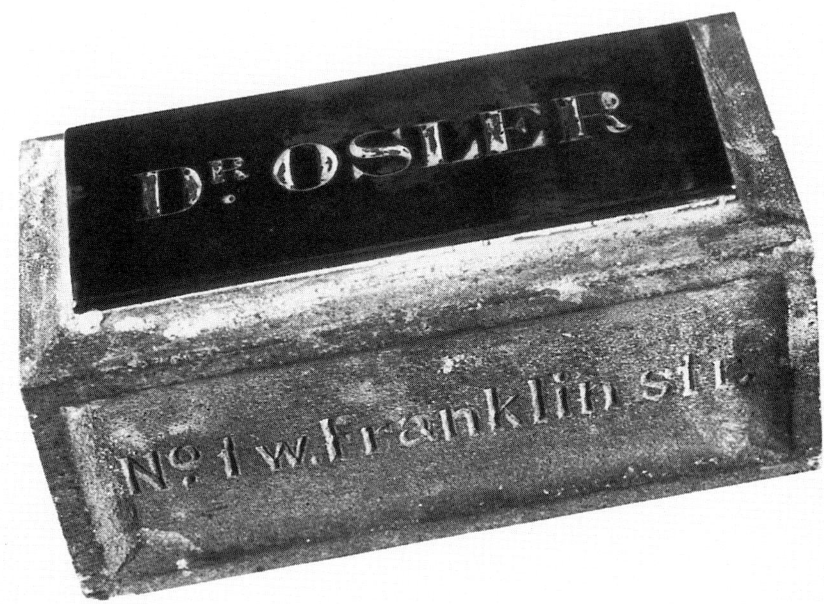

FIGURE 1. Osler's doorplate from 1 West Franklin Street, Baltimore. From the collections of the Historical Library, Yale Medical Library.

emphasized by strong parental role models. Each was high-spirited in boyhood and youth, but found opportunities at home to consort, through books, with the world of ideas and to explore history as a vista evoking feelings of personal identification. Each made a strong marriage that facilitated and supported a life of accomplishment.

But why it should have happened as it did that the young surgical house officer and the Professor of Medicine established the beginnings of such a long and fruitful closeness, is a matter of some interest, a reflection in part of the powerful orientation toward young colleagues held by Osler, and of the charismatic effect he had on his juniors.

Cushing was twenty-seven years old when, in 1896, he came to Baltimore as William Halsted's Assistant Resident in Surgery. Born in Cleveland, he had been to Yale and to the Harvard Medical School, and had spent sixteen months as "House Pupil" at The Massachusetts General Hospital. He had had a wonderful time as a Yale undergraduate, achieving election to Scroll and Key (a matter of considerable importance to him), and, despite his father's vigorous injunctions against drinking, smoking and consorting with those of easy virtue, and above all, engaging in intercollegiate athletics, securing also the shortstop position on the Yale baseball team.

At the Harvard Medical School (M.D. *cum laude* 1895), his drive and brilliance were recognized by his classmates and his gift of originality was already apparent. Thus, during his student years he and his classmate, Amory Codman, developed a system for recording the pulse and respiratory rates of the anesthetized patient as a guide to the surgeon and the anesthetist; these "ether charts", as they were called, were introduced in 1895 (when Cushing was a fourth year student, twenty-five years of age) and were the forerunner of modern operating room records.[2]

During his post-graduate year at The Massachusetts General he was instrumental in purchasing an X-ray tube for the hospital within a year of the announcement of Roentgen's discovery. He brought the tube with him to

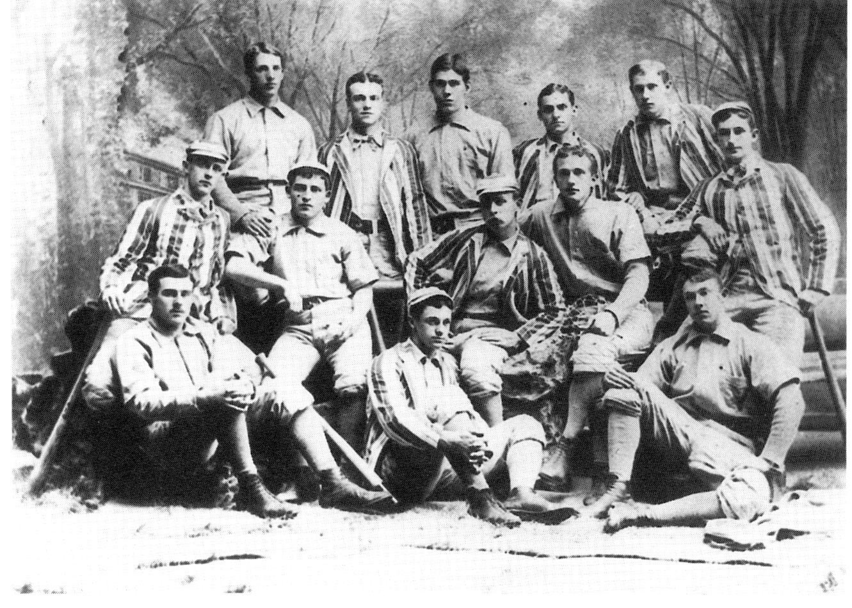

FIGURE 2.   Yale freshman baseball team, 1888. Cushing is in front row, center. From the collections of the Historical Library, Yale Medical Library.

Baltimore the following year, took the first radiographs at The Johns Hopkins Hospital, and, in 1897 and 1898 published two case reports involving the use of X rays.[3,4]

And so, in the fall of 1896, this energetic, attractive and promising young man arrived in Baltimore, filled with ambition, clearly talented, already contributing improvements in clinical care, and destined for a life of high accomplishment. Osler at this time was forty-seven years of age, and had been in his Johns Hopkins professorship for eight years. His renown was already considerable, in fact international; he was the leading American figure in internal medicine and his clinic and textbook were dominant in their fields.

Details of Cushing's contacts with Osler during his early years at Hopkins are sparse, though the small size of the staff and the intense activity that characterized the new institution, including the vigorous young Johns Hopkins Medical Society and the Johns Hopkins Historical Club, must certainly have brought them together frequently. Fulton noted that during Cushing's first two years in Baltimore Osler's influence on him had already become apparent in his (Cushing's) "newly developed interest in books, bookplates, and the acquisition of a library,"[5] interests encouraged by his father. In 1897 Cushing developed appendicitis. Having made the diagnosis and written the admission history himself, he was seen in consultation by Osler before Halsted operated. During his convalescence he designed a family bookplate which included initialed references to the other Doctors Cushing: David (his great-grandfather), Erastus (his grandfather), Henry Kirke (his father), Edward Fitch ("Ned"—his brother), "H.C." himself and, later, Kirke

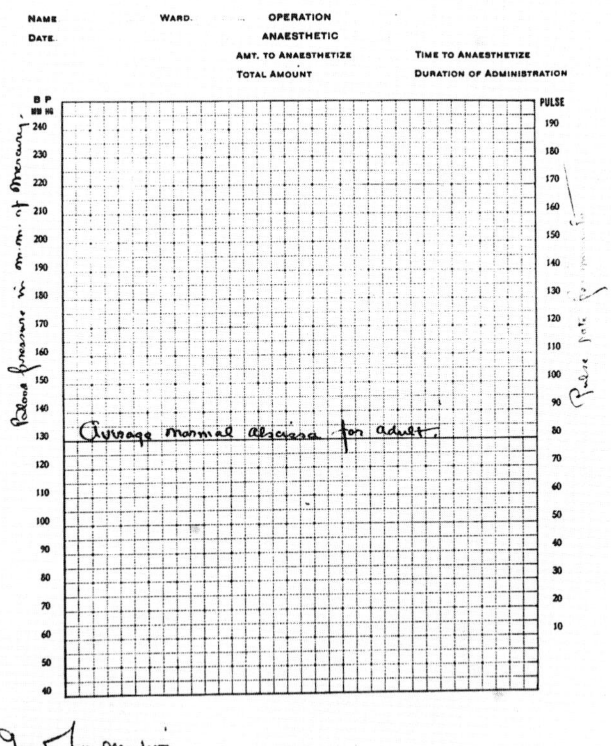

FIGURE 3. Operating room pulse and blood pressure chart. Marginal notes in Cushing's handwriting. From the collections of the Historical Library, Yale Medical Library.

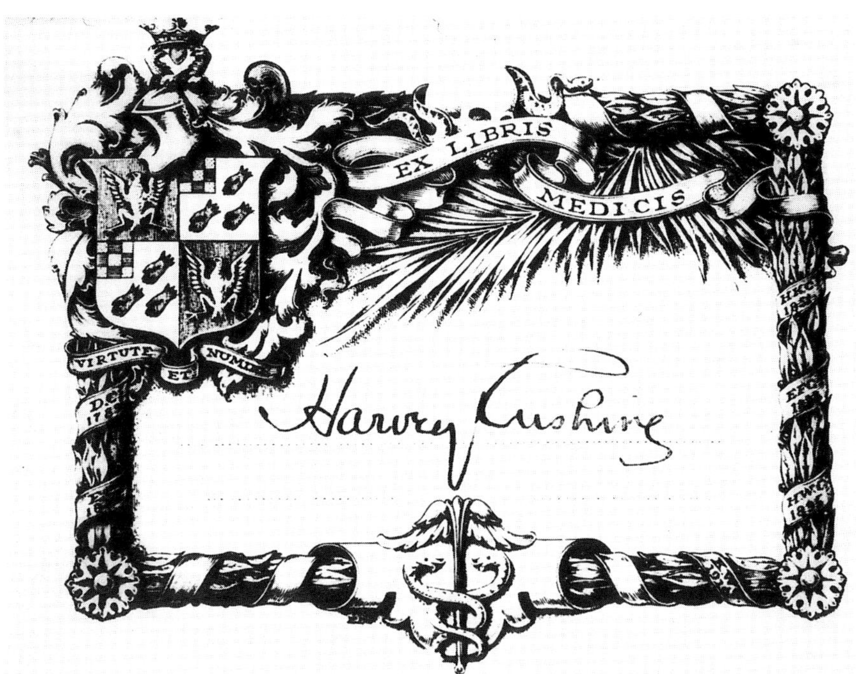

FIGURE 4.   Cushing's bookplate. From the collections of the Historical Library, Yale Medical Library.

and Edward Harvey (nephews), together with the years of their medical degrees.

Early clinical associations with Osler included a case of Banti's Syndrome in which Osler made the diagnosis and recommended splenectomy, which was carried out by Cushing. In addition, he became involved in the Hopkins effort to help with the numerous cases of typhoid fever among U.S. soldiers fighting in the Spanish-American War. He operated upon a number with intestinal perforations, and published two papers on the subject in *The Johns Hopkins Hospital Bulletin* in 1898[6] and *The Johns Hopkins Hospital Reports* in 1900.[7] The first of these brought a note of commendation from Osler and the "kindly admonition" mentioned in the obituary-memoir quoted above. In 1899, two years after his arrival in Baltimore, he introduced his intended, Kate Crowell, of Cleveland, to the Oslers, a clear indication that a close personal relationship already existed with them.

By 1900 Cushing had spent four years at Johns Hopkins, first as Assistant Resident and then as Resident Surgeon, under Halsted. He had become a highly accomplished general surgeon and, in fact, was already a central figure in the Hopkins department. His publications (numbering at this time ten papers), and especially his work on typhoid, had brought him wide recognition, and in 1899 an invitation to join The Department of Surgery at Western Reserve University in Cleveland. Although tempted, he elected to remain in Baltimore. Now, at the age of thirty, committed to an academic surgical career, and with the encouragement of his father and of Osler and Welch, he spent fourteen months in Europe—an experience which transformed him from ". . . a self-assured and somewhat provincial young American with many a deep-rooted prejudice . . . ." into ". . . a cosmopolitan with a greatly broadened point of view on medical matters, and a deep respect for European culture and tradition."[8]

This year of travel was planned around study with Kocher, Horsley and Sherrington, all men with neurological interests, although Cushing remarked

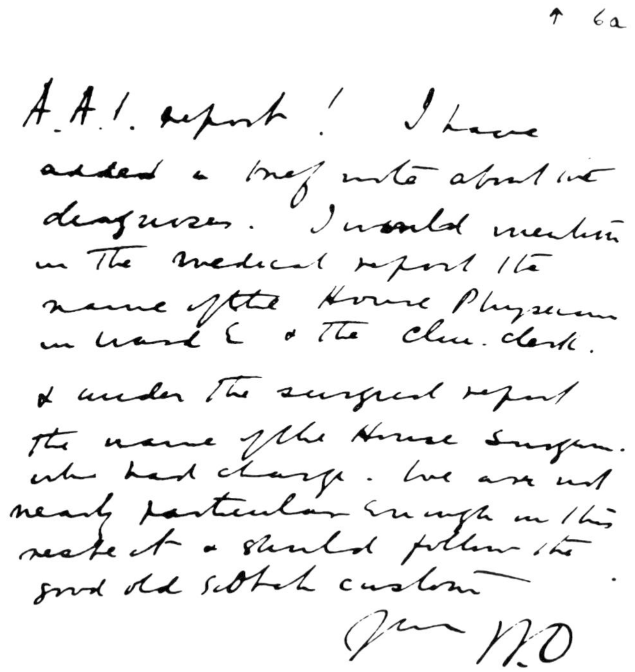
↑ 6a

A.A.1. report! I have
added a brief note about the
diagnoses. I would mention
in the medical report the
name of the House Physician
in Ward E & the clin. clerk.
& under the surgical report
the name of the House Surgeon.
who had charge. We are not
nearly particular enough in this
respect & should follow the
good old Scotch custom
Yours W.O

FIGURE 5. Note from Osler to Cushing, 1898 "A.A.1 report! I have added a brief note about the diagnoses. I would mention in the medical report the name of the House Physician in Ward E and the clin. clerk and under the surgical report the name of the House Surgeon who had charge. We are not nearly particular enough in this respect and should follow the good old Scotch custom. Yours W.O. From the collections of the Historical Library, Yale Medical Library.

twenty years later that at the time he had no idea of ultimately specializing in neurological surgery."[9] He arrived in Liverpool in July, 1900, and was welcomed by Osler, who was spending the summer in England "braindusting." Through Osler's sponsorship he met many of the leading British medical men of the day, and was included in social and professional gatherings to which he would not otherwise have had access. The Oslers included him also in their own activities; lunch at the George and Dragon at Wargrave, rowing on the Thames, a visit to Dorset to escape the sweltering London heat, and through it all, visits to the great London clinics and, over and over again, to the Hunterian Museum at the Royal College of Surgeons. He examined old books with Rolleston, visited the portraits at the College of Physicians and saw the Gold-Headed Cane. He met Jonathan Hutchinson, Horsley, Broadbent and Gowers, and attended the centennial celebration of the Royal College of Surgeons. Thus, the month in England saw his interests broadened, his contacts with medical men of great accomplishment enriched, and his nascent bibliophilia and historical interests beginning to stir, all under the beneficent guidance and stimulus of Osler, who had clearly marked him for special attention.

After the London sojourn Cushing toured France and Switzerland, particularly sites of medical interest. In the process he put into a travel diary notes and a series of beautiful sketches and water colors of LePuy-en-Velay, which give vivid evidence of his capacity for artistic expression and keen observation. Ultimately, in Kronecker's laboratory in Berne, with the requisite blessing from Kocher, Halsted's great friend, he conducted a brilliant series of studies on the effects of increased intracranial pressure on blood pressure and intracranial blood flow. These experiments demonstrated the rise in arterial pressure that accompanies increasing intracranial pressure, and the lethality of intracranial pressures in excess of the arterial level. In other studies he

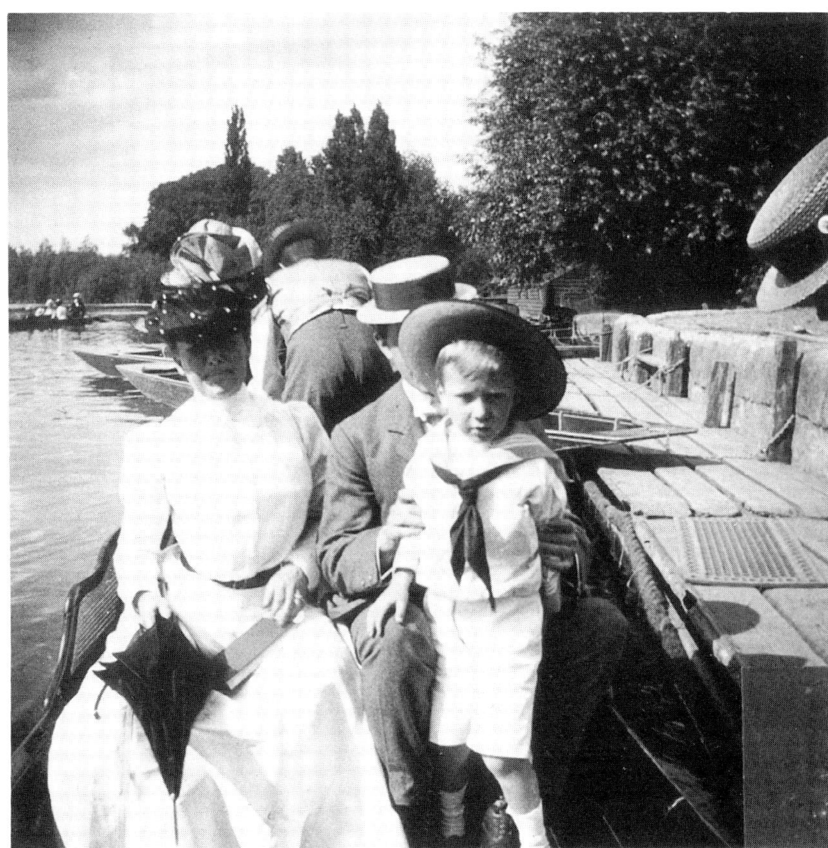

FIGURE 6. Mrs. Osler and Revere, Cushing behind, on the Thames, 1900. From the collections of the Historical Library, Yale Medical Library.

analyzed the effect of saline solutions on frog nerve-muscle preparations. Within four months he not only accumulated a body of highly important data, but found himself included in the social circle of the Berne medical establishment, at least in part, according to Leon Asher, his physiologist friend, because of "his personality and his beautiful dancing."[10] He also grew a moustache which made him look astonishingly like the young Osler!

The trip continued through Italy, where, studying humans with bony defects of the skull in Angelo Mosso's laboratory, he made important additional observations on the relation between systemic arterial pressure and pressure on the vasomotor center. In Florence he was greatly taken with della Robbia's medallions at the Hospital of the Innocents, and in Padua, intellectual seat of Malpighi, Vesalius, Fabricius and Harvey, his historical perceptions were further stimulated and sharpened. At Pavia, in the Ospedale di S. Matteo, he found an adaptation of Riva Rocci's blood pressure apparatus in clinical use, sketched it and brought back to Baltimore a model of the inflatable armlet. Thus, he was instrumental in introducing clinical sphygmomanometry into use in the operating rooms and clinics in this country.[11] He continued through Germany, meeting or visiting with Naunyn, Hofmeister, Erb, Kussmaul, Solley and other greats. The trip ended with a fruitful month with Sherrington working on cerebral localization in the chimpanzee, orangutan and gorilla, a forerunner not only of much of Cushing's future work, but of his warm lifelong friendship with Sherrington. Later he visited William Hunter's

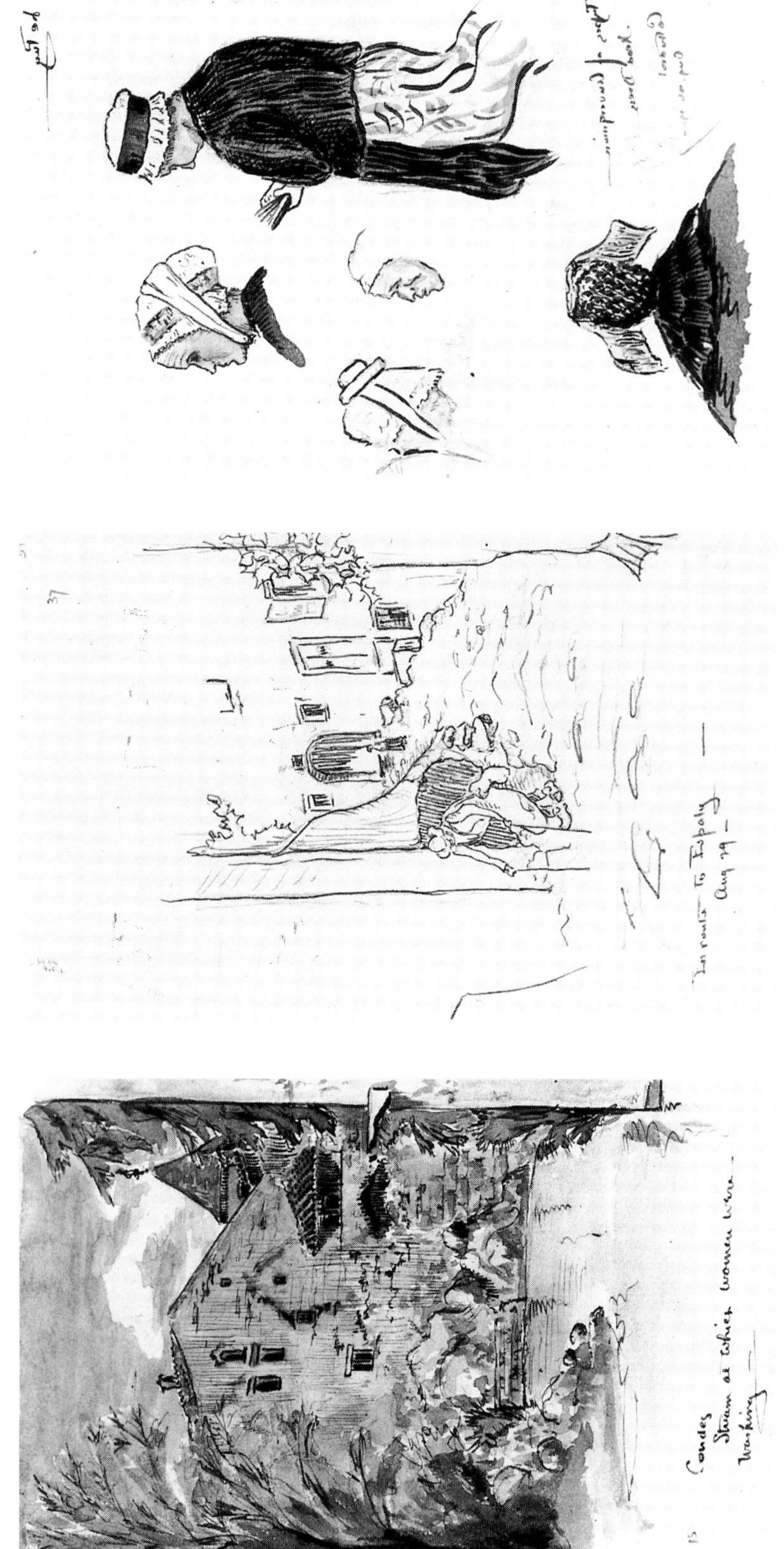

FIGURE 7. Sketches and water colors, Le Puy-en-Velay, 1990. From the collections of the Historical Library, Yale Medical Library.

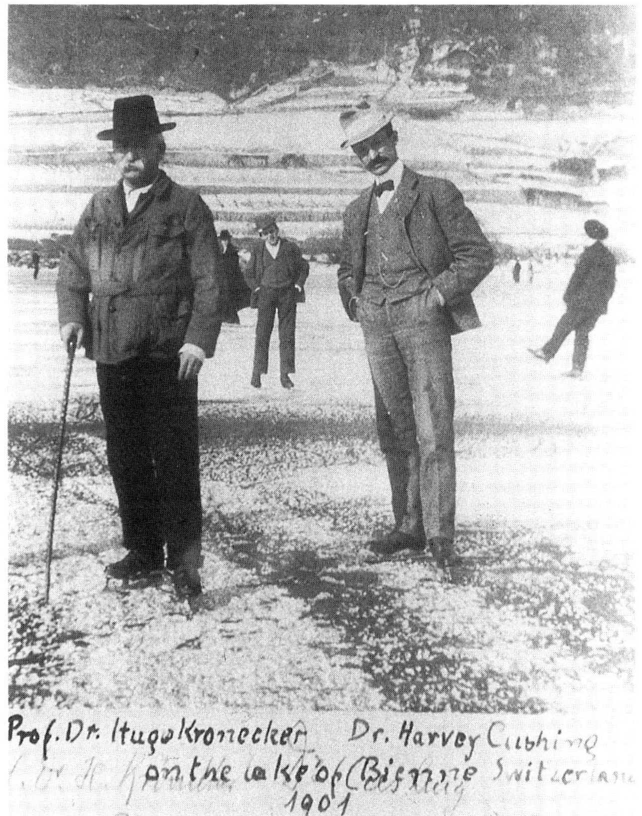

FIGURE 8. On the ice with Hugo Kronecker, 1901. From the collections of the Historical Library, Yale Medical Library.

remarkable museum and great library, an event that Fulton suggested might have crystallized in his mind the idea of forming a library of his own.[12]

The trip over, now acquainted with the wider world of medicine, and with a record of substantial accomplishment in several of the great European laboratories, he returned to Baltimore. The degree to which his experiences in Britain and on the continent were orchestrated or at least facilitated by Osler is unclear, but must have been substantial. In addition, this trip clearly marked the beginning of real intimacy between Cushing and the Oslers. Back at Hopkins he was invited to join the faculty, due, he wrote, "largely . . . to pressure brought to bear by Welch and Osler."[13]

As the friendship grew, so did Osler's influence on Cushing. Fulton felt that the younger man tried to emulate Osler's outgoing personality, as his own relationships with colleagues and subordinates were often difficult.[14] Early in 1902 Osler warned him of the danger of this, further evidence of his concern for the development of Cushing's career:

3/3/02

1 West Franklin St.

". . . you will not mind a reference to one point—the statement is current that you do not get on well with your surgical subordinates and colleagues. I heard of it last year and it was referred to by a strong admirer of yours in New York. The statement also is made that you've criticized before the students the modes of dressings, operations, etc., of members of the staff. This, I need scarcely say, would be absolutely fatal to your success here. The arrangement of the Hospital staff is so peculiar that loyalty to each other, even

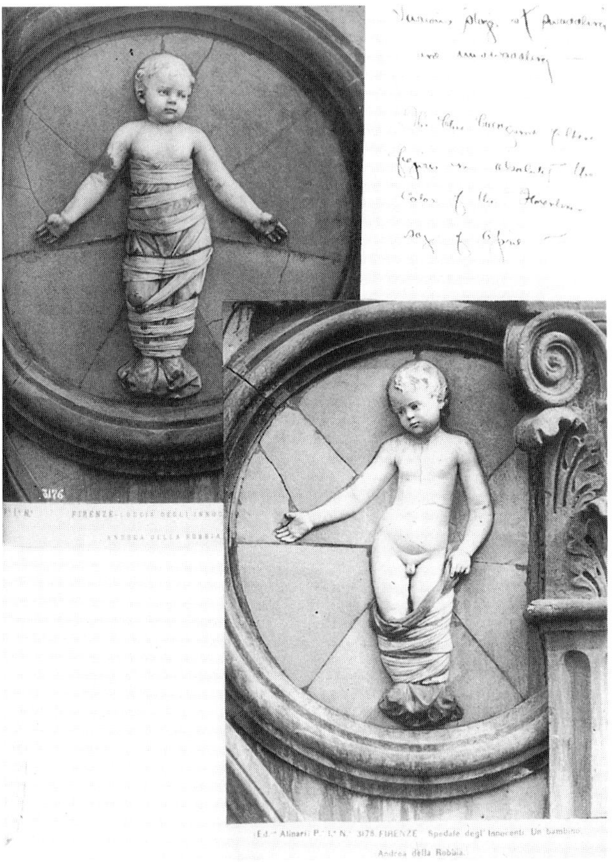

FIGURE 9. Post card showing two of the della Robbia medallions at the Hospital of the Innocents, Florence. From Cushing's travel diary, 1901. The notes, in Cushing's hand say: "Various stages of swaddling and unswaddling. The blue background of these figures is absolutely the color of the Florentine sky of April." From the collections of the Historical Library, Yale Medical Library.

> in the minutest particulars, is an essential. I know you will not mind this from me, and have your interest at heart.
>
> Sincerely yours,
Wm Osler

and, a few days later:

> 1 West Franklin St
> Dear C—Do nothing of the kind! Who is free from faults and failings! It is a simple matter—"Keep your mouth" (as the Psalmist says.)[1]

Later in October, 1901, Cushing moved into the house at 3 West Franklin Street, next door to the Oslers, along with Thomas B. Futcher and Henry Barton Jacobs. Each of them maintained offices in the house and Cushing had a letterhead made up in the style of Osler's. The three were promptly given latch keys to the Osler house and invited to make free use of them, as indeed they did, especially for access to Osler's library. Futcher later married the daughter of R. Palmer Howard, Professor of Medicine at McGill when Osler was a medical student. He practiced in Baltimore until his death in

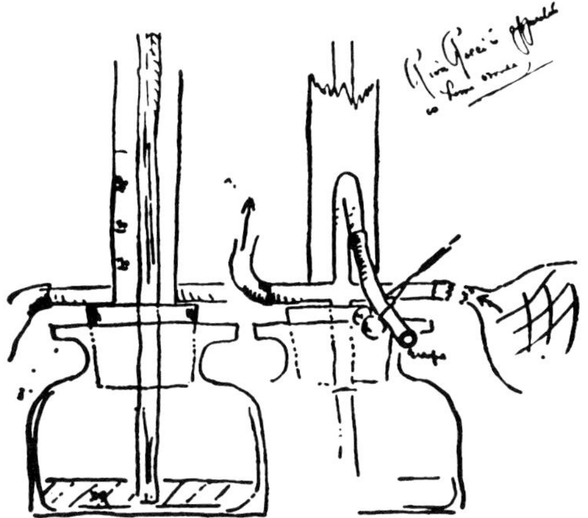

FIGURE 10. From the Alan Mason Chesney Medical Archives, The John Hopkins Medical Institutions.

1938. Jacobs, in 1902, married Alice Frick Garrett. In 1932 he gave to the Welch Medical Library his extraordinary collection of books, prints, tokens, medals and autograph letters relating to the history of medicine, together with funds to provide appropriate space and facilities for the collection. At the dedication ceremonies Cushing delivered a charming allegory about the "latch keyer" days and described how "the man next door" (Osler) began leaving book catalogues at the house; how he, Futcher and Jacobs "each got the infection for which, like the common cold, there is no known preventive;" and how the mysterious brown-wrapped parcels with foreign stamps began to arrive at the house.[15]

Cushing's early faculty years were occupied with clinical problems in general surgery and with the organization and teaching of the famous course in comparative surgery, the "dog surgery" still provided for Hopkins students. Photographs of him at this time show a young man of serious aspect, sometimes rather a dandy, sometimes less so.

In 1902 he and Kate were finally married after a very lengthy courtship and engagement, and took up residence at the 3 West Franklin Street address, where Grace Osler promptly took the new bride under her wing. Osler sent him an occasional consultation.

In 1903 the Cushings' first child, a boy, was born, and named William Harvey, not for the great physiologist, but for Osler and for H.C. himself. Earlier that year Osler started Cushing on a Vesalius essay, loaning him a copy of the *Fabrica*.[16] Cushing determined then to begin to collect Vesaliana and in December, at Osler's Book and Journal Club, he read his first paper on Vesalius, "The Books of Vesalius". Thus began at Osler's instigation a bibliophilic and historical interest leading to one of the great Vesalius collections.

Cushing's interest in medical societies began at about this time, as he became involved in the newly formed Society of Clinical Surgery, with which he remained affiliated. An active member for many years, he served as its President in 1927. Echoes of Osler's strong advocacy of medical societies may perhaps be perceived here, as also in Cushing's membership in the American Neurological Association of which he was president in 1923, The American

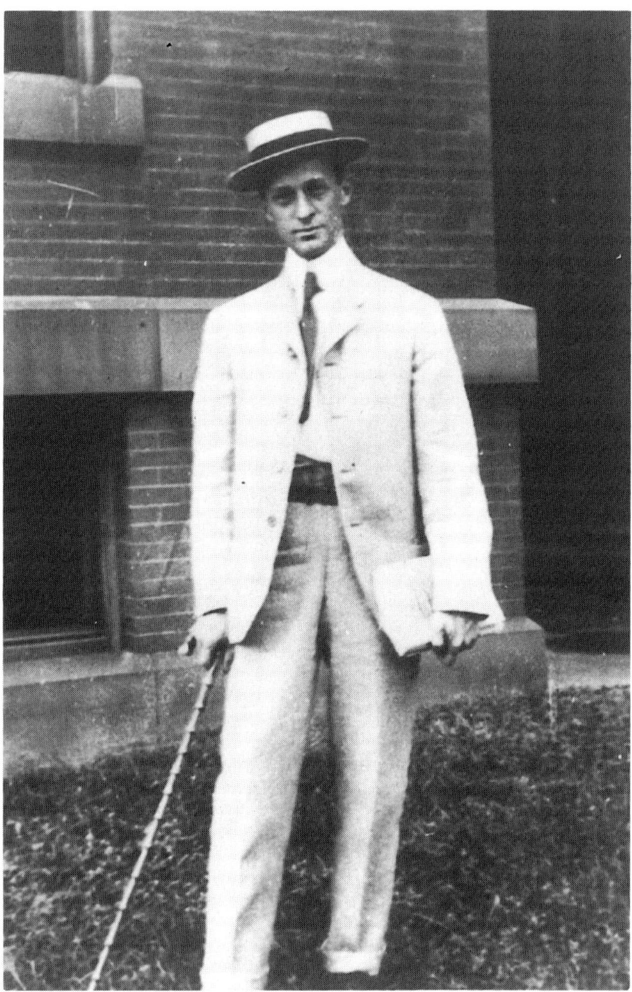

Surgical Association (President, 1927), Association for the Study of Internal
Secretions (President, 1921), and numerous others, domestic and foreign, in
which he held active or honorary memberships. In them he found the unity,
friendship and intellectual refreshment noted by Osler to be the chief values
of the medical society.[17] In 1919 he saw the organization, at his own suggestion, of The Society of Neurological Surgeons, first called The Neurosurgical Club, the first in the specialty and, just as he retired from his chair at
Harvard and the Brigham, the Harvey Cushing Society was given form by some
thirty-five of the younger of his professional offspring, the name having been
adopted with his acquiescence. Thus he came to share with Osler, as a mark
both of distinction and affection, the formation of a society dedicated to his
example and carrying his name.

In July, 1904, Cushing set off for England for a month with Osler,
Futcher and McCrae. A sketch he made, which bears witness to his artistic
talent as well as to his sense of humor, alludes to Osler's habit of cramming the
rack in his berth with books and papers, and working there for four or five
hours each morning. The drawing further suggests the impact of the shipboard cuisine on Cushing's avoirdupois. It was on this trip, at a dinner with

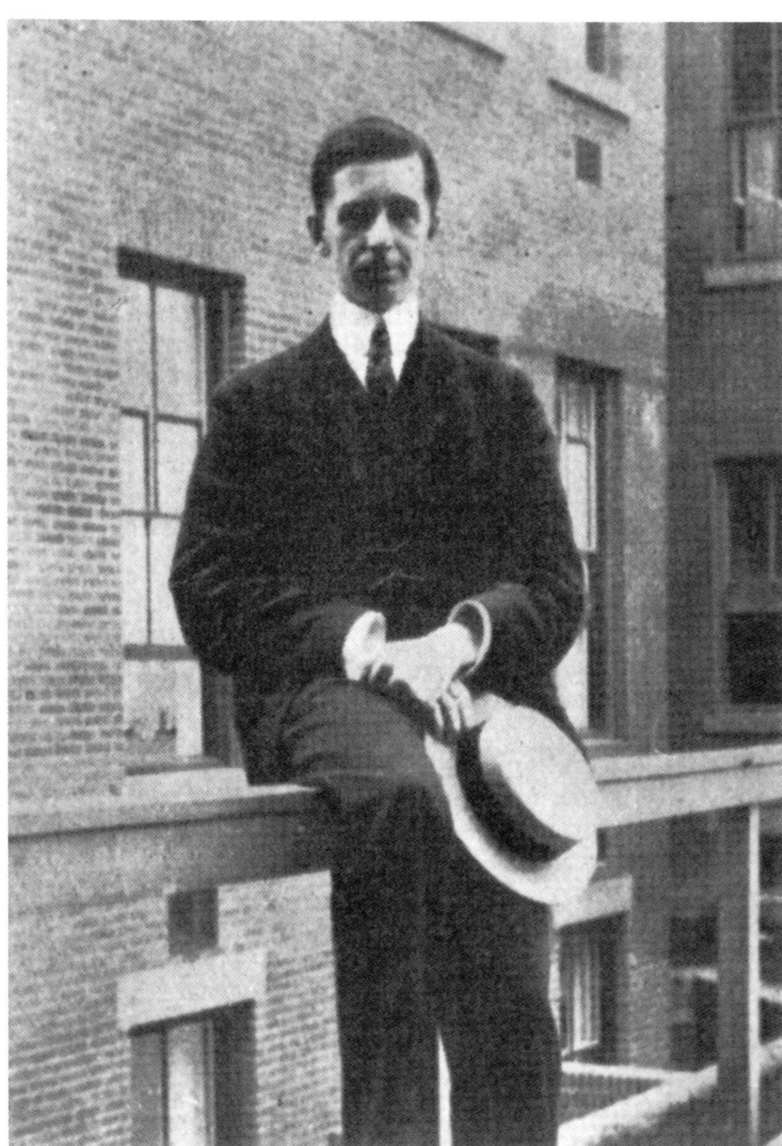

FIGURE 12. Thomas B. Futcher. From the Alan Mason Chesney Medical Archives. The Johns Hopkins Medical Institutions.

Rolleston and his young colleagues, that Osler asked, "Do you think I'm sufficiently senile to become Regius Professor at Oxford?" Other rumors of the Oxford offer came to the ears of Osler's traveling companions, and at one point he showed them the first line of Mrs. Osler's famous cable, "Do not procrastinate. Accept at once," covering over the last phrase, so that they remained uncertain until the return home what his decision was likely to be. In December Cushing read his famous paper, "Dr. Garth: The Kit-Kat Poet,"[18] an early venture into general literature, also undertaken at Osler's instigation. Garth had arranged for the funeral of John Dryden, and had had invitations printed. Cushing searched for years for one of these, but ultimately had to be satisfied with a facsimile.

The early days of 1905 were dominated by Osler's impending departure for Oxford. On February 22, he read his valedictory, the famous, or infamous, "The Fixed Period," and Cushing shared his amazement and distress over the storm that broke in response to it. Such was the reaction that it proved impossible to bring to fruition a plan to build a new library building at the Medical and Chirurgical Faculty of Maryland as a testimonial to Osler, or to purchase and preserve the house at 1 West Franklin Street as a further gesture of respect and affection, both projects in which Cushing had been a leading participant.

The Oslers' departure in May, 1905, was followed in the same year by a Christmas visit to Baltimore, during which the Cushings saw a good deal of them, as they did over the following Christmas when Kate Cushing held a reception for them to which more than three hundred people came. She later wrote her father-in-law that "about forty people stayed on to supper." Shades of the 'Open Arms', as the Osler home in Oxford was to come to be known! In 1907 Cushing's avid interest in medical history was expressed in a vigorous year's program of the Johns Hopkins Historical Club, of which he was

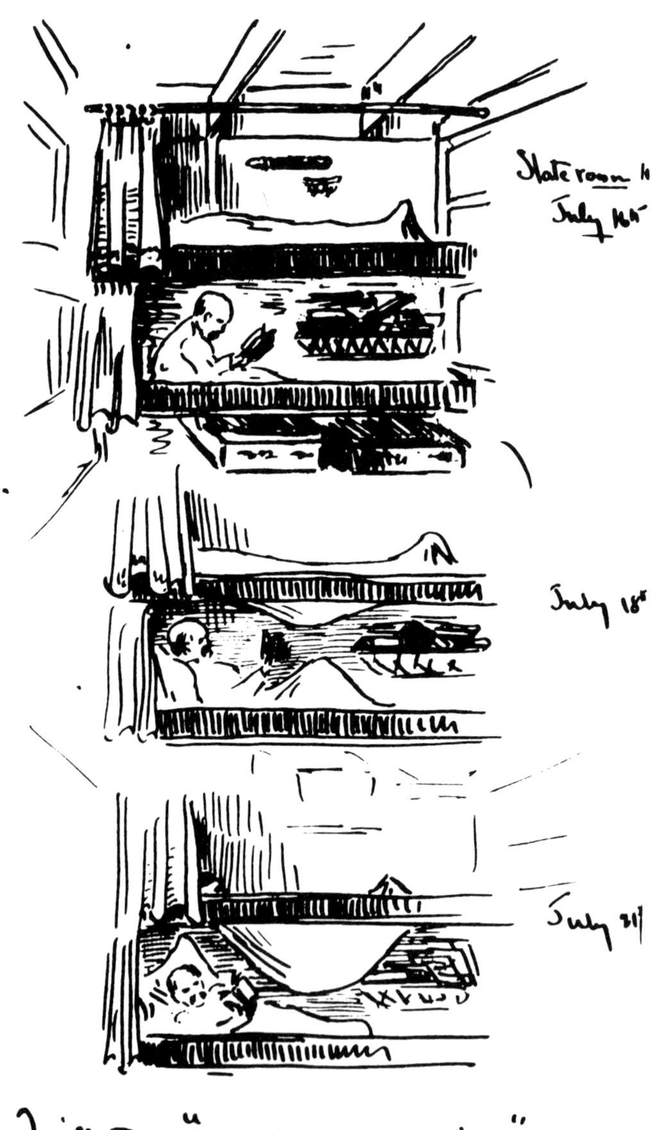

FIGURE 13.   CUSHING'S shipboard sketch, 1904. Rapidly developing obesity in Cushing (upper berth) while Osler works steadily below. From the collections of the Historical Library, Yale Medical Library.

president. At one meeting he read a paper entitled "Notes Concerning John Locke as a Physician," an interest he maintained in later years.

As his activities in neurosurgery increased and came to dominate his research as well as his teaching and his practice, Cushing became to an increasing degree a major figure in the surgical world. This concentration had begun around the turn of the century, with particular focus on trigeminal neuralgia, followed by increasing interest in the surgery of brain tumors and in refinements of operative technique. From 1908 to 1912 he turned his attention more and more to problems of pituitary disease and tumors of the cerebellum. By 1909, at the age of forty, he was publishing steadily in his field, speaking at major medical meetings and presenting invited lectures. Through these busy years his correspondence with Osler went on apace, and he preserved in his papers numerous notes, cards and more extended letters from both of the Oslers, some to Kate, some to himself, some to both. The personal notes from Osler covered a broad terrain, both geographically and in subject matter, but the most constant themes were books and medical history. Almost invariably they closed with love to the Cushing children, now three in number (William, Mary and Betsey).

Cushing at this point had matured not only in the more direct expressions of his professional life, but as a medical historiophile and collector. Thus, a trip to Oxford in the summer of 1909 was notable for examination of the *Fabrica* and *Tabulae Sex* and other Vesalius items at Merton, St. John's and the Bodleian, and in Basle, for a visit to the Vesalianum. Later, in Venice, he examined and photographed the Vesalian items in the Biblioteca Nazionale and the Libreria Vecchia. Later he hunted books in Florence. On this trip he gave invited lectures at the University of Liverpool and at the International Medical Congress in Budapest, but his bibliophilic and historical interests were also given lively expression, much in the fashion of his mentor.

His Johns Hopkins years culminated in the publication of the great pituitary monograph, a milestone in the history of endocrinology. Beginning in 1901 he had been offered the chairs in surgery at the University of Maryland, Jefferson, Washington University, Yale and elsewhere, but declined

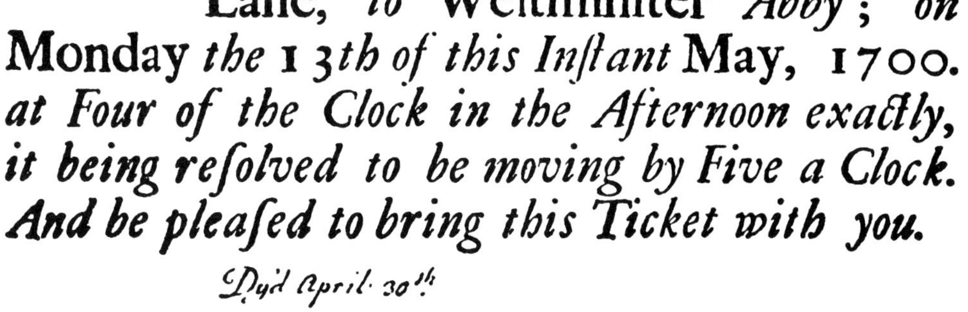

SIR,

YOU are defired to Accompany the Corps of Mr. John Dryden, from the College of Phyficians in Warwick-Lane, to Weftminfter Abby; on Monday the 13th of this Inftant May, 1700. at Four of the Clock in the Afternoon exactly, it being refolved to be moving by Five a Clock. And be pleafed to bring this Ticket with you.

Dryd April 30th

FIGURE 14.   From the collections of the Historical Library, Yale Medical Library.

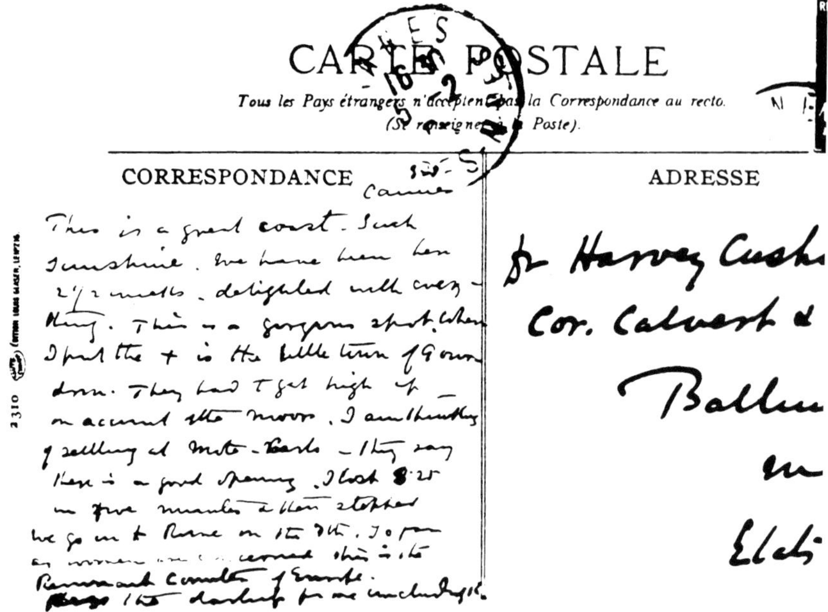

FIGURE 15.   Card from Cannes, probably 1909.
"This is a great coast. Such sunshine. We have been here 2 $^1/_2$ weeks—delighted with everything. This is a gorgeous spot. Where I put the X is the little town of Gourdron. They had to get high up on account of the Moors. I am thinking of settling at Monte Carlo—they say there is a good opening. I lost $25 in five minutes and then stopped. We go to Rome on the 7th. So far as women are concerned this is the remnant counter of Europe. Kiss the darlings for me including K." From the collections of the Historical Library, Yale Medical Library.

them all. Finally, in 1910, when he was forty-one years of age, came the call from Harvard which had been long in his thoughts, and he accepted, with Osler's urging, the Moseley Chair and the position of Surgeon-in-Chief at the new Peter Bent Brigham Hospital. He and Henry Christian, the new Physician-in-Chief, a Johns Hopkins graduate who had trained with Osler, early established the principle of mandatory retirement from the Hospital staff at age sixty-three, a stricture Cushing came to rue when it was applied to him.

Within a year of the opening of the Brigham Hospital the full-time arrangement for clinical teachers was proposed for the Harvard Medical School, and the General Education Board offered the University one and one-half million dollars for the introduction of a full-time system for the chiefs of clinic at the Hospital. Cushing and Christian had put in place an arrangement that permitted the care of private patients and the retention of the fees thus generated. In the ensuing discussions Cushing offered to step down as Surgeon-in-Chief if the University decided to accept the gift, and, in fact, put his resignation in President Lowell's hands. In addition to the financial considerations he doubted, he said, that such an arrangement would "activate" him, and feared it might in fact encourage indolence. He did not think he would become a more active investigator and he was concerned with the preservation of the personal relationship between himself and his patients. Thus, he occupied a position closer by far to Osler's original one than to Flexner's. In the event, Harvard declined both the gift and Cushing's resignation.[19]

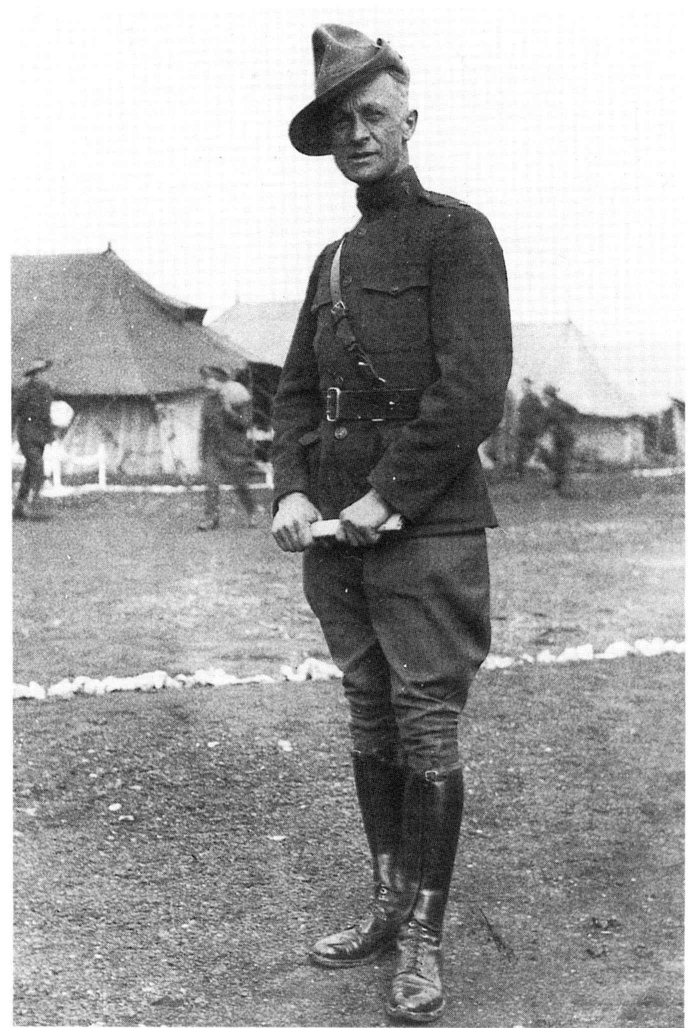

FIGURE 16. Cushing at the *Ambulance Americaine*, Paris, 1915. From the collections of the Historical Library, Yale Medical Library.

In 1913, in London for the International Medical Congress, he gave one of the three principal addresses. Cushing's speech contained a call for reform in medical education and for recognition of the role surgery had come to play in medicine. He called for directors of hospital units in continuous service, without practice outside the institution, rather than "visiting" appointees, and urged bringing the students to the bedside. This amounted to "a frontal attack upon the vested interests of the British hospital system, in which a student could pass an examination in surgery . . . without ever having entered a surgical operating theatre."[20] Along the way he delivered a vigorous attack on the antivivisectionists, a battle he had joined on numerous prior occasions. As might be expected, his remarks on medical education and training and on the decline of animal experimentation in Britain drew fire, and Osler rose to his defence in a letter to *The Times*.

The war in Europe found Cushing, in December, 1914, organizing a Harvard medical unit which sailed on March 18, 1915. It served with distinction in Neuilly with the *Ambulance Americaine* for two months or so, an interval in which Cushing saw many head and spinal cord injuries. Two years later, in May, 1917, he sailed to France again, this time with Base Hospital No. 5, a Harvard Unit, which he had largely organized. His extraordinary war journals contain a detailed daily record of his experiences, extending to some nine volumes of one thousand pages each. In addition he kept clinical records on each of the many cases on whom he personally operated.

The War involved the Oslers from the start. Lady Osler organized numerous supporting activities in Oxford—clothing for the troops in France and for those dislocated by the fighting; help with hospital arrangements in Oxford, and so on. Sir William, having been made an honorary colonel in 1908, when the "territorials" were organized, was never called up. Nevertheless, he was almost feverishly active, serving as Physician-in-Chief of the Queen's Canadian Military Hospital near Folkestone, and as consultant to a number of other Canadian and American military hospitals. He attempted, without success, to introduce mandatory typhoid vaccination for the Army, the effort being beaten back through the combined efforts of the antivivisectionists and the antivaccinationists, both deeply opposed to any compulsory legislation of this nature.[21]

The Oslers' mounting concern for their son, Revere, is apparent in their notes and letters of the time. Initially in the Quartermaster Corps, the boy transferred to the artillery to be nearer the action. Osler himself had a premonition from the first, according to Cushing, that the war would bring him personal sorrow. When the blow fell, on August 30, 1917, Cushing was a half-hour away from Revere, and, with Crile, helped while Darrach and Brewer operated in an effort to repair the shrapnel wounds of the abdomen. He wired a warning to Oxford and, when Revere died the next morning, Cushing saw him carried to his grave covered by a Union Jack. He wrote, "A strange scene—the great-great-grandson of Paul Revere under a British flag, and awaiting him a group of some six or eight American Army medical officers—saddened with the thoughts of his father."[22] Correspondence from the Oslers over the next few days revealed their heartbreak, of course, but also something of what Cushing meant to them. Osler's notes of a year and two years later echoed the same feelings:

> 13 Norham Gardens
> Oxford
>
> 8/31/17
> "Dear Harvey—What a comfort to feel that you were with the laddie at the end and that someone who loved him and that he loved was near. We are heart-broken but shall face the ordeal bravely. With deepest gratitude, yours affectly—Wm Osler."
>
> (From the Osler Library of the History of Medicine, McGill University)

To Cushing from Lady Osler:

> 13 Norham Gardens,
> Oxford
>
> 8/31/17
> "Dearest Harvey—Our one comfort is that you were with him. No one in the world could have done as much and no one been fonder of him. I can only think what an agony it was to you when you saw him come in . . . Dear Revere,

he was living for his leave—a letter last evening told what we would do—I hope he knew you and could talk to you—it is very hard—and we are getting old. There was a fine life in store for the boy—but it couldn't be. I always expected this to happen—but I never could be ready . . . . What a marvel it is that we have you all to help us—and your children . . . .
Our love,
Tante Grace"

(From the Osler Library of the History of Medicine, McGill University)

To Mrs. Cushing:

13 Norham Gardens,
Oxford
Aug 31, 1917

"Dear Kate,
    The sole comfort in our sorrow is that Harvey was with the dear laddie at the end. Was there ever anything more fortunate! Of all men he is the one we should have chosen to be near Revere at the end. We cannot tell you what a consolation it is to us. Grace keeps up bravely and we are going to bear our sorrow with patience, but we are just heartbroken as you may suppose. He had grown more and more lovable as the years passed and he and I had so much in common.
    Blessings on you all.
Yours affectionately
Wm Osler"

(From the Osler Library of the History of Medicine, McGill University)

To Mrs. Cushing from Lady Osler:

Oxford
September 1st, p.m.

"O Kate, dear Kate, my darling fair baby has gone—just laid in that wet cold Belgium. I thank God for two things—your Harvey was with him and he has gone to a peaceful spot. I feel sure of that—and we are rather old and may go too, very soon—we hope so—just fancy Harvey being with him—we are waiting and waiting for his letter and I'm sure he will come here on his first leave—and perhaps bring some messages he couldn't write. I can only see Revere lying on his stretcher with Harvey holding his dear, dirty hand. It is our comfort—our only comfort today to think Harvey was there and you'll be glad too."

and later:

Aug 30th (?)
13 Norham Gardens,
Oxford

"Dear Harvey

    Just a year ago poor Isaac was taken and the one bright spot in the tragedy was that you were with him. It has been a hard year but we have stood it better than we could have expected. . . ."

(From the Osler Library of the History of Medicine, McGill University)

From Jersey:

    "A line of love and thankful remembrance for all you did for the dear laddie two years ago. I think of what it must have meant to him to open his eyes and see his dear friend beside him. How hard it must have been for you! But to us it is and has been an inexpressible comfort. Who was the nurse? I do not believe we ever had her name. Best love to you all. Yours ever, Wm Osler.''

(From the Osler Library of the History of Medicine, McGill University)

After the war Cushing returned to the pace and the program of activities to which he was accustomed. Within six months of his return from Europe he wrote and published anonymously a history of Base Hospital No. 5.[23]

He had already attempted, in 1917 and 1918, to establish a National Institute for the Investigation of Disorders of the Nervous System, through the help of the General Education Board, and was prepared to give up the Moseley Chair to join it. After protracted negotiations the proposal died, as Fulton said, "of inanition," having failed to attract support from the Rockefeller and Carnegie Foundations as well as the War Department, all of whom he had approached.

During 1919 he helped to put together the Osler seventieth birthday volumes and in May he sent Osler, as a birthday gift, Clemenceau's thesis for his doctorate in medicine, of which, as it turned out, Osler already had a copy.

Cushing had become increasingly concerned about Osler's health after Revere's death. Lady Osler had written that he was sleeping badly and losing weight. During Osler's final illness Cushing was kept aware of the situation, and was finally advised by cable of his death on December 29. The brief memoir quoted at the beginning of this paper was written shortly thereafter, but even before, four days after Osler's death, he wrote an obituary notice which appeared in the *Boston Evening Transcript*.[24] It was a moving tribute to Osler's personal qualities, written in Cushing's clear and powerful style, and it persuaded Lady Osler that he should be entrusted with the biography rather than William S. Thayer, of Baltimore, as she had originally planned. In her letter she alluded to the unique closeness of their relationship. "I know of only one man worthy and able to do it and that is *you*, and printed by the (Oxford) Press—I can say no more. I leave the answer to you. There is no one here who knows everything—medicine, brain, home, friends, heart, endurance, in fact all that he was—you know all."[1] And a day later, after hearing Sir Humphrey Rolleston's enthusiastic reaction to the idea, she wrote again, "I have come home with my mind and heart full of it and am sending this second note to you to ask if you will think seriously of it. I am convinced there is no one else who understands as you do."[1] Fulton noted, "clearly this was a request which H.C. could not decline. Osler had meant everything to him for twenty years. He had been a spiritual father and had had a keener understanding of Cushing's own restless nature than almost anyone. He had done much to inculcate in H.C. his love of literature, history, and his undying interest in Vesalius."[25] Cushing accepted.

Although he had originally estimated that the research would take about a year and the writing six months, in the event his labors on the biography took some four years; they were characterized by his unfailing thoroughness and his desire for detail. He read biographies and discussed biographical writing with Boston friends. He spent months in Oxford, canvassed friends and colleagues of Sir William for letters and details, peppered Lady Osler for minutia, sometimes to her exasperation, and depended heavily on her letters. Finally, in 1924, he had a manuscript of one million words, edited later, at the insistence of the Oxford University Press, to about 650,000. Lady Osler received her first bound copy of *The Life of Sir William Osler* in March, 1925, and the book was officially published on April 16.

That the book was a labor of love there can be no doubt, and the avalanche of praise that greeted it, including the Pulitzer Prize in 1926 and the acclaim of Osler's friends, must have been substantial indeed. Even more, the satisfaction of having done this for his friend and mentor, for his "spiritual father," and for Lady Osler, must have warmed his heart and eased his mourning. It is of interest that Cushing left himself out of the biography completely, except by inference or circumlocution. He had read Henry Festing Jones' life of Samuel Butler before writing the biography, and had been irritated by the way in which Jones had brought himself into the story; Fulton felt this had lent weight to the decision to efface himself from the 'Osler.'

Criticism came too, though, importantly, from his old friend Welch, who reviewed the book for the *Saturday Review of Literature*. Welch felt that Osler's objections to the full-time system had been overdrawn. Certain Philadelphians felt that he had been unfair to William Pepper. But on balance the book was immensely successful, not only as a literary effort, but, as time proved, by the degree to which it accomplished the purpose expressed in the dedication: "To medical students, in the hope that something of Osler's spirit may be conveyed to those of a generation that has not known him; and particularly to those in America, lest it be forgotten who it was that made it possible for them to work at the bedside in the wards." Indeed, the greatest contribution made by the biography has been the degree to which it has helped to keep Osler a palpable and powerful presence among his professional descendants.

While writing the book Cushing continued to be productive not only in his clinical work, but in teaching and writing. Between January, 1920, and the end of 1924, when the final chapters of the biography went to press, he published fifty major papers and reports. He had by this time a personal series of more than one thousand brain tumors operated upon, and had begun to classify and analyze the clinical behavior of the various types, an effort never previously undertaken.

Honors came to him in abundance in these years. In 1922 he was offered Halsted's chair, but responded that he could not face another transplantation. He continued to write on historical subjects, and organized a program at Harvard in 1923 in celebration of the centenary of Pasteur's birth. His connections with British medicine continued to grow. In 1922 he was made a "Perpetual Student" at St. Bartholomew's Hospital in London and in the same year gave the Cavendish Lecture in which he introduced the term 'meningioma.' At a dinner preceding the lecture Sir Arthur Keith, proposing the health of the Cavendish Lecturer, said no man was better fitted to cement the brotherhood of the medical professions in the two great English-speaking countries. In this one may infer that he was filling at least this pair of Osler's shoes.

A sadder echo of Sir William's life came in 1926, when Cushing's son Bill was killed in an automobile accident in Connecticut. Thomson[26] has noted how heavy a blow this was to Cushing, for he and the boy had had a relationship that was often tempestuous and difficult. In the last two years of William's life a degree of rapprochement had been developed, though the full fruition of this was denied them both. As a result, Cushing's grief was undoubtedly the greater. In 1927 he established the William Harvey Cushing Research Fellowship in Surgery in memory of his son.

Although he had maintained his scientific productivity at a high level (thirty-five papers in 1926, '27 and '28), he continued to speak and write in a philosophical vein. Many of the papers of this genre were developed from speeches, some delivered to graduating classes in medicine, and thus ad-

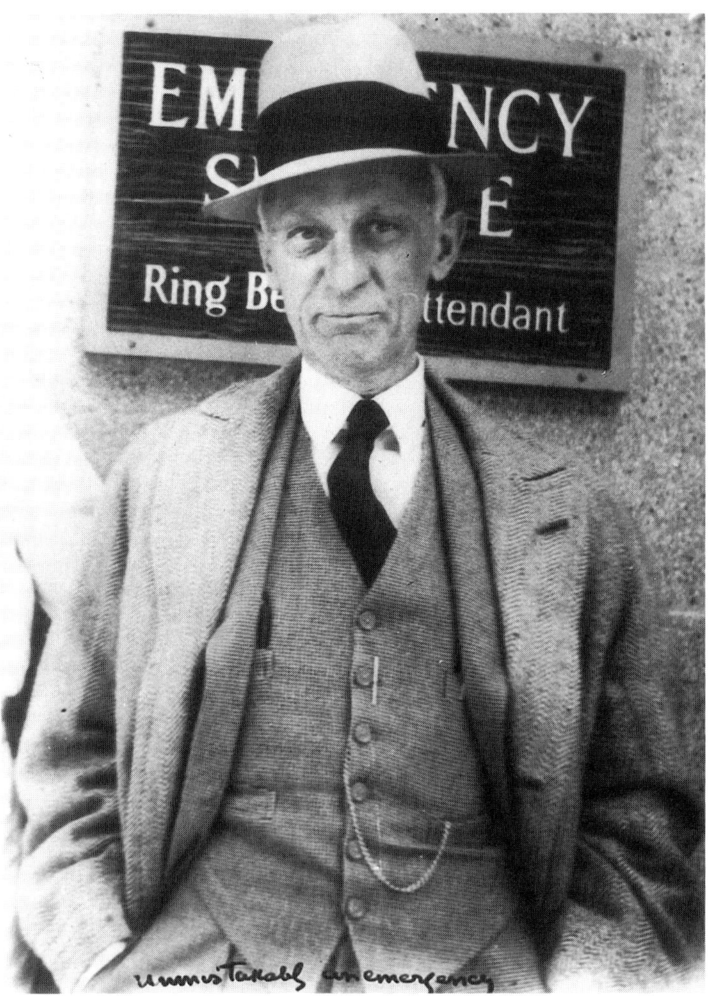

FIGURE 17.   Cushing at the emergency entrance of the New Haven Hospital; taken between 1935 and 1939. He has written at the bottom, "Unmistakably an emergency." Courtesy of Elizabeth H. Thomson.

dressed to the young, some marking the openings of libraries or other scholarly facilities, and some celebrating important anniversaries such as the Lister centenary. His style was at least as felicitous as Osler's, his topics often the same timeless ones, and his allusions to the dignity and importance of the practicing doctor as heartfelt and respectful. The impression emerges, on reading these reports, that Cushing, although clearly having modeled himself on his mentor, was not so much imitating him as representing, in effect, an extension, a continuation of Osler and Osler's influence on those broad areas of medical education, practice and research which both viewed as vital. One of his general addresses, "The Medical Career," was presented at Dartmouth College in 1928. It contains a recommended reading list for students considering medicine as a career, a list reminiscent of Osler's Bedside Library for Medical Students; and it is surely more than coincidence that Cushing's first volume of collected essays carried the Latin title of the index paper— *Consecratio Medici.* Shades of *Aequanimitas,* and of the Master!

He could lighten his literary efforts with an amusing anecdote. For example, in the Dartmouth speech he described a visit by President Wheelock of Dartmouth to a lecture given at the medical school by Nathan Smith in 1798. Wheelock was so impressed, Cushing relates, that " . . . at the ensuing evening prayers in the old chapel he gave thanks as follows: '0 Lord, we thank Thee for the Oxygen Gas; we thank Thee for the Hydrogen Gas; and for all the gases. We thank Thee for the Cerebrum; we thank Thee for the Cerebellum; and for the Medulla Oblongata. Amen' ".[27]

In May, 1929, the Osler Library at McGill was dedicated, and Cushing was present. He had been invited, to his delight, to represent the Osler Club of London. (Mrs. Cushing was forbidden by him to attend because she had defied his injunctions against smoking cigarettes[28]). He wrote later that Thayer's remarks at the dedication ceremonies were "inspired—the best thing I have ever heard him give." Cushing was especially pleased with Thayer's tribute to W. W. Francis, who had spent nine years revising Osler's library cards and preparing the catalogue (*Bibliotheca Osleriana*) for press, and who made ready the library for shipment to Montreal after Lady Osler's death

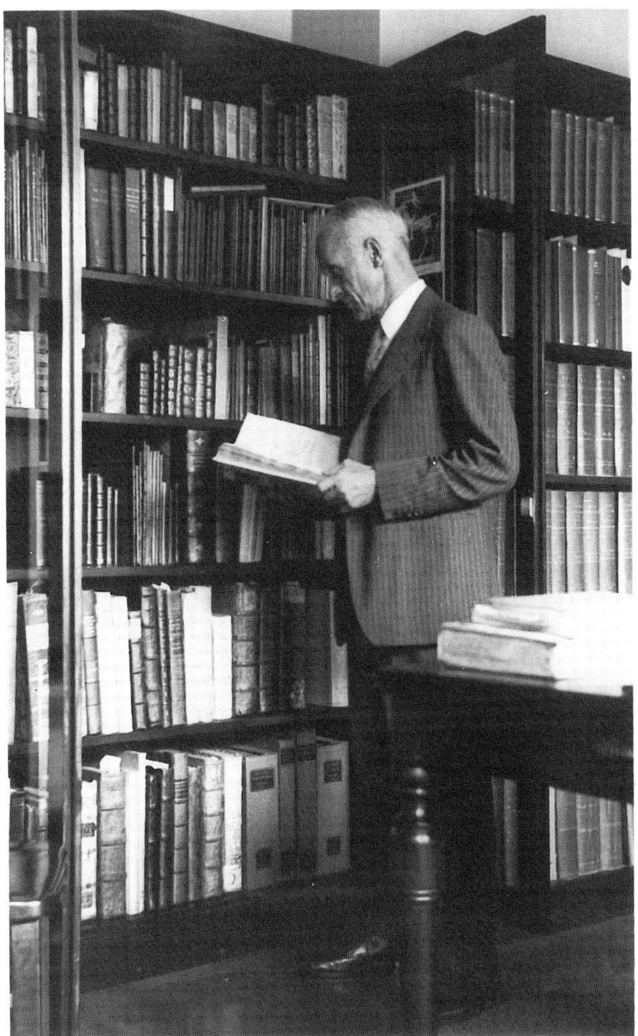

FIGURE 18. Cushing at Yale, late 1930s. From the collections of the Historical Library, Yale Medical Library.

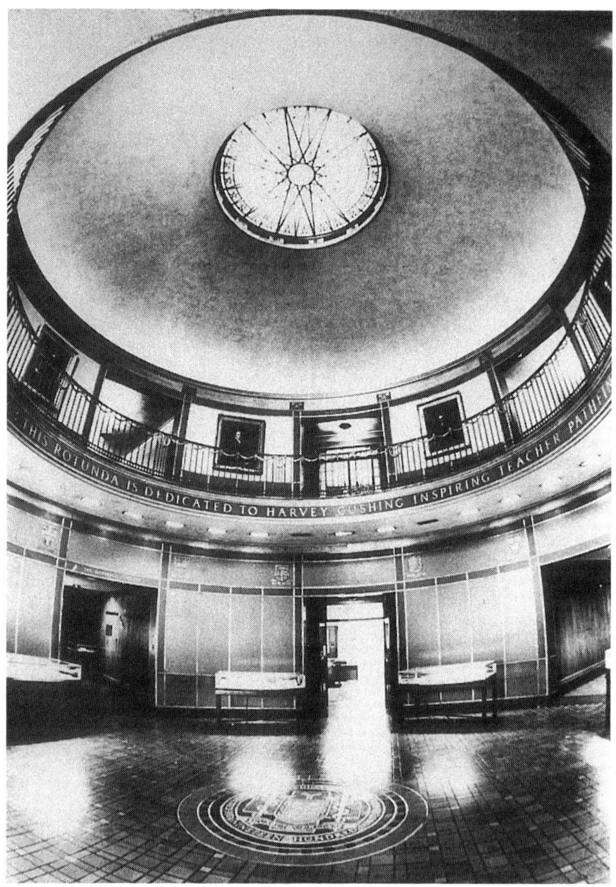

FIGURE 19. Rotunda of the Yale Medical Library. The arms of the universities which awarded him honorary degrees are reproduced on the walls. From the collections of the Historical Library, Yale Medical Library.

in August, 1928. This trip appears to have been a seminal event in Cushing's thinking about the eventual disposal of his own books.

In 1929, in honor of his sixtieth birthday the *Archives of Surgery* published a Cushing *festschrift* consisting of papers by many of his former trainees. It was in a sense, an echo of the Osler seventieth birthday volumes. Welch at about this time began to importune him to come back to Hopkins as his (Welch's) successor in the Chair in the History of Medicine and Yale invited him to consider returning to New Haven as Professor of Neurology or Neurosurgery. Two years later, on the eve of his retirement at the Brigham, Harvard offered him a Professorship of the History of Medicine.

He retired at Harvard on September 1, 1933, twenty years to the day after his arrival, and left Boston a month later for the New Haven chair in neurology he had decided upon. The next seven years, his last, were spent there in continuing scholarly activity, including work on his great meningioma monograph and the brain tumor registry. He became involved in an active national debate on compulsory health insurance and attempted to moderate the adamant stand taken by the American Medical Association. Later he published several extracts from his nine-thousand-page war journal, and attempted, through his family contacts with President Roosevelt, to secure appropriate housing for the Surgeon General's Library. He was active in the Elizabethan

Club, a literary society at Yale. In 1938 he returned to Oxford for the last time to receive, in the ambience he had come to know through Osler, the D.Sc. *honoris causa.*

The great projects of his final years were bibliophilic ones, the disposition of his library and the Vesalius bio-bibliography. He had originally planned to have his books sold at auction after his death, but when he began to think of leaving his collection to Yale he conceived of joining his to those of Arnold Klebs and John Fulton, to form the basis of a medical historical collection at the Medical School—and so it came to pass as he had wished, and the architectural plans for a suitable facility were drawn, though he did not live to see it built. Here now, accessible to students as he insisted they should be, and in company with the equally well-loved collections of his two friends, reside his papers and journals, his desk and chair and, in the high-ceilinged, panelled reading room, the great collection of Vesaliana. Over the fireplace, lit by the rays of the afternoon sun coming in through high clerestory windows, the Calcar Vesalius portrait, and under it, cut in the stone of the mantel, George Stewart's lines, beginning, "Here, silent, speak the great of other years . . .", and ending, " . . . but you, be you but brave and diligent, may freely take and know the rich companionship of others' ordered thought", an eloquent injunction, and a fitting epitaph for William Osler's friend.

Acknowledgments

The author gratefully acknowledges the generosity of time, resources and spirit of the staffs of the Historical Library, Yale Medical Library (especially Elizabeth Thomson, Ferenc Gyorgyey and Susan Allon); the Alan Mason Chesney Medical Archives of the Johns Hopkins Medical Institutions (especially Harold Kanarek); the Osler Library of the History of Medicine at McGill University; and Dr. Palmer Futcher. A special word of thanks is due Mrs. Betsey Cushing Whitney for her encouragement and her friendship.

References

1. Cushing-Osler correspondence. Yale Medical Historical Library.
2. Fulton, J.F. *Harvey Cushing—A Biography.* Springfield, Illinois: Charles C. Thomas, 1946, pp. 93–96.
3. Cushing, H. Hematomyelia from gunshot wounds of the cervical spine. *Johns Hopkins Hosp. Bull.* 8:195–196, 1897.
4. Cushing, H. Haematomyelia from gunshot wounds of the spine. A report of two cases, with recovery following symptoms of hemilesion of the cord. *Am. J. Med. Sci.* 115:654–683, 1898.
5. Fulton, op cit p 135.
6. Cushing, H. Laparotomy for intestinal perforation in typhoid fever. A report of four cases with a discussion of the diagnostic signs of perforation. *Johns Hopkins Hosp. Bull.* 9:257–269, 1898.
7. Cushing, C. Laparotomy for intestinal perforation in typhoid fever. A report of four cases occurring in 1898. *Johns Hopkins Hosp. Reports* 8:209–240, 1900.
8. Fulton, op cit p 161

9. Fulton, op cit p 162.

10. Asher, L., quoted by Fulton, op cit p 182.

11. Cushing, H. On routine determinations of arterial tension in operating room and clinic. *Boston Med Surg J.148*:250–256, 1903.

12. Fulton, op cit p 201.

13. Cushing, H., quoted by Fulton, op cit p 204.

14. Fulton, op cit p 205.

15. Cushing, H., in: Dedication of the Henry Barton Jacobs Room. *Bull. Johns Hopkins Hosp.50*:305–317, 1932.

16. Fulton, op cit p 230.

17. Osler, W. On the educational value of the Medical Society. *Boston Med. Surg J 148*:275, 1903.

18. Cushing, H. Dr. Garth: The Kit-Kat poet (1661–1718) in: Cushing, H. *Consecratio Medici and other Papers* Boston: Little, Brown and Company, 1928, pp. 14–48.

19. Fulton, op cit pp 377–384.

20. Fulton, op cit, pp 368–369.

21. Cushing, H. *The Life of Sir William Osler.* New York: The Oxford University Press, 1940, p 1113.

22. Fulton, op cit p 425.

23. Cushing, H. (published anonymously) *The Story of U.S. Base Hospital No. 5 by a member of the Unit.* Cambridge: The University Press, 1919.

24. Cushing, H. (Published anonymously). William Osler, The Man. *Boston Evening Transcript,* Jan 3, 1920.

25. Fulton, op cit p 458.

26. Thomson, E.H. *Harvey Cushing—Surgeon, Author, Artist.* New York: Neale Watson Academic Publications, Inc., 1981, p 223.

27. Cushing, H. The Medical Career, *in: The Medical Career and Other Papers.* Boston: Little, Brown and Company, 1940, p 22.

28. Whitney, Mrs. Betsey Cushing: Personal communication to the author, 1983.

Concerning Osler and Agnew: A Note on Historical Discrepancies

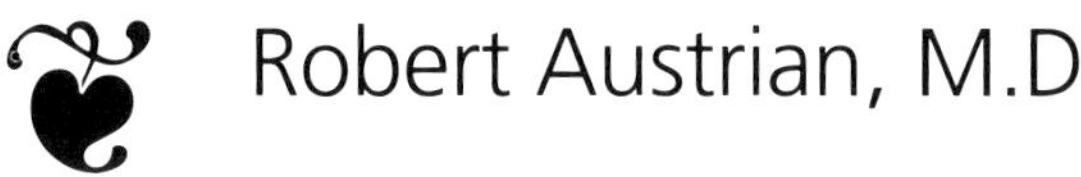 Robert Austrian, M.D.

Having passed Weir Mitchell's test on the disposition of cherry pits in London the summer before, an unwed William Osler came to Philadelphia in October, 1884, and took up residence shortly thereafter at 131 South 15th Street, the present site of the Union League Club[1].

Soon after his arrival, Osler received an invitation from D. Hayes Agnew to attend Sunday services with him at the Second Presbyterian Church. Agnew, aged 66 at the time, and one of Philadelphia's leading surgeons, had had an interesting career[2]. Born in Lancaster County, Pennsylvania, the only child of a physician, Agnew enrolled in the Medical Department of the University of Pennsylvania in 1836 and received his medical degree in 1838. For a time after graduation he practiced medicine with his father in Nobleville, Pennsylvania; and, between 1843 and 1846, he devoted a major portion of his energies to a family iron foundry which subsequently failed. Relieved of this diversionary activity, Agnew renewed his interest in medicine, dissecting bodies sent to him from Philadelphia. His practice of placing the bones of cadavers in a near-by pond where the remaining adherent soft tissue was removed by eels caused some consternation when the local residents who ate fish from the pond discovered what was taking place.

Agnew moved to Philadelphia, where he spent the remainder of his life, in 1848. From 1852 to 1862, he ran the Philadelphia School of Anatomy, obtaining experience of undoubted crucial importance to his subsequent development as a surgeon. He received an appointment to the faculty of the University of Pennsylvania as Demonstrator of Anatomy and Lecturer in Clinical Surgery in 1863, and eight years later was named Professor of Surgery at the same school, a post held till his retirement.

In addition to his commitment to teaching, Agnew had a large and

Read at the annual meeting of the American Osler Society, April 27, 1984.

Reprinted with permission from *Transactions and Studies of the College of Physicians of Philadelphia*, 6:275, 1984 successful practice. Among his patients was the President of the United States. On July 2, 1881, James A. Garfield was shot in the back by a deranged Charles J. Guiteau. Agnew was called to Washington at midnight July 3rd, and made the 135 mile trip from Philadelphia to Washington in 171 minutes on a special train. The President, who had recovered from shock by then, was seen by several physicians, including Agnew, among whom it was agreed that surgical intervention was contraindicated. Despite temporary initial improvement in the President's condition, he failed to recover fully, and his illness ran a protracted course over the next two months, the result of smoldering infection which ultimately seemed to disseminate, leading to his demise. For his professional services, Agnew received $5,000 from the Congress after he had declined to submit a bill.

Among his attributes, Agnew was noted for his unusual piety. According to D. F. Willard: "He never operated on the Sabbath except in accident cases. On one occasion he astonished one of the younger members of the profession with whom it became necessary to make a trip into the country on a Sunday by fixing the hour at 6 A.M. It is almost unnecessary to say that he returned in time to be in his accustomed pew."[3] So it was when William Osler arrived at the Second Presbyterian Church in the autumn of 1884. I have discovered two versions of this episode early in Osler's five year sojourn in Philadelphia, one by Osler's biographer, Harvey Cushing, the other by George Dock, Osler's resident in Philadelphia and later Chairman of the Departments of Medicine at the University of Michigan, Tulane and Washington University in St. Louis. According to the former's account:

> Though his advent had been much heralded, little was known about him, as is evident from a story told of old Dr. D. H. Agnew, a devout person of Scotch-Irish ancestry, who wrote and asked if Dr. and Mrs. Osler would not share his pew in the Second Presbyterian Church the following Sunday. When Osler was ushered in unaccompanied, Agnew whispered regrets that he was alone, whereupon Osler's mischievous half got the better of him. He merely raised his eyebrows and finger, which was interpreted by Agnew—and circulated—that the new-comer's wife was "expecting."

By contrast, Dock[4] recounts:

> In the medical school and also among the staff of Jefferson Medical College and the profession in general, as well as among clever and well informed men of every line of activity, Osler at once showed his unusual capacity for making friends and admirers, and his attraction for bright and inquiring minds. Although he sometimes spoke of his shyness, he was always cordial and unassuming. To a prominent woman who asked him whether he called it Osler or Ossler, he replied; 'I will answer to Hi! or to any loud cry.' His irrepressible playfulness was shown the first Sunday after he arrived when Dr. D. Hayes Agnew, the most pious and venerable member of the faculty, asked him to church, which Osler of course accepted. On arriving in the pew Dr. Agnew asked him why he did not bring Mrs. Osler. "Mrs. Osler is a Buddhist and would not come' was the startling reply."

Four years later, according to Cushing, Osler was to be concerned once again with Agnew, for 1888 marked the fiftieth anniversary of the latter's receipt of a diploma from the Medical Department of the University of Pennsylvania. Cushing's biography states:

> So it was he (Osler), rather than some Philadelphian of longer standing, who is found on a committee with James Tyson, J. William White and a student representative of each class, preparing to celebrate the fiftieth

anniversary of D. Hayes Agnew's graduation in medicine—a form of jubilee much more common in continental than American faculties. Agnew, then nearing the end of his indefatigable career, was a surgical colleague not only at Blockley and the Orthopedic Hospital but also held a chair at the University and well deserved the sort of tribute Osler had seen paid to Frerichs and Rokitansky and others during his sojourn in Europe.

To what event did Cushing refer? In Dr. J. Howe Adams' *History of the Life of D. Hayes Agnew, M.D., LL.D.,* a biography I can find no more appropriate word to characterize than "adoring", there is no mention of Osler in the detailed chapter of 20 pages devoted to the "Jubilee of Dr. Agnew." According to Adams' account of the tribute paid Agnew by the medical profession and to the documents in a remarkable and unique scrap-book in the library of the College of Physicians of Philadelphia[5], the gala affair held at the Academy of Music on April 6 was organized by a committee of eight chaired by S. Weir Mitchell, which did not include Osler. Neither did the Committee of Arrangements, numbering twelve and headed by J.M. DaCosta. The only reference to Osler which I found was in the diagram of the seating for the dinner. The subscription price was $12.00, of which $2.00 were to defray the cost of a portrait for the College, the remainder the dinner.

The absence of any reference to Osler's participation in planning the celebration cited led to a further search for the basis of Cushing's statement. At the end of Adams' chapter on "The Jubilee of Dr. Agnew," there is brief mention of a celebration of the fiftieth anniversary of his graduation held on April 24, 1888, by the Medical Department of the University of Pennsylvania. In the scrap-book of J. William White for that year in the University's Archives, a circular letter dated March 1, signed by Tyson, Osler, White and a representative of each of the three medical classes was found. It proposes a gathering to be held at the University's Chapel on April 24, to be followed by a supper, the subscription price being fixed at $3.00. It is this event to which Cushing makes reference. His implied neglect of Agnew by the local profession seems to me somewhat misleading, for the affair which Osler helped to organize clearly followed that arranged by the physicians of Philadelphia and was, in a sense, more provincial in its scope.

The year 1888 saw not only the celebration of Agnew's jubilee but also brought word of the impending resignations of both Osler and Agnew from the faculty of the University of Pennsylvania. On October 18th, Osler wrote a brief note, the holograph of which is in the University's Archives, to Provost William Pepper:

> I hereby tender my resignation of the Chair of Clinical Medicine in the Medical Faculty.
>
> > Very truly yours
> > Wm Osler

One week later, Pepper received this letter from Agnew:

> My Dear Doctor—
> At the termination of the present term I propose to withdraw from the Chair of Surgery, in the medical department of the University, and consequently deem it proper to communicate to you at this early period, my intentions, even before sending my resignation to the Board of Trustees.
> When a man passes his seventy first year his future is filled with so many (contingencies) that I do not think it proper that he should jeopardize the welfare of a great institution by longer continuing to hold so important a chair as that of surgery.

In taking the above step, one of the most delightful thoughts which enters my mind is the fact, that during my connexion with the University, not a single event has occurred to disturb the most cordial relations between the members of the faculty and myself.

Very respectfully your friend
D Hayes Agnew

The foregoing communication preceded by a month Agnew's formal letter of resignation dated November 29, 1888.

Osler and Agnew were destined to meet one last time formally as members of the faculty of the Department of Medicine at its 115th Annual Commencement held at the Academy of Music on Wednesday, May 1, 1889, with music provided by Wannemacher's Military Band. The occasion was a notable one in the lives of both men. The Valedictory Address, given by Osler, was his memorable essay "Aequanimitas." It was followed by presentation to the University of Thomas Eakins' famous portrait of Agnew known now as "The Agnew Clinic." The events of the day are recorded in *The Evening Telegraph*.[6]

The next event on the programme was the presentation of a portrait of Dr. Agnew to the University by the three classes of the Medical Department. Dr. Joseph Allison Scott, of the graduating class, in a few appropriate words made the presentation. "This is our Agnew Day," he said, "and well may we be deeply impressed by its solemnity, for it is the last time we shall see our beloved Professor before us in his official capacity." At a sign from Dr. Scott the veil was slipped from the portrait, showing a life-size likeness of Dr. Agnew, standing in the midst of his students and demonstrating to them an operation. All the figures in the group were taken from life. To the right of Dr. Agnew, in the foreground of the picture is seen Dr. J. William White, with forceps and scalpel, performing the operation in a case of cancer of the breast, assisted by Drs. Kirby and J. Leidy, Jr., resident physicians of the University Hospital. Grouped above these on the terraced seats of the clinic room, the faces of Messrs. Adams, Davis, Lincoln, Woodward, Toulmin, Tunis, Posey, Scott and Keifer can be recognized. The painting is 7×11 feet, without the frame. The artist was Mr. Thomas Eakins.

The portrait was received on behalf of the trustees by Dr. S. Weir Mitchell, Chairman of the Trustees' Medical Committee. Dr. Mitchell said that he had been advised of the office devolving upon him but an hour before, else he should have prepared a sermon more worthy of such a noble text. He thanked the students for presenting such a magnificant gift to their Alma Mater, and said that those who had listened to Dr. Agnew's words for three years saw his portrait not only on the canvas before them, but had it hung in the gallery of their hearts. "And when you are plunged into the difficulties and trials of professional life, think what this man has done, and try at least to do the same. What a model for a physician to copy after; clear of brain, tender of heart, resolute of hand, firm of conscience. Whenever you become involved in doubt and uncertainty, think what Dr. Agnew would have done, and you will be sure to do the right thing." When Dr. Mitchell sat down there was a loud call of "Agnew" from all parts of the house. The venerable surgeon had taken his seat to the left of Dr. Pepper, and, in response to the call, he slowly rose and stepped to the front of the stage. This was the signal for a universal burst of applause and deafening clapping of hands. Probably at none of the University's 114 previous commencements has there been such an exhibition of enthusiasm and excitement. When the noise had subsided Dr. Agnew turned smilingly to his counterpart in oil and said that, though he had often heard of speaking likenesses, this did not hold in the present instance, and so he would have to do the speaking himself. 'You have all heard,' he said, 'of the woman who wanted to be free from all trouble and turmoil of this life and accordingly built for herself a palace fitted out with every modern luxury and elegance. But she soon became so tired of her comforts that she went back into her old kitchen to smell grease. If, now that I have retired into comparative ease, life becomes unbearable to me, I shall still have the consolation of going across the river to hear the boys yell.' At this, Dr. Agnew 'heard the boys yell' where he stood and such was the din that he was unable to proceed for several minutes. When the 'Meds'' had quieted down he addressed a few words of earnest advice and exhortation to them and was just returning to his chair when he was overcome with emotion and fell back into the arms of Dr. McVickar. He recovered himself immediately, and before Dr. Pepper could go on with the programme, he again rose and, turning to the students, said in a firm and distinct voice ''I wish you all success in your profession.''

Writing of this episode, Adams makes the only reference to Osler I have found in his biography of Agnew. Of the latter he writes:

> He had been suffering all the morning from a very acute attack of indigestion, which brought on a considerable amount of dizziness. This with the glare and heat of the foot-lights over which he was standing, the moving sea of upturned faces, and possibly, with some natural emotion under the circumstances caused this momentary indisposition. It gave the students a chance to study that imperturbability of manner under the most startling circumstances which Professor William Osler, in the valedictory address a few minutes before, had declared so necessary in the young physician.

In this fashion, two notable figures in the history of American medicine bade their farewells to the University of Pennsylvania. It has been a source of interest and entertainment in reviewing the histories of these two prominent physicians to discover the discrepancies in the recounting of events in which their lives touched. It calls to mind a tale by one this century's more perceptive authors, James Thurber; and, at the risk of introducing a note of unseemly levity, I should like to close these remarks by presenting to you his fable of ''The Sheep in Wolf's Clothing''[7].

> Not very long ago there were two sheep who put on wolf's clothing and went among the wolves as spies to see what was going on. They arrived on a fete day when all the wolves were singing in the taverns or dancing in the street. The first sheep said to his companion ''Wolves are just like us for they gambol and frisk. Everyday is fete day in Wolfland.' He made some notes on a piece of paper (which a spy should never do) and he headed them ''My Twenty-Four Hours in Wolfland'' for he had decided not to be a spy any longer but to write a book on Wolfland and also some articles for the *Sheep's Home Companion*. The other sheep guessed what he was planning to do, so he slipped away and began to write a book called ''My Ten Hours in Wolfland.'' The first sheep suspected what was up when he found his friend had gone, so he wired a book to his publisher called ''My Five Hours in Wolfland,'' and it was announced for publication first. The other sheep immediately sold his manuscript to a newspaper syndicate for serialization.
>
> Both sheep gave the same message to their fellows: wolves were just like sheep, for they gamboled and frisked and every day was fete day in Wolfland. The citizens of Sheepland were convinced by all this, so they drew in their sentinels and they let down their barriers. When the wolves descended on them one night, howling and slavering, the sheep were as easy to kill as flies on a windowpane.
>
> *Moral: Don't get it right, just get it written.*

References

1. Cushing, H. *The Life of Sir William Osler*. Chapters XI and XII. Oxford at the Clarendon Press. 1925. Vol.1, pp. 233–310.
2. Adams, J.H. *History of the Life of D. Hayes Agnew, M.D., LL.D.* F.A. Davis Co., Publishers, Philadelphia, 1892.
3. Willard, D.F. D. Hayes Agnew, M.D., LL.D. Biographical sketch by his pupil, friend and assistant, De Forest Willard. Read by invitation before the Philadelphia County Medical Society April 13, 1892. p. 13.
4. Dock, G. Dr. William Osler in Philadelphia 1884–1889. *Bulletin No. II of the International Association of Medical Museums and Journal of Technical Methods*. Sir William Osler Memorial Number Appreciation and Reminiscences. Maude Abbott, Ed. 1926. Montreal. Privately issued. pp. 208–212.
5. The Agnew Dinner. Library of the College of Physicians of Philadelphia.
6. *The Evening Telegraph* (Philadelphia). Medicine and Dentistry. The commencement of the Medical and Dental Departments of the University of Pennsylvania—List of the prizes and graduates. Wednesday, May 1, 1889.
7. Thurber, J. The Sheep in Wolf's Clothing. In: *Fables for Our Time and Famous Poems Illustrated*. Harper & Brothers Publishers. New York, 1940. p. 39.

Thomas McCrae: A Life Patterned After Osler

 Frederick B. Wagner, Jr., M.D.

A striking testimony to the force of Osler's personality was his power to induce distinguished men like Thomas McCrae (Fig 1) to pattern their lives after him.

McCrae was born in Guelph, Ontario, on December 16, 1870. His father was Lieutenant Colonel David McCrae and his mother Janet Eckford—both Scottish. The McCrae family was of "Old Galloway, fighting stock." The father, Colonel McCrae, during World War I when he was 70 years of age recruited and trained a field battery in Scotland which he subsequently took to England. Because of his age he was not permitted to accompany his battery to France, which caused him considerable chagrin. Mrs. McCrae, characterized as a "rare woman" endowed her sons John and Thomas with a good sense of humor.

John McCrae although a physician, served in the artillery during the Boer War and also in W.W.I as an artillery officer. He subsequently was transferred to the medical service and died in France of pneumonia complicated by meningitis. To English speaking people on both sides of the Atlantic he is immortalized as the author of "In Flanders Fields."

Thomas McCrae attended the University of Toronto from which he received his A.B. degree in 1891. Continuing as a Fellow in Biology from 1892 to 1894 he received his M.B. in 1895 and his M.D. in 1903. In 1927 an honorary D.Sc. was awarded him by his Alma Mater. In 1901 he became a member of the Royal College of Physicians of London and in 1907 a Fellow. These Royal College degrees were achieved only after thorough academic preparation and by passing strict examinations. In all probability, McCrae had Osler's *Principles & Practice of Medicine* with him in England and used it to assist him in preparation for the examinations.

After graduating in medicine he served an internship in the Toronto General Hospital. In 1899 he studied at the University of Gottingen in Germany. On his return he went to Johns Hopkins, like a succession of other

Read at the annual meeting of the American Osler Society, May 10, 1990.

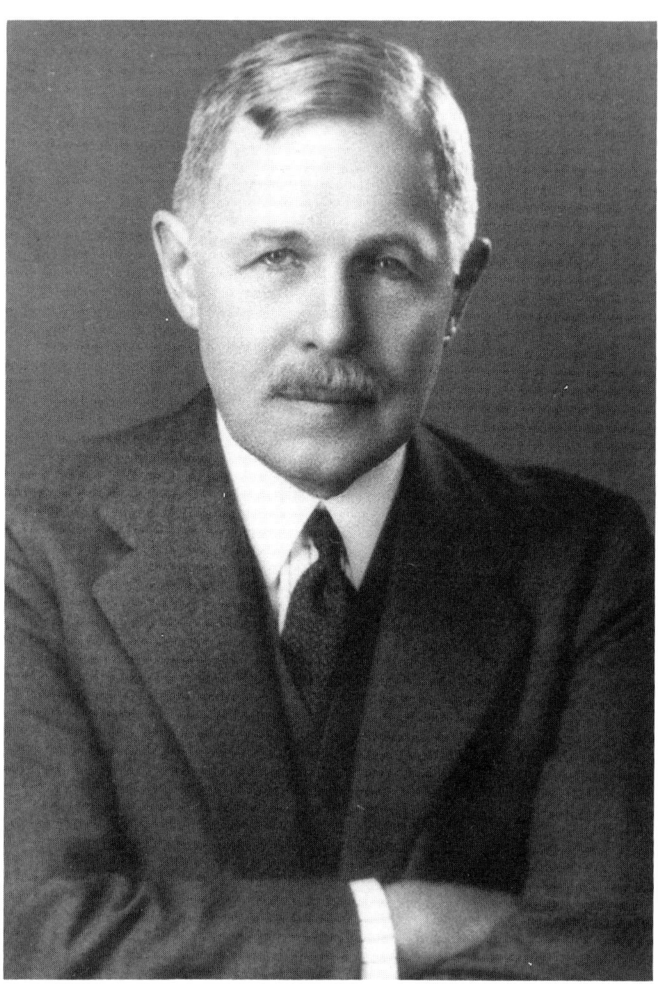

later distinguished Toronto graduates such as Barker, Cullen, Parsons, Futcher, MacCallum, and his brother John. In those days one Toronto graduate a year usually had the opportunity of an appointment on the House Staff of the Hopkins Hospital. A preliminary period during the summer was spent in the Garrett Children's Hospital with work starting in the autumn at the Hopkins Hospital. McCrae called on Osler with letters of introduction coupled with apprehension about the interview. In place of meeting a grave professor he was received with a slap on the back and a greeting of "Hello, old Canuck." That was the ending to any future apprehension.

After McCrae's first position as resident medical officer in 1900, he became an Instructor in Medicine in 1901 and Associate Professor of Medicine in 1906. It was in Baltimore that he became an intimate associate of William Osler, a professional connection and friendship that lasted until Sir William's death in 1919.

Early on and throughout his career, McCrae revealed an interest in the history of medicine. Examples of his articles in this field were: *History of the Gold-Headed Cane; Benjamin Jest, A Pre-Jennerian Vaccinator; The History of St. Bartholomew's Hospital; Life of George Cheyne; Influence of William Osler on Medicine in America; John and William Hunter; The Early History of the Association of American*

Physicians; and *Memoir of Sir William Osler.* He also served as an Associate Editor of the *Annals of Medical History.*

Although he was a warm and friendly person, McCrae indulged in few social activities, in order to spare time for reading and writing on clinical subjects. His interest was not in basic research, but he wrote more than 110 articles on a wide spectrum of clinical subjects almost entirely under his sole authorship. Osler was aware of McCrae's talent and industry in medical writing, enlisting his help in editing later editions of his *Principles and Practice of Medicine.* After Osler's death McCrae became a co-editor of the 1922 revised edition in which Lady Osler received one half of the royalties. Thereafter he was the sole editor for the revised tenth edition in 1925, the eleventh in 1930 and the twelfth in 1935, the year of his death.

In July, 1904, Osler wrote in a letter: "I have been beguiled into editing a seven (!!) volume System of Medicine (McCrae to do the dirty work)." The actual title of this monumental work was *Modern Medicine: Its Theory and Practice.* Although Osler carried out the lion's share in planning and writing, in which none of the credit can be denied him, McCrae was of vital help in the very first edition, with Volumes 1–7 appearing between 1907 and 1910. He was a co-editor with Osler in the second edition in which Volumes 1–5 appeared between 1913–1915. The third edition was re-edited by McCrae in Volumes 1–6 which appeared during 1925 and 1928.

In 1908 McCrae married Osler's niece, Amy Gwyn, who survived him after 27 years of congenial married life. They had no children, and since his brother John never married, Thomas was the last of the American McCraes.

Although successfully and contentedly entrenched in Baltimore, there arose in 1912 a turning point in McCrae's career. In that year he was elected Professor of Medicine in the Jefferson Medical College of Philadelphia, succeeding James Cornelius Wilson, a staunch friend of Osler. In 1913 he was elected an Attending Physician to the Pennsylvania Hospital, where excellent use could be made of the wealth of material for teaching students in the wards. He came to Philadelphia as an alien and comparative stranger, but his sterling qualities soon won for him many devoted friends and admiring acquaintances. His ability as a teacher and his practical sense in application of his medical knowledge and experience were soon recognized.

In McCrae's weekly clinics in the hospital amphitheater (Fig 2) he strove to demonstrate the average types of cases a physician might encounter in his daily practice. He used x-ray and laboratory reports sparingly, insisting that the student use his eyes, ears and hands in the exercise of his mind. Dr. Stiles D. Ezell, a Jefferson graduate in the class of 1932, kept a record of McCrae's presentations of cases in the session of 1930/31. There were 16 of lung infections, 6 of syphilitic lesions of the cardiovascular system, 3 of liver cirrhosis, 3 of peptic ulcer, 2 of myeloid leukemia, 2 of carcinoma of the stomach, 1 of carcinoma of the head of the pancreas, 1 of carcinoma of the bronchus, 1 of dementia praecox, 1 of malaria, 2 of acute nephritis, one of spondylitis, 1 of tabes dorsalis, 1 of exophthalmic goiter and 3 of diabetes mellitus. Many of the pulmonary cases involved pleuritis with effusion, as well as pneumonia. He also showed acute rheumatic fever, endocarditis and aneurysms. On the wards McCrae demonstrated an even greater variety of cases (Figure 3).

A distinct honor came to McCrae in 1924 when he delivered the Lumleian Lectures at the Royal College of Physicians of London on *Foreign Bodies In The Bronchi.* In 1934 he was made an Honorary Foreign Member of the Association of Physicians of Great Britain and Ireland. The only other

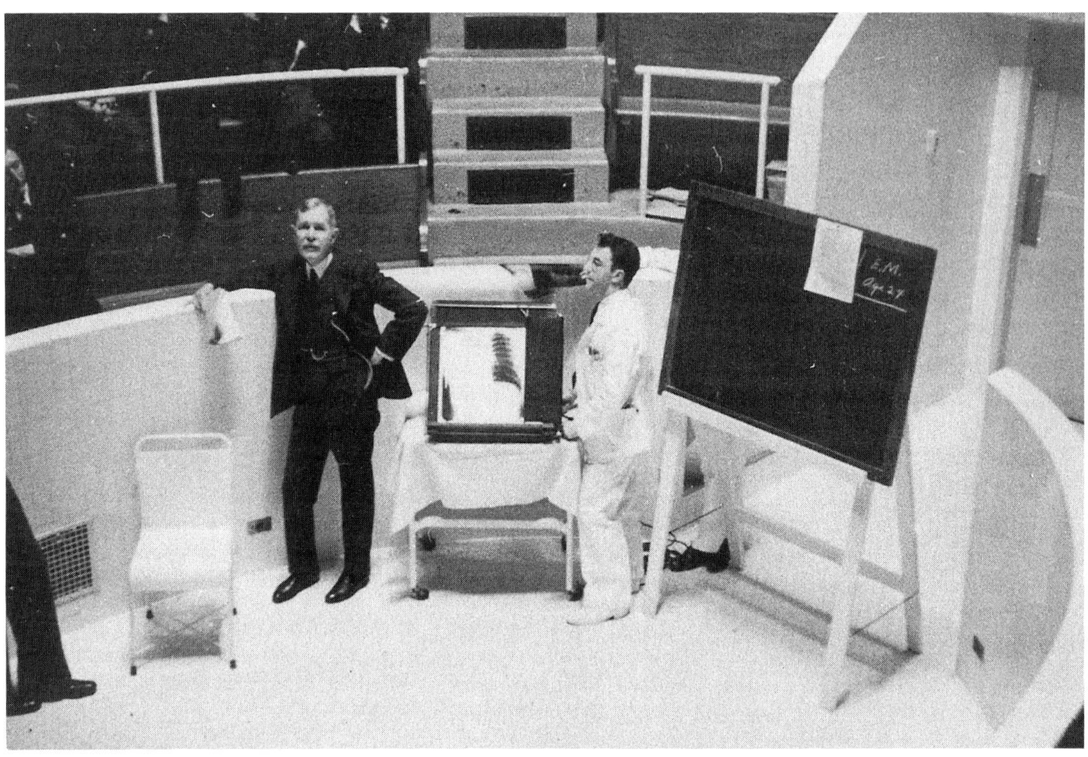

FIGURE 2   McCrae Clinic in amphitheater of Jefferson Hospital (ca. 1930).

previous foreign recipients had been Chauffard, Widal, Thayer and Van den Bergh. Although not a "joiner" in the ordinary sense of the word, he kept an active interest in all the societies to which he belonged. In the College of Physicians of Philadelphia, like Osler before him, he was for years a member of the Library Committee and was elected several times to the Council. He was Chairman of the Section of Practice of Medicine in the American Medical Association 1914/15 and from 1916 to 1925 the Secretary of the Association of American Physicians as well as the President in 1930. He also belonged to the American Philosophical Society and the Charaka Club of New York City (composed of physicians who were bibliophiles) in which Osler had been a member.

McCrae was a slave to duty all of his academic life and rarely indulged in extraneous relaxation. He never permitted anything, however alluring, to distract him from his work. His vacations were spent in travel, reading and writing much in the style of Osler. His recreations were distinctly intellectual. He possessed a thoughtfulness and compassion for others which were revealed in his notes of congratulations or condolence. The Archives of Jefferson Medical College contains a series of 20 letters he wrote between 1932 and 1934 to Dr. Robert Charr (a Jefferson graduate in the class of 1931) who was stricken with pulmonary tuberculosis. Charr was a Korean of brilliant teaching ability, unusual charisma and fine humor. The letters revealed that McCrae repeatedly sent small amounts of money to Charr with the usual comment "to keep things going." He also sent books to Charr while he was in White Haven Sanatorium. When Charr returned the books, McCrae wrote that he should have kept them since "Mrs. McCrae is always glad to reduce the number of books in the house." Also, when Charr later tried to repay McCrae for his checks, the latter deposited them to Charr's account in a savings bank. After McCrae's death Mrs. McCrae answered Charr's letter of sympathy with the remark that "I think he would rather be remembered for his kindness than his skill."

Near the end of May, 1935, Professor McCrae completed his last ward round in Jefferson Hospital. On that occasion he was in a wheelchair and pushed toward the Annex where he usually left the hospital by the Sansom street door. After a short conference with his two interns, he waved a casual goodbye. It was little realized or even suspected that this would be his last presence in the hospital. For many months he had used a wheelchair and it was generally known that he had instability in his legs. Details of this last illness have been described by his brother-in-law, Dr. Norman Gwyn. "For the last two years Dr. McCrae had been suffering from symptoms which baffled the best clinical brains in the country. He had first noticed mild sensations on the outer side of both feet. These changes at the time seemed trivial, amounting to nothing more than a slight feeling of coldness. At times they might completely disappear, at times under stress of work or particularly when the atmospheric

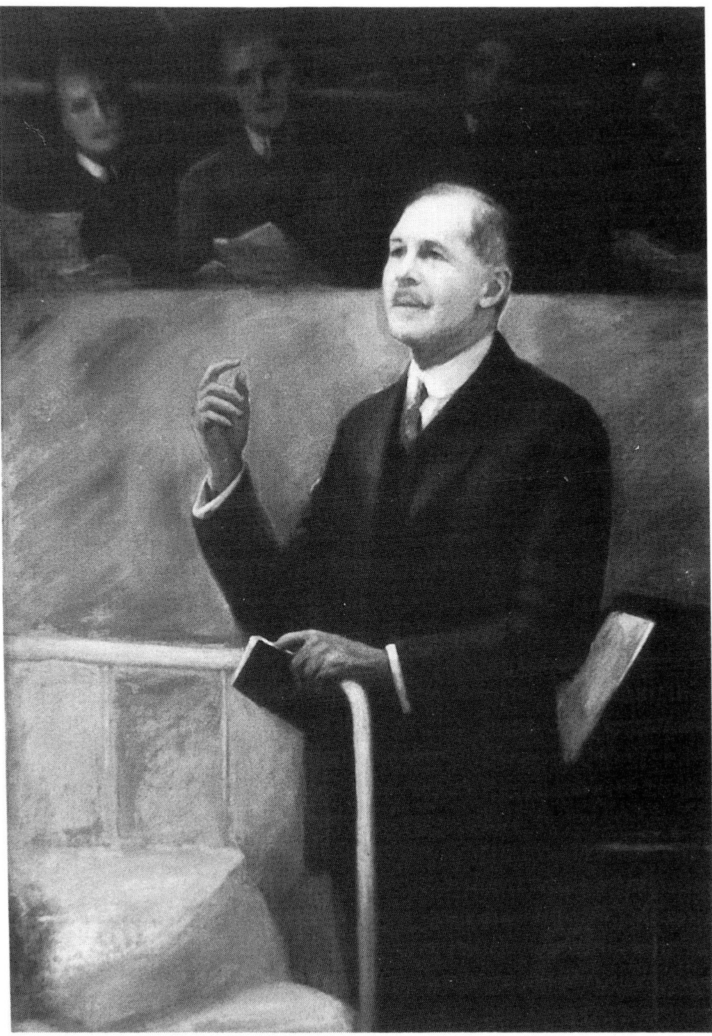

FIGURE 3   McCrae teaching at bedside. Portrait painted posthumously (1936).

pressure were high, these sensations would become more marked. Following these early symptoms he noted more particularly heaviness of both legs and a feeling as if the tissues of the legs were being distended, and very quickly after this a marked loss of power from the hips down began to assert itself.

As time went on, other sensory manifestations appeared, such as dulling of the tactile senses in irregular areas of both legs, disturbance of muscle sense and upsetting of the proper perception of heat and cold. Vibration sense was interfered with but at no time was there any sensation of pain which he could call distressing. Power of the legs gradually failed and was associated with some degree of atrophy of the muscles below the knees and a general flaccidity rather than rigidity. At no time until within the last two weeks were there any very positive changes in the reflexes: the knee jerks, however disappeared toward the end and at one time an examiner reported a Babinski.

Without detailing the course of the illness further, one can say that the general opinion of all examiners was that the symptoms were due to a neuritis, the origin of which remained obscure. So suggestive of a peripheral neuritis was the course of the disease that three months before his demise Dr. McCrae submitted himself to a de-leading treatment.

With the failure of all methods of treatment to attain any results, with loss of power in the legs becoming increasingly evident, and with the cause of the symptom completely hidden, it was deemed wise to explore the spinal canal looking more particularly for tumor or something giving rise to pressure or disturbance in the region of the cauda equina. In the carrying out of this procedure, Dr. Mohler and attending physicians had the concurrence of Dr. McCrae's neurological consultants in Philadelphia: Dr. Burns, of Jefferson, Dr. Strecker of the University of Pennsylvania, and of Dr. C.P. Frazier, the neurological surgeon at the hospital of the University of Pennsylvania. Dr. Harvey Cushing of Yale, Dr. Tilney, and Dr. Foster Kennedy of New York had also agreed that an exploratory operation should be carried out. A lipiodol injection had seemed to show some hesitation of the drug in the lower dorsal and upper lumbar area and this portion of the spinal canal was accordingly exposed. All that could be said after a most careful examination was that the strands of the cauda equina showed a curiously beaded appearance as if, perhaps, they had been constricted here and there by some inflammatory process.

McCrae's postoperative course was complicated by meningitis which resulted in death after several days. Post mortem examination of the spinal cord revealed a large collection of varicosities beginning at the level of the second and third dorsal vertebrae and stretching downward for several inches inside the dura. From the extent and nature of these dilated veins which could be found penetrating deeply into the spinal cord it was hypothesized that hemorrhages might have occurred from time to time and resulted in a progression of the symptoms.

McCrae was honored at Jefferson by being made the first Magee professor of medicine in 1917. His portrait was presented by the class of 1925. In 1937, two years after his death, a portrait depicting his characteristic teaching at the bedside was presented by friends and students. This great physician, teacher and author is remembered for his dignity, humor, humility, and dedication to his profession. His ability to impart to the students his own knowledge of medicine and care for the patient, created in them respect and admiration which lasted a life time.

Medicine, War, and Poppies:
John McCrae and William Osler

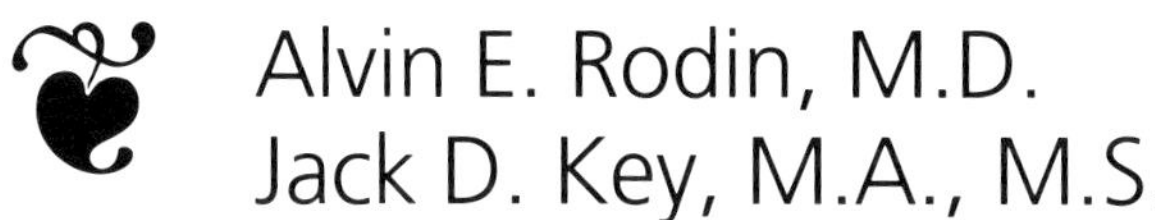

Alvin E. Rodin, M.D.
Jack D. Key, M.A., M.S.

Sir William Osler's widespread fame and influence are such that some of the physicians whose lives he touched, have become more generally appreciated than they would otherwise have been. Examples include Maude Abbott, George Adami, James Bovell, WW Francis, Robert Palmer Howard, Geoffrey Keynes, and Thomas Browne; not to mention the more prominent members of the American Osler Society. Worthy of inclusion in this august group of dedicated physicians is John McCrae, whose poem "In Flanders Fields" is familiar to many who cannot even name its author (Fig 1).[1]

Two Biographies

The first of three direct encounters of John McCrae with William Osler, as cited in Cushing's biography of Osler, was in October, 1899 when McCrae became, for a brief period, a member of his house staff at Johns Hopkins.[2] Although they may not have met before, they had a similar cultural milieu, both being born into respectable middle class families and raised in Upper Canada, now Southern Ontario. Osler was born in 1849, 23 years before McCrae's birth in 1872; but they died within one year of each other, Osler, in 1919, outliving McCrae by one year.[3] Thus, Osler's life span bridged the transition from the prescientific to the scientific practice of medicine to a somewhat greater extent than did that of McCrae.

Both William Osler and John McCrae were born within 50 miles of Toronto. Osler's birthplace was the rural village of Bond Head, where a

Read before the annual meeting of the American Osler Society, April 27, 1989.

Reprinted with permission from *The Journal of the US Army Medical Department*, June/July, 1990

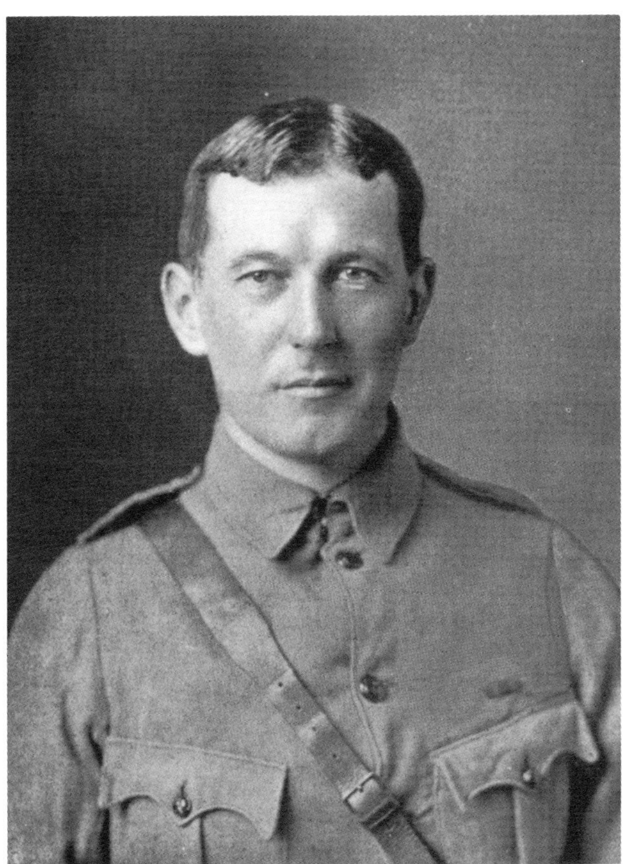

memorial cairn was dedicated to him in 1961. McCrae's birthplace was in the more urban town of Guelph, where a memorial has been erected to his memory. The Osler family moved to the more populous Dundas when William was seven years old. Osler's family was Anglican and his father a minister. McCrae's religious background was strict Scottish Presbyterianism. His older brother Thomas, was to become co-editor of Osler's renowned textbook. Their father farmed and also became the manager of the Guelph Woolen Mills. Neither family was predominantly medical. However, Osler's paternal uncle, Edward, was a member of the Royal College of Surgeons of London. McCrae's father joined the militia to repel Fenian raids from the United States. He then served as a regular officer in the artillery for several years. This propensity towards the military was also to be exhibited by his son John.

Less information is available on the education of John McCrae than that of William Osler. Both received an extensive liberal arts education, McCrae at the Guelph Collegiate Institute and Osler at Weston near Toronto. Higher education in the liberal arts and natural sciences was obtained by both at the University of Toronto—by McCrae at Knox College and by Osler at Trinity College. According to their biographers, they each considered a theological vocation before choosing medicine as a career.

Osler enrolled in the Toronto Medical School in 1868, and McCrae in 1894 (Fig 2).[4] The latter completed his medical education there, graduating with a gold medal. Osler, however, transferred to McGill University for his clinical training after two years of basic science studies. Both men indulged in writing while still medical students, but each in a different genre. By the time of Osler's graduation in 1872, he had to his credit seven scientifically oriented publications. In contrast, McCrae had published 16 poems and several short stories by the time of his graduation in 1898.[5] Osler had two years of postgraduate training in Europe. He then returned as a McGill faculty member, first to teach physiology and pathology, and then as a clinician and pathologist. In 1889, Osler accepted the position as head of medicine at Johns Hopkins. It was there that McCrae went, after graduation in 1898, as one of Osler's house staff. However, he abruptly left to enlist in the Canadian Armed Forces for service in the Boer War.

John McCrae's involvement with the military began long before the Boer War. At the age of 14 he joined his school's Highland Cadet Corps, became a bugler in his father's reserve battery at the age of 15, and enrolled as a gunner at 18. He did not hesitate to leave his choice position at Johns Hopkins to defend the British Empire in the Boer War. McCrae functioned, not as a medical officer, but as military line officer in the Canadian Field Artillery, and took part in several major battles (Fig 3). He was promoted from lieutenant to captain before returning to Canada in 1901 (to be promoted to major by the time of his resignation from the military in 1904). McCrae then studied pathology at McGill for four years, unlike Osler who was largely self-trained in this field. His training was under a leading pathologist of the time, JG Adami,

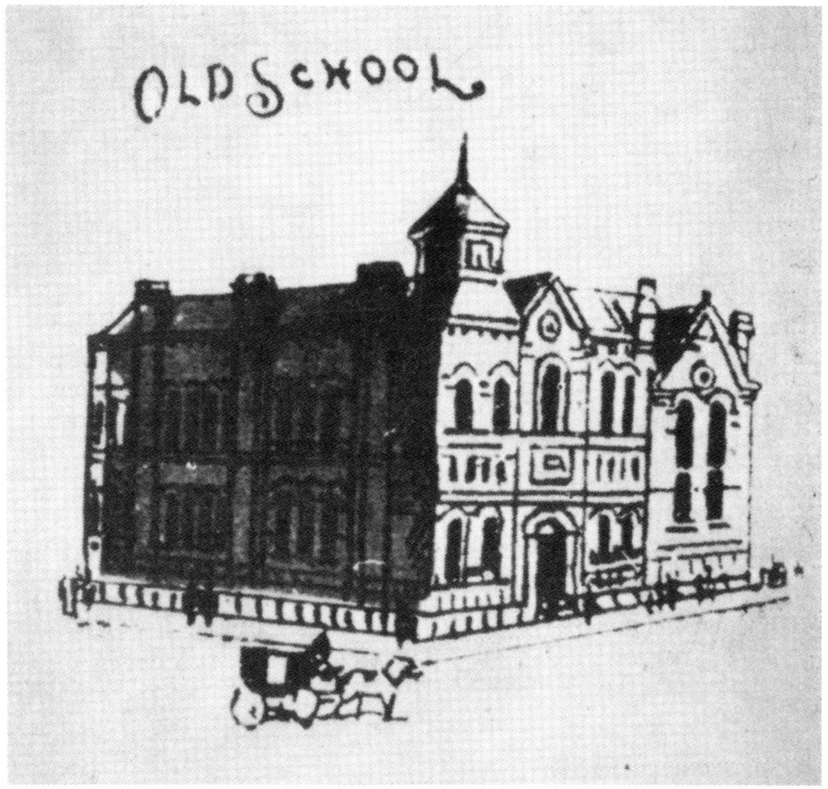

FIGURE 2   The old Medical School Building, Toronto University, 19th century.[4]

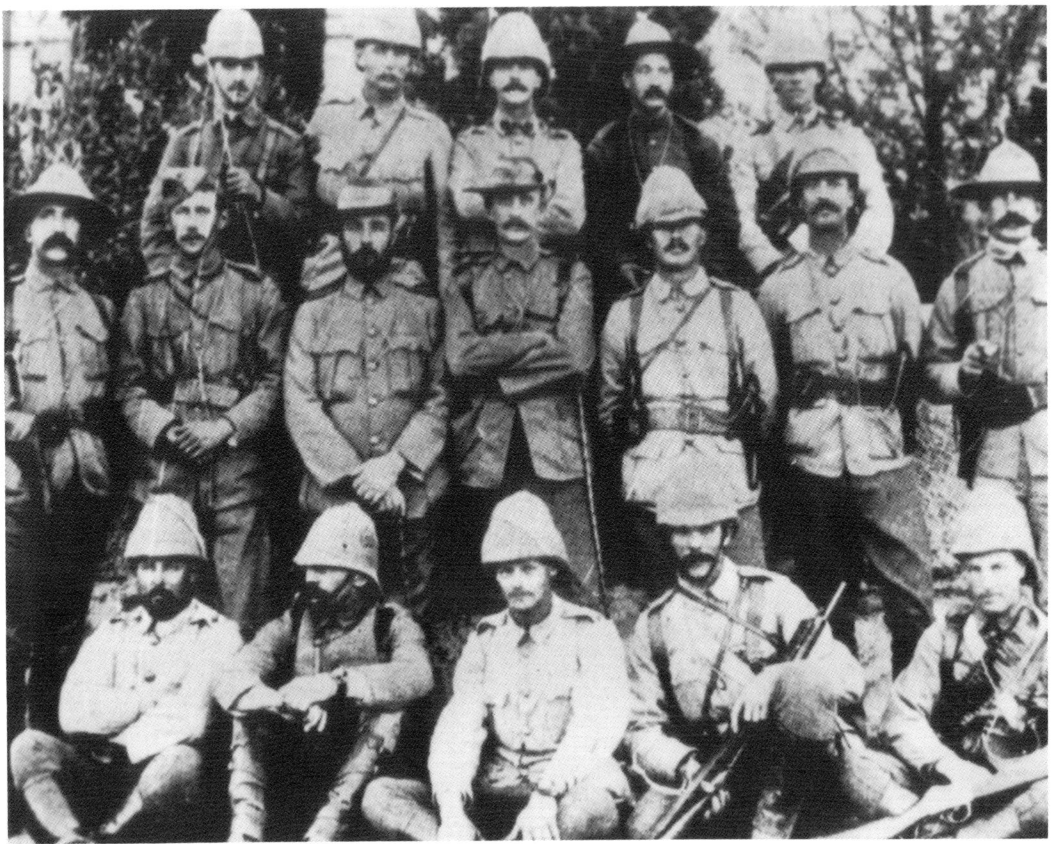

FIGURE 3   John McCrae in the Boer War (middle row, second from left).[3]

Professor of Pathology at McGill University, a position held by Osler over ten years previously.

Osler's direct involvement in the practice of pathology ceased within a year or so after leaving Montreal for Philadelphia.[6] McCrae, however made it his permanent medical specialty, becoming pathologist to the Montreal General Hospital in 1901, a position that Osler had held until 1882. McCrae taught both bacteriology and pathology to medical students, and, like Osler had done, gave demonstrations of pathologic specimens on Saturdays. He also gave lectures in pathology at the University of Vermont Medical College at Burlington. McCrae's continuing poetic proclivity, which surfaced while a medical student, is evident by his inscription in the autopsy book of the hospital, written on Jan 3, 1902:[7]

> "Here begynneth y' Booke of y' Deade, wherin is fayrely set foorth ye last state
> of four Hundred and seventeen persones, th' have departed from lyfe;
> wherein be tabled diverse and straunge and fearsome condicions th' have
> ledde to y' same final ende: God have them of his grace."

Another McCrae/Osler connection is to be found in the pathology specimen collection at McGill. Twenty years after Osler had left Montreal, he added a specimen from an autopsy, performed by McCrae, to the museum which he had established.[6] It is an excellent example of two aneurysms of the ascending aorta, one of a sinus of Valsalva and the other of the aortic wall with rupture into the mediastinum. McCrae's protocol of the autopsy is quite similar to those of Osler a generation before, except for containing microscopic descriptions of the aorta, heart, liver and kidney. Although Osler did not record microscopic studies in his own protocols, they were performed in some cases, being added to later presentations. This addition to the museum is indicative of Osler's intensive and prolonged dedication to morphologic aspects of disease.

McCrae's medical activities were not limited to pathology. In 1904, he began the practice of clinical medicine, as had Osler while at McGill; but, unlike Osler, McCrae also continued to practice pathology. In that year, he studied medicine in England for several months. During this time, he became a licentiate of the Royal College of Physicians by examination, as had Osler before him in 1873. In 1908, he was appointed physician to the Royal Alexandra Hospital for Infectious Diseases, reminiscent of Osler's involvement with the smallpox ward at the Montreal General Hospital. Also in Osler's footsteps was McCrae's appointment in 1909 as lecturer at McGill, but in medicine rather than pathology.

John McCrae did not write as many (nor as seminal) medical articles as

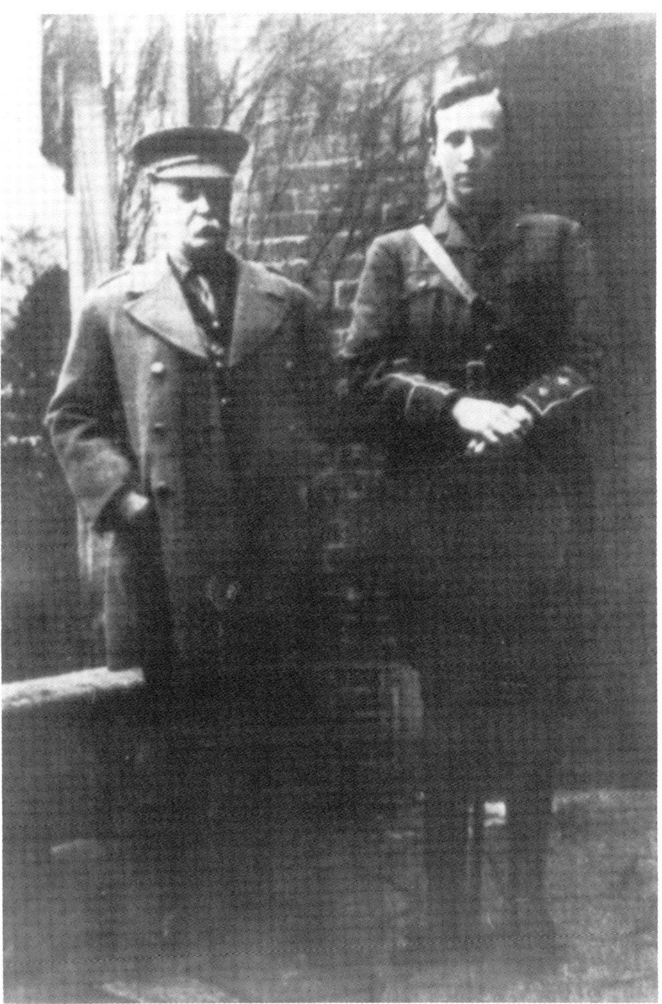

FIGURE 4   Colonel William Osler and Lieutenant Edward Revere Osler in 1916.[33]

did Osler. Both produced manuals for medical students. McCrae collaborated with Adami on *A Textbook of Pathology for Students of Medicine* in 1912; and Osler had prepared a manual called *Student's Notes: I Normal Histology For Laboratory and Class Use* in 1882.[8,9] It was John McCrae's brother, Thomas, who became Osler's collaborator for *The Principles and Practice of Medicine,* beginning with the eighth edition.[10] Another area of interest for both John McCrae and William Osler was quackery. In 1909, McCrae wrote a long paper on quacks in medicine, titled "The Pirates of Medicine."[11] His literary bent, if not his expertise on the subject, is evident in the allegorical summary of this article:

> "I have spoken of a few of the pirates of medicine, and though the ships are at times prosperous, the keels that carry the regular flag win ultimately. We are not all line-of-battle ships; but a little one-gun sloop with the ensign is more honourable than a 40-gun frigate that is a buccaneer."

Although Osler did not publish articles on medical charlatans as such, his *Bibliotheca* contains 49 books related to the subject.[12]

In 1914 John McCrae was 42 years old and a respected senior physician in Montreal. In the same year, Osler was in his mid-sixties and a very highly regarded Regius Professor at Oxford, with a world-wide reputation. McCrae was elected a member of the Association of American Physicians, Osler having been one of the founders of this group in 1885. With the onset of the first World War, McCrae again joined the Canadian Artillery Unit, but this time as brigade surgeon with the rank of major. As in all wars before the antibiotic era, morbidity and mortality from infectious disease often outranked that from trauma. Vaccination of troops for typhoid was still not compulsory, even 20 years after its development by Almouth Wright.[13] The Canadian contingent made certain that the front line troops were vaccinated by sending the few who

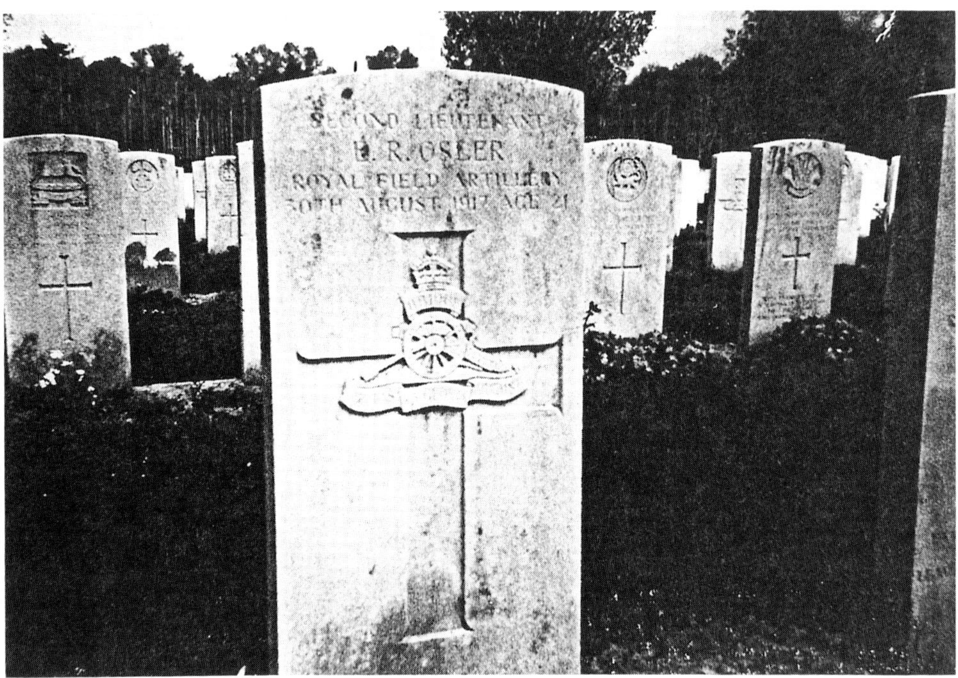

FIGURE 5 Revere Osler's headstone (Courtesy of Dr. Robert Devloo).

refused to be, back to the base depot. Osler was one of the leading exponents of vaccination, stating that "In war the microbe kills more than the bullet."[14]

The Canadian Field Artillery brigade took part in many battles during Word War I. Some occurred in Flanders, a historic region in the southwest area of the Low Countries. The best known of these battles occurred in April–May 1915, near Ypres (Ieper), a city in the Belgian province of West Flanders. It was here that troops, including McCrae, were exposed to poison gas. Following this he visited the Oslers at Open Arms in Oxford. Cushing describes McCrae as a "broken man who had given all with his Canadian battery."[2] Lady Osler described this visit in a letter to her sister:

> "Sunday afternoon Jack McCrae came . . . He looked thin and worn, but was intensely interesting; 31 days in the trenches with eight days rest . . . His clothes were awful . . . The nerve strain, he says, is beyond any sensation possible to describe. When they had to stand on the roadside waiting for orders and saw the French Colonials and civilians rushing away from the gas when it was first turned on, he says it was Hades absolutely; and they stood fast, expecting the Germans on top. After that, orders came to push ahead and attack, and they were at it day and night, saving the situation as we know."

The Oslers were visited at Open Arms by many other Canadians, as well as Americans during the war. Among them was McCrae's former pathology teacher, George Adami from McGill. On this visit Adami was elected a member of the Royal College of Physicians, of which McCrae and Osler had become licentiates much earlier.

Following his battlefield experiences, McCrae was posted as lieutenant-colonel in charge of medicine at the Canadian General Hospital.[3] This was a 520-bed hospital equipped and operated by McGill University and located a few miles from Boulogne-sur-Mer. The hospital unit arrived in France in the summer of 1915. Attached to it was Osler's son, Lieutenant Edward Revere who served as orderly officer and Assistant Quartermaster (Fig 4).[2] In September, William Osler visited the hospital. Colonel McCrae took him on a tour of the front, visiting dressing stations and observing the bombardment of airplanes by German aircraft guns. Quite prophetic for McCrae and Revere is Osler's description of "Everywhere great squares of graves—marked with names of the men of the Regiments."

In March 1916, Revere Osler obtained a transfer from the Canadian Hospital to the British Army, to join the Royal Field Artillery in Flanders. He reached the Front at the Somme in October and was involved in several battles. In May of 1917, Revere came home for a ten-day leave. On Aug 29, while serving in Ypres (Ieper) Salient, he was seriously wounded by an exploding shell and sustained multiple injuries of the chest, abdomen and thigh. In spite of surgery and a blood transfusion, he died the next morning, at the age of 21.

Revere Osler was buried in the Dozinghem British Military Cemetery, located about eight miles northwest of Ypres. His final resting place is Plot 4, Row F (Fig 5). Its simple headstone lies with thousands of others, in great squares of graves, row on row. William Osler's grief was deep and intensely personal. He recorded it in a letter. "The Fates do not allow the good fortune that has followed me to go to the grave—call no man happy till he dies . . . A sweeter laddie never lived, with a gentle loving nature . . . We are heartbroken, but thankful to have the precious memory of his loving life."[2]

Five months later, in 1918, John McCrae was still at the Canadian General Hospital in Boulogne.[3] His only relief from the laborious and

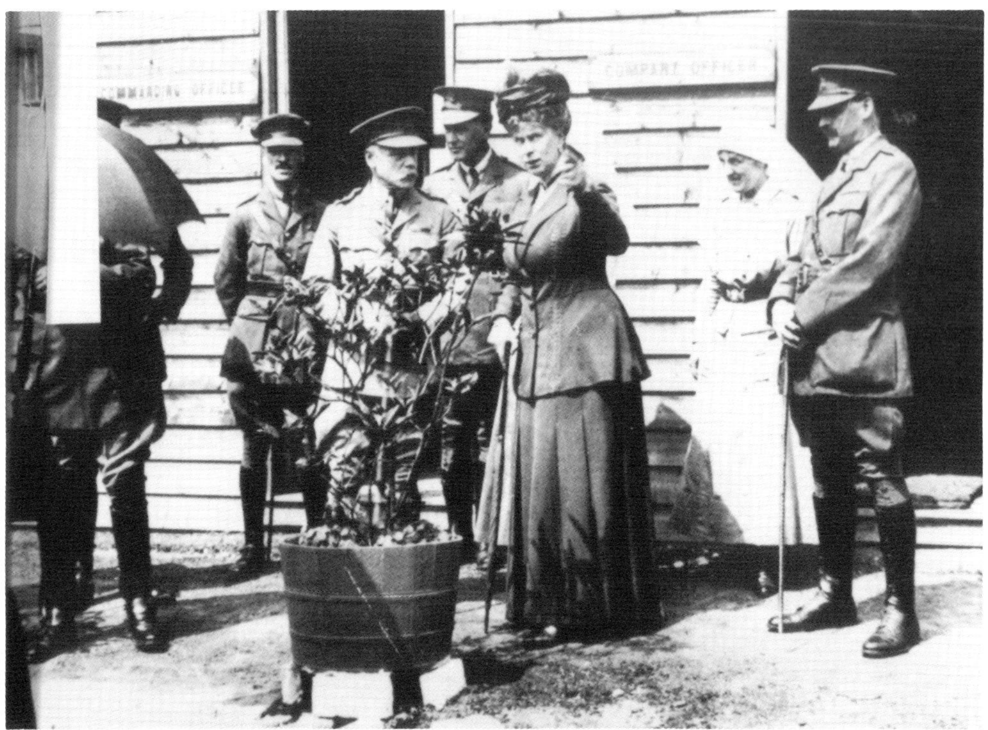

FIGURE 6   Queen Mary with McCrae on her right, at Boulogne.[3]

time-consuming activities had been the four-day visit with the Oslers at Open Arms, and visits by prominent individuals, such as Queen Mary (Fig 6). McCrae's optimism and health suffered from the work load imposed by the large number of casualties. In addition, his asthma, from which he had suffered since childhood, worsened greatly probably due to the chlorine gas inhaled at Ypres.

On Jan 24, McCrae was appointed consulting physician to the First British Army—a considerable honor. On the same day he developed pneumonia. Four days later, on Jan 28, McCrae died of meningitis. John McCrae was buried with full military honors in the small town of Wimereux, three miles north of Boulogne (Fig 7). The British Military Cemetery in Wimereux contains the graves of 2,847 soldiers, including 216 Canadians.[15] McCrae's headstone reads simply: "Lieutenant Colonel / J. McCrae / Can. Army Medical Corps / 28th January, 1918" (Fig 8). In 1984, the Province of West Flanders erected a plaque commemorating McCrae and his poem on the wall of the cemetery.

As in the case of John McCrae, William Osler was afflicted with respiratory disease, but his was in the form of bronchial infections rather than asthma. Episodes of bronchial attacks which began in 1897 at the age of 48, had gradually increased in severity.[2] His terminal illness began with a severe chill on Sep 28, 1919 followed by pyrexia and acute pleurisy. A culture yielded *Hemophilus influenza,* and pus was aspirated from a large abscess cavity. The terminal event on Dec 29, was the rupture of an abscess with hemorrhage into the pleural cavity. Autopsy revealed bronchiectasis, pneumonia, lung abscesses, and empyema.[16] The stresses of the war and the loss of Revere undoubtedly had contributed towards his lowered resistance.

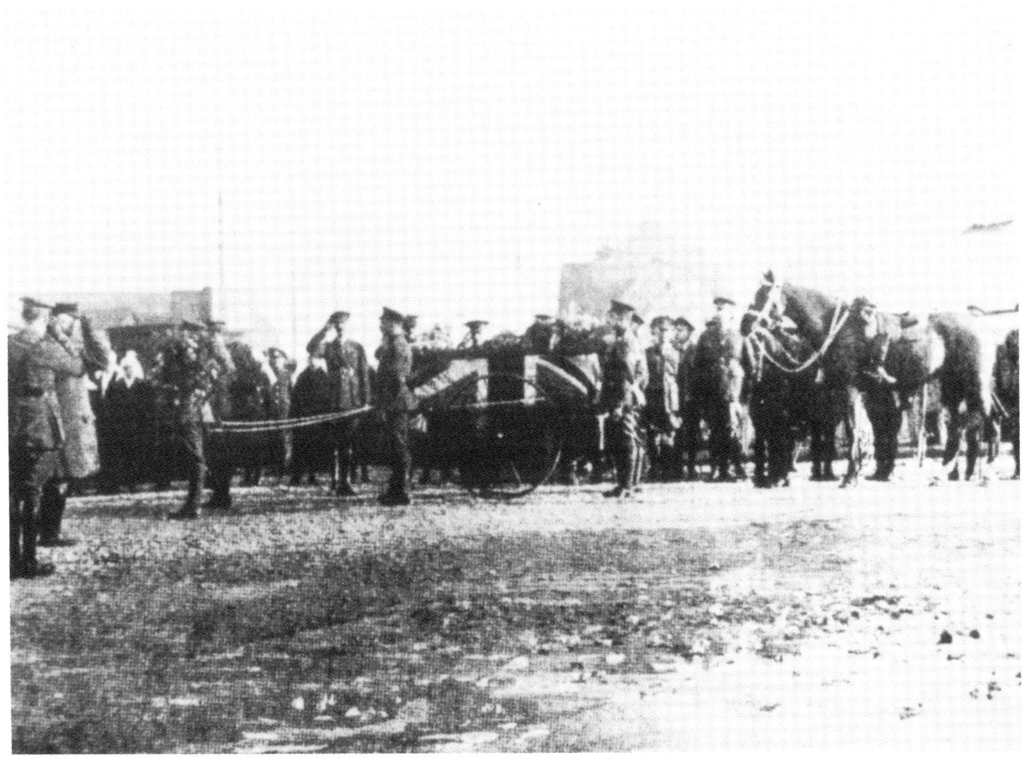

FIGURE 7   John McCrae's funeral, January 29th, 1918.[3]

Discussion

Both William Osler and John McCrae were, in essence, pathologists and clinicians. Only Osler, however, made lasting contributions to the advancement of medicine, both to its science and to its humanitarian practice. Both also have scientific publications to their credit. Osler's are well known but McCrae's 45 papers are not. The latter include subjects such as scarlet fever, burns, cretinism, and the use of subcutaneous oxygen in pneumonia.[17] Like Osler, McCrae wrote several papers on typhoid. According to McCrae's biographer, Sir Andrew Macphail, his medical writings "testified to his industry rather than to invention and discovery."[18] Unlike Osler, McCrae wrote and published poetry, of which only one poem is well known today—"In Flanders Fields."

"In Flanders Fields" was written while McCrae was on the battleground of Ypres in May, 1915, $2^1/2$ years before his death.[19] It was inspired by the traumatic death of Lieutenant Alexis Helmer.[3] McCrae wrote the poem in a dugout of the Field Dressing Station at the bottom of the small butte of the field command post of the First Canadian Field Artillery Brigade at Essex Farm, $1^1/2$ miles north of Ypres (where Revere Osler was first treated for his wounds almost two years later) (Fig 9). In 1984, the government of the province of West Flanders erected a plaque commemorating this literary event.[20] It is located by the entry to the Essex Farm Cemetery. On the plaque is carved the crest of the Province of West Flanders and a poppy.

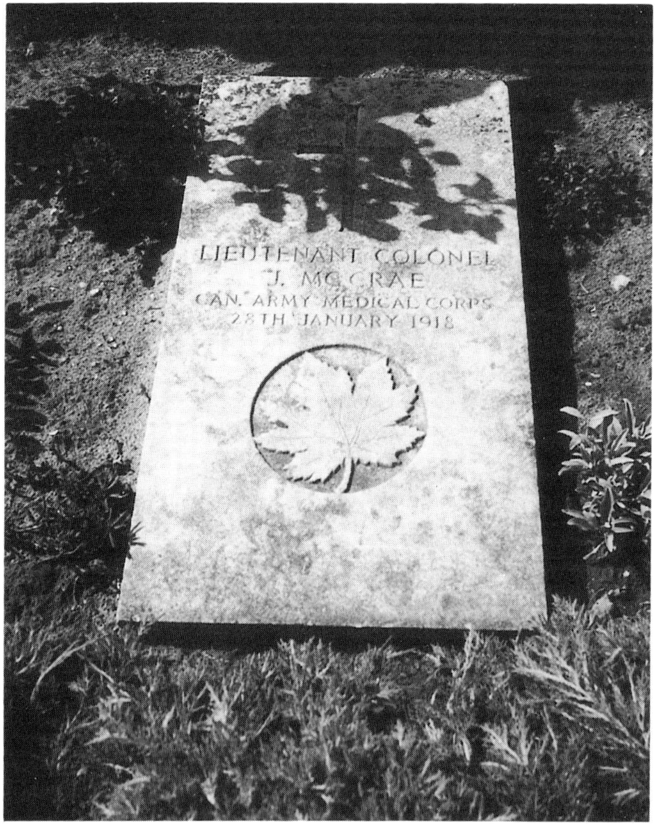

FIGURE 8   John McCrae's headstone (Courtesy of Dr. Robert Devloo).

The poem of only 15 lines captured the hearts and imagination of the then war beleaguered western world, and subsequently became a timeless classic. (Fig 10):[21]

"In Flanders fields the poppies blow
Between the crosses, row on row,
That mark our place; and in the sky
The larks, still bravely singing, fly
Scarce heard amidst the guns below.

We are the Dead. Short days ago
We lived, felt dawn, saw sunset glow,
Loved, and were loved, and now we lie
In Flanders Fields.

Take up our quarrel with the foe:
To you from falling hands we throw
The torch; be yours to hold it high.
If ye break faith with us who die
We shall not sleep, though poppies grow
In Flanders Fields."

McCrae first sent this poem to the *Spectator* which rejected it.[3] He then submitted it to *Punch,* in which it was published on Dec 8, 1915. Although not comparable to the works of more highly regarded poets, it immediately captured the mood of the British public. The poem, and thereby the war, was romanticized, as evidenced by an ornate printing in 1921. By the time of McCrae's death, "In Flanders Fields" had become the most popular war poem in the English language. It is responsible for the poppy becoming the symbol of memorial days in the United States, Canada, and Great Britain. However, only artificial poppies are used on these occasions because opium is derived from *Papaver somniferous,* the opium poppy.

"In Flanders Fields" was not the only poem written by John McCrae. Andrew Macphail compiled 29 of McCrae's poems.[18] The first was published in 1894 while McCrae was still a medical student, and the last in 1917 while he was in France. Quite striking is that 19 (70%) of his poems have the same theme—a preoccupation with death. H.E. MacDermont has commented on the fact that John McCrae was both a pathologist and a poet. "Who more than the pathologist is tempted to soliloquize on death? And when he happens also to have in him the elements of a poet, who rather than he should yield to the temptation? In John McCrae there was just that combination of training with illumination of mind."[7] This comment implies that McCrae's training and experience as a pathologist directed his poetic gift to the topic of death. But, if his close exposure to the dead in a professional capacity had influenced his poetry, then one would expect the theme of death not to have entered his poetry until the beginning of his apprenticeship in pathology in 1899. However, death is the theme in eight of 16 poems published before 1899, and in 11 of 14 published after 1898.[22]

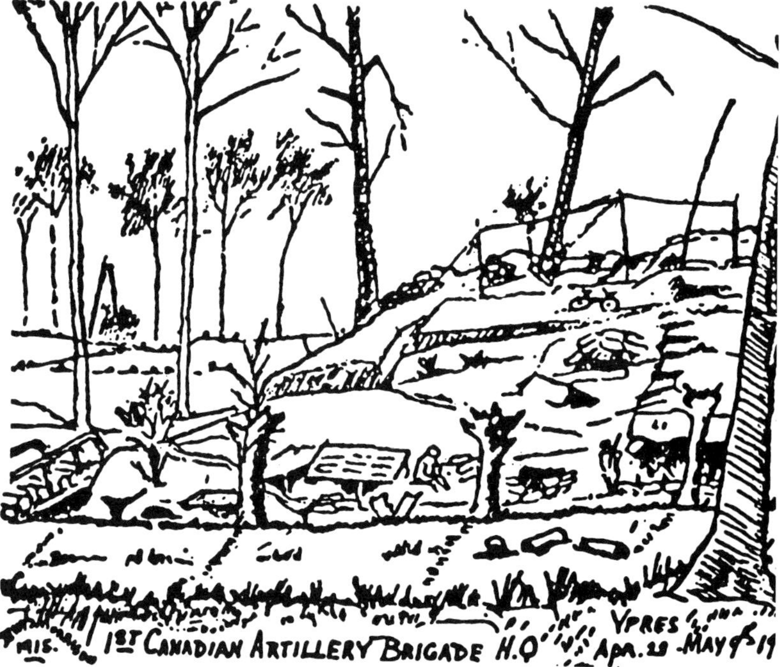

FIGURE 9   Drawing of the field command post of the First Canadian Field Artillery Brigade at Essex Farm (by Maj Gen Sir Edward WB Morrison in the latter part of 1915).

McCrae's 19 poems, which are oriented to death, all exhibit the same orientation—that death represents the rest and calm which come after a life of stress in an evil and difficult world. For example, there is reiteration of the phrase "Sweet Rest of Death" in his 1897 poem "Slumber Songs." In the "Dying of Pere Pierre" of 1904, McCrae suggests that death is far more wonderful than life because of the splendors of the Heavens and of God. Because the predominating theme in McCrae's poetry was exhibited both before and after his training in pathology, it is quite possible that his preoccupation with death may have influenced his choice of medical specialty as well as his poetry. The influence of a physician's attitude towards death on his professional activities is well recognized.

Although William Osler did not exhibit as pervading a concern with death as did McCrae, he did consider several of its aspects. The best known of these is found in his 1905 valedictory address at Johns Hopkins University.[23] Its notoriety is based on only two sentences:

> "The teacher's life should have three periods, study until twenty-five, investigation until forty, profession until sixty, at which age I would have him retired on a double allowance. Whether Anthony Trollope's suggestion of a college and chloroform should be carried out or not I have become a little dubious, as my own time is getting short."

What was meant to be a humorous and whimsical reference to his own aging was taken up by the press as a serious recommendation for euthanasia for all on achieving the age 60 (a procedure that was designated as "being Oslerized").[24] More meaningful and significant views on death are found in Osler's Ingersoll Lecture of 1904 on *Science and Immortality*.[25] Without overtly stating that there is a life after death, Osler speaks warmly of the "ever small and select, (group who) lay hold with the anchor of faith upon eternal life as the controlling influence in this one." Yet, based on his own experience with dying patients, he stated that "The great majority gave no sign one way or the other; like their birth, their death was a sleep and a forgetting."

Two further quotations from the lecture suggest that Osler's scientific mind may have inhibited him from acknowledging a belief in life after death. On the one hand he stated that "amid the turbid ebb and flow of human misery, a belief in . . . the life of the world to come is the rock of safety to which many of the noblest . . . of fellows have clung." On the other hand he asserted that "of the things that are unseen science knows nothing, and has at present no means of knowing anything." Such a desire to believe in spite of inability to do so is also apparent in his statement on spiritualism in the same lecture:

> ". . . there may be a vast supra-conscious sphere of astral life, the manifestations of which are only now and then in evidence,—a sphere in which, where all the nerve of sense is numb, in unconjectured bliss or in the abyss of tenfold complicated change, the spirit itself may commune with others, . . . and do diverse wonders of which we are told in the volumes of the Society for Psychical Research, . . ."

Further interest in spiritualism is apparent by the presence of 12 related items in his *Bibliotheca Osleriania,* including a book on the subject by Oliver Lodge, the great British physicist, and a definitive statement by Arthur Conan Doyle on his own acceptance of spiritualism.[12,26,27] Cushing, however, states that Osler had scant patience with spiritualism. Unlike Osler, John McCrae's writings had no reference to spiritualism, and his approach to death was more patriotic and religious.

Summary

In summary, John McCrae's contributions to medicine were considerably less than those of William Osler and even those of Thomas McCrae, both of whom had held the rank of professor of medicine at Philadelphia and at Johns Hopkins. Nonetheless, Garrison's *History of Medicine,* lists John McCrae and not his brother Thomas among physicians in America who had done good work in teaching and practice.[28] The first name could well have been an error, John being much more generally known because of the popularity of his poem "In Flanders Fields." Although Cushing's biography of Osler discusses Thomas considerably more than John, his evaluation of John McCrae is high—"others can best judge whether as soldier, physician, or poet he ranks highest . . . his immortal poem . . . tells better than could a volume, how the men felt in Flanders during those tragic days of April–May 1915."[2]

Both Osler and McCrae were excellent teachers who were highly praised by their students. They differed, however, in personality. Osler's was extroverted and accompanied by a keen sense of humor. Although McCrae is stated to have shown students the human side of medicine, he has been characterized as having "much of the soldier in his make-up. His carriage, his approach and his appearance before an audience marked him of soldierly character . . . He was a man of few words but of decided action."[29] However, McCrae's poem "In Flanders Fields," speaks eloquently for the sensitivity of the inner man. He was by nature a quiet, but pleasant man—a person of high principles, imbued with strong spiritual values, and optimism. He also exhibited considerable affinity for both children and animals.

As to war, Osler's attitude was more pragmatic than that of McCrae.[30] Osler considered that war, "this furious monster with so many heads and arms is yet man—feeble, calamitous and miserable man; 'tis but an ant hill disturbed and provoked."[31] This is in striking contrast to the idealization of war in McCrae's poem, "In Flanders Fields."[1]

Both McCrae and Osler were honored by Canadian commemorative stamps issued on the 50th anniversaries of their deaths.[32] The McCrae stamp was issued in 1968, primarily for his poem "In Flanders Fields."[1] The Osler stamp was issued in 1969 for his activities as a teacher, innovator and practitioner, as exemplified by the seven volumes of *A System of Medicine* which he edited with John McCrae's brother, Thomas.[33] Both McCraes were contributors. A final honor is the recognition in Montreal of the contributions of William Osler and John McCrae—Osler's is in the form of a plaque in the main corridor of the Montreal General Hospital, and McCrae's is in the form of a memorial window on the second floor of the Strathcona Anatomy and Dentistry Building at McGill University.[34,35]

The lives of both of these "kindred spirits" can be summed up in the following quotation from a speech given by John McCrae to students:[18]

"What I spent, I had: What I saved, I lost: What I gave, I have; . . . It will be in your power every day to store up for yourselves treasures that will come back to you in the consciousness of duty well done, of kind acts performed, things that having given away freely you yet possess."

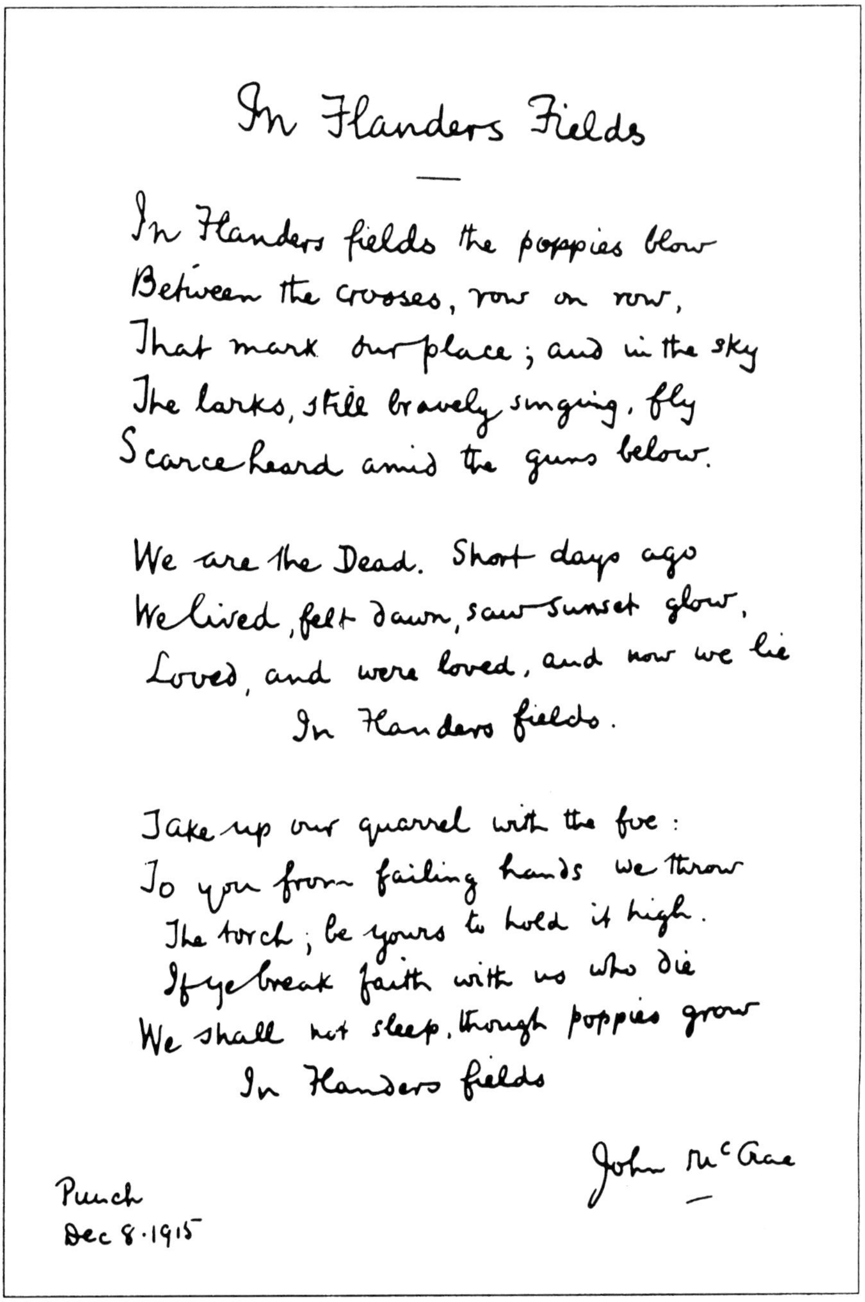

In Flanders Fields

—

In Flanders fields the poppies blow
Between the crosses, row on row,
That mark our place; and in the sky
The larks, still bravely singing, fly
Scarce heard amid the guns below.

We are the Dead. Short days ago
We lived, felt dawn, saw sunset glow,
Loved, and were loved, and now we lie
In Flanders fields.

Take up our quarrel with the foe:
To you from failing hands we throw
The torch; be yours to hold it high.
If ye break faith with us who die
We shall not sleep, though poppies grow
In Flanders fields

John McCrae

Punch
Dec 8·1915

FIGURE 10 "In Flanders Fields" in John McCrae's own handwriting.[18]

References

1. McCrae J: In Flanders Fields. *Punch,* December 8, 1915.
2. Cushing H: *The Life of Sir William Osler,* vol 1 & 2. Oxford, Clarendon Press, 1925.
3. Prescott JF: *In Flanders Fields. The Story of John McCrae.* Erin, Ontario, Boston Mills Press, 1985.
4. James (Professor): The history of the Toronto General Hospital and medical school. *Middlesex Hosp J* 57:74–76, 1957.

5. Charles J: *John McCrae.* Ottawa, Canada, Veterans Affairs, Government of Canada, 1988.

6. Rodin AE: *Oslerian Pathology. An Assessment and Annotated Atlas of Museum Specimens.* Lawrence, Kansas, Coronado Press, 1981.

7. MacDermot HE: John McCrae's autopsy book. *Can Med Assoc J* 40:495, 1939.

8. Adami JG, McCrae J: *A Textbook of Pathology for Students of Medicine.* Philadelphia, Lea & Ferbiger, 1912.

9. Osler W: *Students Notes. Normal Histology for Laboratory and Class Use.* Montreal, Dawson Bros, 1882.

10. Osler W: *The Principles and Practice of Medicine,* ed 8. Revised with assistance of Thomas McCrae. New York, D Appelton, 1912.

11. McCrae J: The pirates of medicine. *Montreal Med J* 38:523, 1909.

12. Osler W: *Bibliotheca Osleriana.* Oxford, Clarendon Press, 1929.

13. Wright AE: On the results obtained by antityphoid inoculation. *Lancet* 2:651–654, 1902.

14. Osler W: *Bacilli and Bullets.* London, Oxford University Press, 1914.

15. Coombs REB: *Before Endeavours Fade. A Guide to the Battlefields of the First World War.* London, England, Battle of Britain Prints Int, 1983.

16. Robb-Smith AHT: Did Sir William Osler have carcinoma of the lung? *Chest* 66: 712–716, 1974.

17. Prescott JF: The extensive medical writings of soldier-poet John McCrae. *Can Med Assoc J* 122:110–114, 1980.

18. McCrae J: *In Flanders Fields and Other Poems, with an Essay on Character by Sir Andrew Macphail.* Toronto, William Biggs, 1919.

19. Swinton WE: Physicians in literature. Part I: John McCrae, physician, soldier, poet. *Can Med Assoc J* 113:900–902, 1975.

20. Devloo R: Personal Communication to JD Key. July 18, 1988.

21. Angevine DM: John McCrae: pathologist, poet, soldier, a man among men, 1872–1918. *Arch Path* 88:455–458, 1969.

22. Rodin, AE: John McCrae, poet-pathologist. *Can Med Assoc J* 88:204–205, 1963.

23. Osler W: *The Fixed Period: in* Aequanimitas, ed 3. Philadelphia, Blakiston Co, 1932, pp 375–393.

24. Roland CG: The infamous Wlliam Osler. *JAMA* 193:98–100, 1965.

25. Osler W: *Science and Immortality.* Boston. Houghton, Mifflin & Co. 1904.

26. Lodge OJ: *Raymond, or Life and Death, With Examples of the Evidence for Survival of Memory and Affection after Death,* ed 3. London, 1916.

27. Doyle AC: The new revelation. *Metropolitan,* January 1918, pp 5–10, 68, 75.

28. Garrison FH: *An Introduction to the History of Medicine,* ed 4. Philadelphia, WB Saunders, 1929, p 636.

29. Klotz O: John McCrae B.A., M.D., M.R.C.P. (London), Lieutenant-Colonel, C.A.M.C. *Am J Med Sci* 155:469–472, 1918.

30. Henderson AR: War comes to the peacemaker: William Osler, 1914–1918. *Military Med* 136:227–233, 1971.

31. Osler W: *Science and the War.* Oxford, Clarendon Press, 1915.

32. Kyle RA, Shampo MA: *Medicine and Stamps,* vol 2. Huntington, NY, Krieger, 1980, pp 142, 156.

33. Golden RL, Roland CG (eds): *Sir William Osler. An Annotated Bibliography with Illustrations.* San Francisco, Norman Pub, 1988.

34. Internat Assoc Med Museums: Sir William Osler Memorial Number. Appreciations and Reminiscences. Montreal, privately issued, 1926.

35. Bensley EH: Flanders poppies. *Glaxo* 28:34, 1964.

Sir William Osler, Sir William Gowers and Medical Phonography

Thomas A. Horrocks, M.A., M.S.L.S. and
Richard L. Golden, M.D.

In the January 25, 1908 issue of the *British Medical Journal* there appeared the following communication addressed to the editor from the officers of a medical society bearing a very unusual name:

> Sir,—It has been many years since the Society of Medical Phonographers was last mentioned in your columns, and we shall be glad if you will allow us to direct attention to the fact that it still exists, and still issues its medical periodical in lithographed phonetic shorthand. We believe that many students and members of the profession are ignorant of the Society and its efforts to promote the effective use of shorthand in medicine, both in practical work and in research.

The letter closed with an offer to furnish "particulars of the society to any members of the profession, or students, who may desire to join it."[1] The letter was signed by the officers of the Society, including its President, Sir William Gowers, the distinguished British neurologist, who was the founder of the Society and the most famous crusader on behalf of medical phonography, or the use of shorthand in medicine.

Shorthand, a method of writing rapidly by substituting characters, abbreviations, or symbols for letters, words, or phrases has been in use, in one form or another, since antiquity. In fact, Gowers was not the first physician to be closely associated with shorthand, for it was a physician, Timothy Bright (1550–1615) who introduced shorthand into England during the sixteenth

Read at the annual meeting of the American Osler Society, April 26, 1989.

Reprinted with additions, with permission from *Fugitive Leaves from The Historical Collections*, Third Series, *3*:1–5, 1988 century. Bright's crude system, consisting of straight lines, circles, and half–circles, appeared in his book *Characterie. An Arte of Shorte, Swift, and Secrete Writing by Character,* published in London in 1588. There is no evidence to suggest, however, that Bright applied his invention to his medical practice.[2]

Other shorthand systems were devised during the next three centuries, many of them short–lived. One of the most popular systems developed during the nineteenth century, and one which was used well into this century, was designed by Sir Isaac Pitman (1813–1897), a British educator. Convinced that other systems of shorthand did not contain enough of the phonetic principle, Pitman developed his own system, which he called "phonography," which was based on the sounds of words rather than on the conventional spellings. Pitman's system was introduced in 1837 in his book *Stenographic Sound–Hand.*[3]

Phonography met with extraordinary success, causing Pitman to give up his private school in Bath to devote himself to the promotion of his shorthand system. Queen Victoria knighted him in 1884.[4] As we shall see, Pitman's system of shorthand profoundly affected the career of a young medical apprentice by the name of William Richard Gowers.

Gowers was born on March 20, 1845. His medical training began at the age of sixteen when he was apprenticed to Dr. Thomas Simpson at Goggeshall

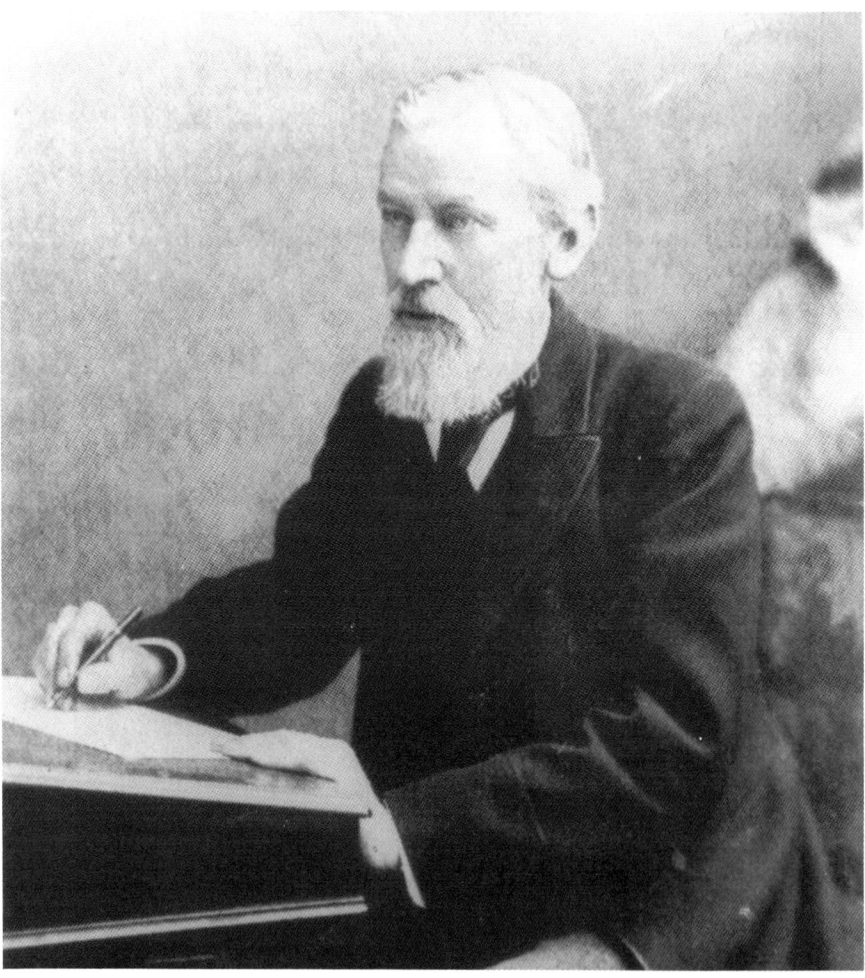

FIGURE 1   Sir William Gowers (1845–1915).

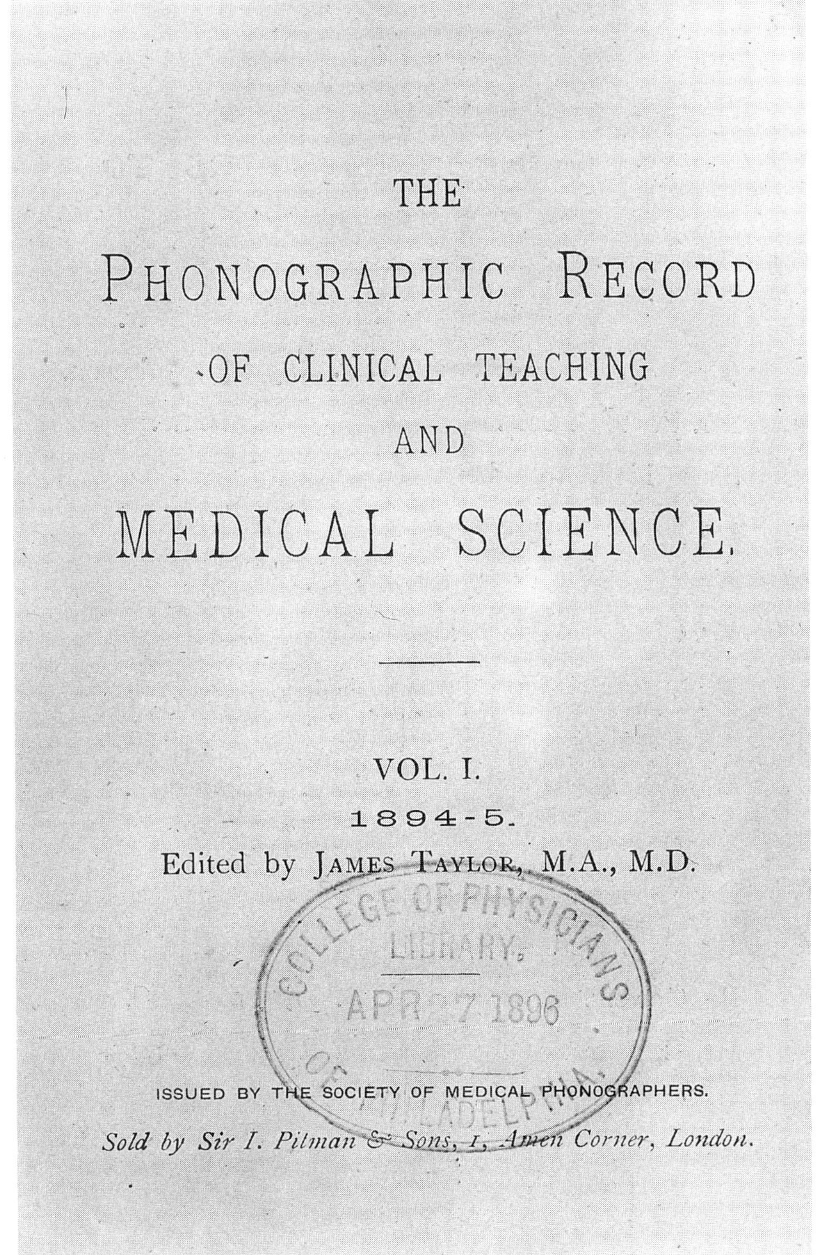

FIGURE 2 *The Phonographic Record of Teaching and Medical Science,* Volume I (1894–1895), the journal of The Society of Medical Phonographers.

in Essex.[5] In 1863, after two years with Dr. Simpson, Gowers went on to complete his medical studies at University College Hospital in London, where he received his M.D. in 1870. During his student days at University College, Gowers was not only a pupil of, but an assistant to Sir William Jenner (1815–98).

Upon graduation from medical school, Gowers was appointed the first Medical Registrar at the National Hospital for the Paralysed and Epileptic in Queen square.[6] Three years later he was promoted to Assistant Physician, and in 1880 he was named Physician to the Hospital. While at Queen Square, Gowers worked with many of the leading figures of British neurology,

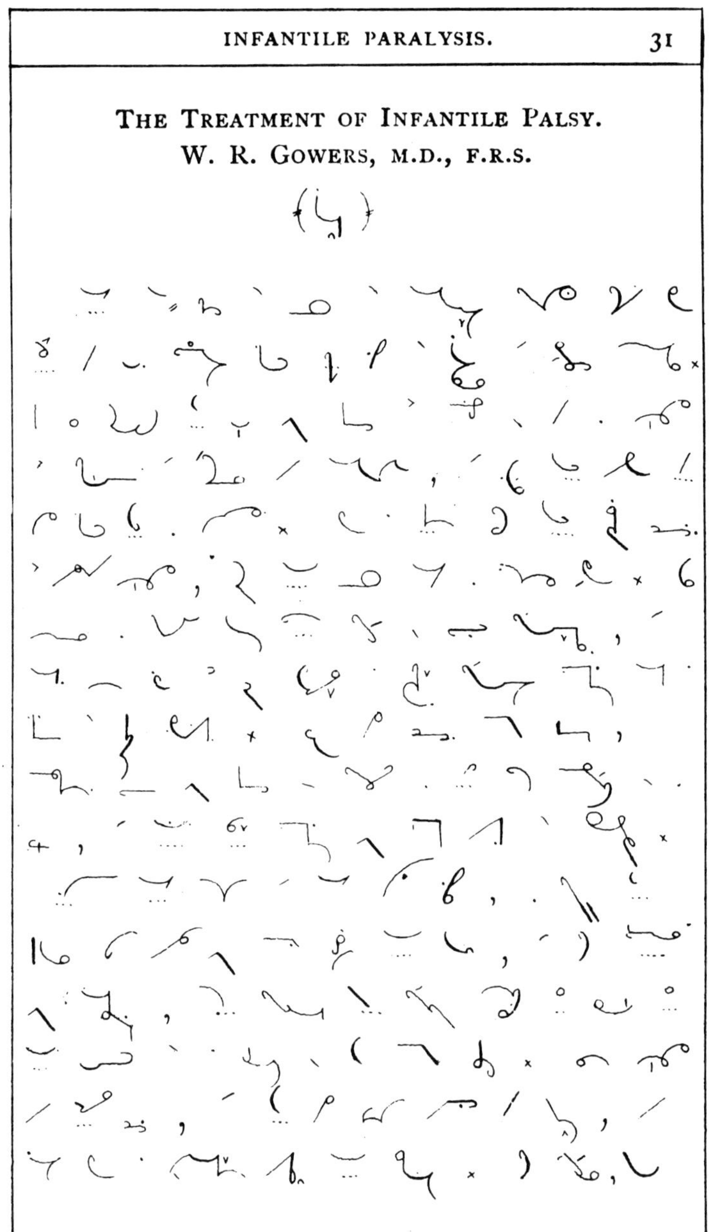

FIGURE 3   Gowers published many articles in *The Phonographic Record*. This is the first page of one he wrote on infantile palsy, which appeared in the first volume of this unusual journal.

including John Hughlings Jackson (1835–1911), David Ferrier (1843–1928), and Victor Horsley (1857–1916). During his years at Queen Square Gowers served on the staff at University College Hospital, and developed a large private consulting practice as well.[7]

Gowers' notable achievements in medicine include the designing of a hemocytometer and a hemoglobinometer, and the discovery of Gowers' Tract.[8] He became the leading authority on various nervous disorders through a number of classic studies, such as *Diagnosis of Diseases of the Spinal Cord* (London, 1880),[9] *Epilepsy and Other Chronic Convulsive Disorders* (London, 1881),[10] *Diagnosis of Diseases of the Brain* (London 1885),[11] and his *magnum opus, Manual of Diseases of the Nervous System* (London, 1886–1888).[12] The last mentioned work, translated into seven languages, became known as the "Bible of Neurology."

It is in connection with Gowers' "Bible of Neurology" that we return to his life-long passion for shorthand. Gowers firmly believed that his *Manual* could not have been written without the aid of shorthand. Once, when entertaining a friend at his home, Gowers pointed to the hundreds of volumes of notes which formed the basis for his great work, stating "[t]here are my personal notes in shorthand on more than twenty thousand cases of nervous diseases. A human lifetime would scarcely be long enough to allow them to be taken in ordinary writing."[13]

Gowers apparently taught himself Pitman's phonography during his years with Dr. Simpson. His appreciation of the system grew as he became more adept at it. To Gowers, the simplicity of the system and the fact that it produced greater results were the most attractive features of phonography. In one of his many promotional tracts on the advantages of its use, Gowers claims that shorthand

> is a lever which multiplies the effects of labor for every work in which it is used . . . It is a lever which at once increases speed and power. It doubles record while far more than halving its labour, and it allows twice the time for thought and observation. It influences quality to a greater degree than quantity.[14]

These attributes, Gowers believed, made phonography invaluable to the physician and especially to the medical student, and it was to the latter group particularly that Gowers directed his crusade for the adoption of shorthand. In proclaiming its many benefits to the student, Gowers stated that shorthand "enables the student to make a perfect epitome of his lectures, more useful than any textbook, and yet give more attention to the subject than if he took no notes."[15] As a student himself, Gowers had found that his shorthand notes "contained more than twice as much of the substance of the lecture." Moreover, he claimed, his notes never needed to be rewritten.[16] As proof of the value of shorthand to the student, Gowers proudly offered his own academic record, which included "the gold medal at the M.D. examination," although he never used a textbook. There were no textbooks, he claimed, that were comparable to his shorthand notes.[17]

Convinced that students should be instructed in the art, Gowers strongly advocated making phonography an extra mark-bearing subject in the preliminary examination for the profession. Although students could learn shorthand during vacation, Gowers advised them to learn it before they entered medical school. A student with shorthand skills, Gowers claimed, "starts on a higher level, with the means of a more rapid rise to thorough practical power."[18]

Although he urged students to learn and use shorthand from the beginnings of their careers, Gowers stressed that it was never too late to acquire proficiency in this area. He also called on practitioners, even those in the field for many years, to learn shorthand. And what he advocated to the profession, he expected from his resident and assistants. He even persuaded his wife and children to take up shorthand.[19]

During his later years, Gowers' interest in shorthand became an obses-

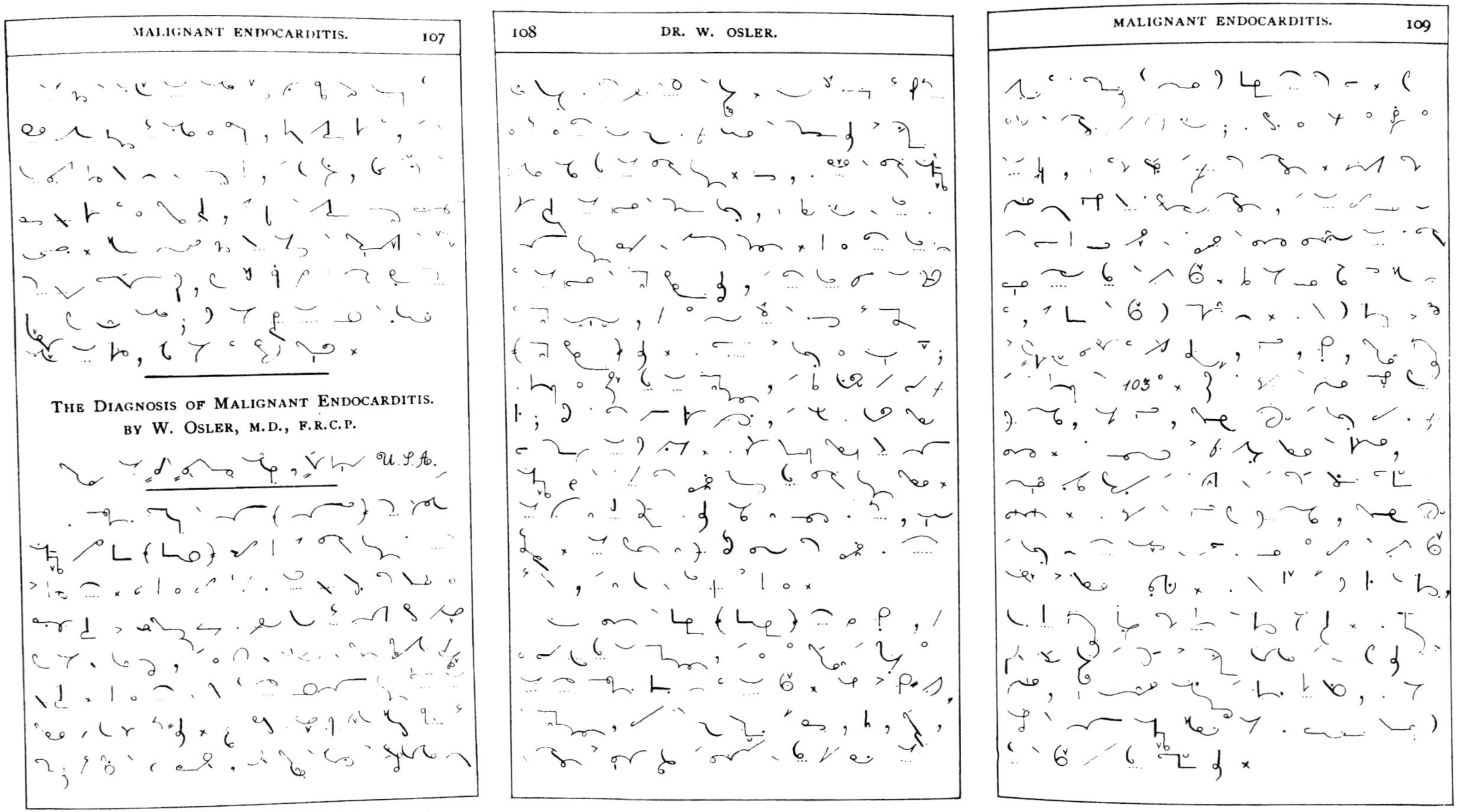

FIGURE 4 Article on "Malignant Endocarditis" that Osler submitted to *The Phonographic Record.*

sion. Over half of his one hundred or so works during the years 1894 to 1902 were published in shorthand. Almost all appeared in a peculiar medical journal, *The Phonographic Record of Clinical Teaching and Medical Science,* which was the official organ of an equally peculiar medical organization, the Society of Medical Phonographers.[20]

Gowers founded the Society of Medical Phonographers in December of 1894.[21] It was the culmination of his many efforts on behalf of shorthand in medicine. Not surprisingly, he was the Society's first President, and served as co-editor of *The Phonographic Record* for a long time. The objectives of the Society were, naturally, "to promote the use of shorthand in medicine, especially by the publication in Shorthand of useful medical literature . . . and to form a bond of union among medical phonographers."[22]

In his inaugural address before the Society Gowers expressed hope that "the influence of our society may ultimately extend the use of shorthand in many branches of intellectual work." As individuals in these various fields of endeavor began to use shorthand, the effect on their work could only be positive, stated Gowers, because

> If a man habitually observes more precisely, and more carefully, he must become a better observer, able to perceive more accurately, more minutely, more adequately, and to attain precision more readily. This influence moreover, whatever its degree, must be progressive. We might take as our motto the words "Writing maketh an exact man."[23]

Through the achievement of its goals, the Society would, according to Gowers, ultimately benefit those in need of the medical profession, because shorthand is most beneficial to society "when it facilitates, increases, makes more effectual the work that is for others."[24]

The Society of Medical Phonographers exhibited signs of growth during its early years. Originally consisting of sixty members, the society's rolls grew to 230 in less than two years.[25] Membership in the Society was open to all practitioners and students with an interest in shorthand. A number of members were Fellows of the Royal College of Physicians and the Royal College of Surgeons.

Beside promoting the use of shorthand in medical schools and in the profession in general, the main efforts of the society were directed toward publication. In addition to its periodical, *The Phonographic Record,* the Society issued a number of instructional pamphlets, including *The Use of Shorthand by the Student* and *The Use of Shorthand by the Practitioner.* The Society also published *The Phonographic Medical Library* series, consisting of a number of small monographs, printed in shorthand, on various topics. As one might expect, the first contribution to this series was a work by Gowers on *The Diagnosis of the Nature of Organic Brain Diseases* (London, 1897).[26]

The major concern of the society, however was the publication of the *Phonographic Record.* The objective of this unusual periodical was "to promote the use of shorthand among Medical Students and Practitioners, by affording the means of increasing, at the same time, their familiarity with the art and their professional knowledge."[27] Contributors to the first volume included some notable authors, such as Sir William Jenner, Frederick Treves (1853–1923), and Gowers' good friend, William Osler. Osler's contribution was an article on "The Diagnosis of Malignant Endocarditis," which was recently translated for the first time.[28]

Osler was a great admirer of Gowers; he once referred to the eminent neurologist as a "brilliant ornament of British medicine." Their long friendship began in 1878 when Osler visited England to accept his membership in the Royal College of Physicians and to work at clinical medicine.[29] Osler never failed to pay Gowers a visit during his subsequent trips to England and he dedicated the English edition of his book *On Chorea and Choreiform Affections,* published in 1894, to Gowers.[30]

It was probably more out of friendship to Gowers and a desire to assist his phonographic crusade than a personal commitment to shorthand, however, that Osler contributed his article on endocarditis to the *Phonographic Record.* There is no evidence to suggest that Osler was a member of the Society of Medical Phonographers. While Osler's article on endocarditis was his only original contribution to Gowers' shorthand journal, there were two of his articles reprinted in the *Phonographic Record,* one of which shows us that while Osler may not have been a vocal supporter of shorthand in medicine, he nevertheless recognized its value to the clinician and, we might add, it tells us also that Osler never learned shorthand. The article in question is really nothing more than an excerpt from *Ephemerides,* which originally appeared in the *Montreal Medical Journal* in 1894.[31] Gowers, with or without Osler's approval, lifted the paragraph and included it in the 1906 volume of the *Phonographic Record,* and entitled it "Professor Osler on the Value of Shorthand to Medical Men." Here is the complete text as it appears in the *Phonographic Record.*

> For several years I have adopted the plan of dictating at odd times abstracts of the histories of special cases and filing them in order ready for publication. In this way, when noting carefully during the session of 1892-3 all the cases of abdominal tumour which came before me for diagnosis, I had, in October 1893, when I began the series of lectures which have been published, all the cases type-written and ready. It has always been a regret to me that I had not learned stenography, which Sir William Gowers has found so serviceable, and the use of which in medical work he has advocated so warmly.[32]

This passage appears to be Osler's last words on medical phonography. But what about Gowers? Unfortunately, his hopes and dreams for the Society's success were not to be realized. The initial appeal of the Society soon waned and by 1910 it was moribund. Despite the "plug" by Osler just referred to and appeals to the medical profession, such as the letter quoted at the beginning of this paper, the Society steadily lost members while attracting little interest. It ceased operations in 1912, with the publication of the seventeenth and last volume of the *Phonographic Record.*[22]

Undoubtedly discouraged by the failure of the Society, Gowers offered nothing more to the cause of medical phonography. Plagued by poor health and progressive invalidism, his personal crusade was over. He died on May 4, 1915. Appropriately, his last contribution to medicine appeared in the *Phonographic Record.*[34]

To one of his pupils, Gowers was a "star of first magnitude" in the field of neurology, and we have already referred to Osler's glowing compliment.[35] These may have been tributes to his professional achievements only, for he was not a popular figure. Reserved, dogmatic, and often intolerant of views contrary to his own, Gowers' personality did not attract a large circle of friends. He was respected by all for his valuable contributions to medicine, yet there were some who considered him foolish for wasting, as they thought, so much time on medical phonography.

It must have been frustrating for Gowers to see his campaign for medical phonography produce so little response, for there was certainly no groundswell of support for his program. The neurologist Foster Kennedy (1884–1952) once related an anecdote illustrating Gowers' obssesion with shorthand and his impatience with those who did not share his enthusiasm. Gowers, Kennedy wrote

> was once seen—and it probably happened often—to stop his coachman in crowded Southampton Row, having fastened his eye on a likely-looking young man hurrying on his lawful occassions (sic) along the pavement. Gowers climbed out of his carriage, white beard waving, stumbled up to him—his gait was unsteady—clutched him by the arm, and glaring at him with his frightening flaming fierce blue eyes said, "Young man, do you write shorthand?" To which the shocked man answered, "No, I don't." Whereupon Gowers dropped his arm, saying bitterly, "You're a fool, and will fail in life." He then clambered abruptly back into his carriage.[36]

To Gowers, it was incomprehensible that anyone should not strive to become "an exact man."

References

1. *British Medical Journal* (1908):1:235.
2. Geoffrey Keynes, *Dr. Timothie Bright 1550–1615* (London: the Wellcome Historical Library, 1962); William J. Carlton, *Timothie Bright: Doctor of Physicke* (London: Elliot Stock, 1911); *Dictionary of National Biography* 6 (New York: Macmillan and Company, 1886):266–67.
3. *The Dictionary of National Biography,* Supplement vol. 3 (New York: The Macmillan Company, 1901):266–67.
4. Ibid.
5. Macdonald Critchley, *Sir William Gowers 1845–1915: A Biographical Appreciation* (London: William Heinemann, 1949), p. 14.
6. Lawrence C. McHenry, *Garrison's History of Neurology* (Springfield, Illinois: Charles C. Thomas, 1969), p. 312.
7. Critchley, *Sir William Gowers,* p. 85.
8. Gowers first referred to this tract in his book, *Diagnosis of Diseases of the Spinal Cord,* which was published in 1880.
9. W.R. Gowers, *Diagnosis of Diseases of the Spinal Cord* (London: Churchill, 1880).
10. W.R. Gowers, *Epilepsy and Other Chronic Convulsive Disorders, Their Causes, Symptoms and Treatment* (London: Churchill 1881).
11. W.R. Gowers, *Lectures on Diagnosis of Diseases of the Brain* (London: Churchill, 1885).
12. W.R. Gowers, *Manual of Diseases of the Nervous System* 2 vols. (London: Churchill, 1886–88).
13. F.W. Langdon, "Sir William Gowers, M.D., F.R.C.P., F.R.S., an Appreciation," *The Lancet-Clinic* 114 (1915):143.
14. W.R. Gowers, "What is Shorthand?" *The Medical Magazine* 4 (1895):8–9.
15. W.R. Gowers, "The Inaugural Address on the Art of Writing in Relation to Medical and Scientific Work," *British Medical Journal* (1895):2:818.
16. W.R. Gowers, "Shorthand and Students," (letter) *British Medical Journal* (1897):1:113.
17. Ibid.
18. Gowers, "Inaugural Address . . . ," p. 818.

19. Critchley, *Sir William Gowers,* p. 61.
20. Ibid., pp. 105–110.
21. W.R. Gowers, "Inaugural Address . . . ," p. 817. See also, Critchley, *Sir William Gowers,* p. 61.
22. *Phonographic Record of Clinical Teaching and Medical Science* 4 (1898). The bylaws of the Society were published in the front of this volume.
23. W.R. Gowers, "Inaugural Address . . . ,' p. 817. Gowers borrowed his "motto" from Francis Bacon, who wrote that; "Reading maketh a full man, conference a ready man, and writing an exact man." John Bartlett (comp.), *Familiar Quotations* 13th ed. (Boston: Little Brown and Company, 1955):168.
24. Ibid., p. 819.
25. *Phonographic Record of Clinical Teaching and Medical Science* 2 (1896):48.
26. W.R. Gowers, *The Diagnosis of the Nature of Organic Brain Disease* (The Phonographic Medical Library, vol. 1) (London: Pitman, 1897).
27. *Phonographic Record of Clinical Teaching and Medical Science* 1 (1895):32.
28. Richard L. Golden and Thomas A. Horrocks, "William Osler's Views on Malignant Endocarditis From an 'Unknown' Report," *The American Journal of Cardiology* 16 (1989):241–43.
29. W.Osler, "The Medical Clinic: A Retrospect and a Forecast," *British Medical Journal* (1914):1:10–16.
30. Harvey Cushing, *The Life of Sir William Osler* 2 vols. (Oxford: Clarendon Press, 1925), I, p. 402.
31. Osler's comments on the value of shorthand to medical students appeared in volume 12 (1906) of *The Phonographic Record.* It is also reprinted in C.N.B. Camac's *Counsels and Ideals From the Writings of William Osler* 2nd ed. (Oxford: Oxford University Press, 1921), p. 217.
32. Ibid.
33. Critchley, *Sir William Gowers,* p. 63.
34. W.R. Gowers, "The Neurology of the Eyelids," *Phonographic Record of Clinical Teaching and Medical Science* 16 (1910):6.
35. F.W. Langdon, "Sir William Gowers . . . ," p. 142.
36. Foster Kennedy: "William Gowers (1845–1915)," in *The Founders of Neurology,* compiled and edited by Webb Haymaker and Francis Schiller. 2nd ed. (Springfield, Illinois: Charles C. Thomas, 1970), p. 444.

SECTION IV

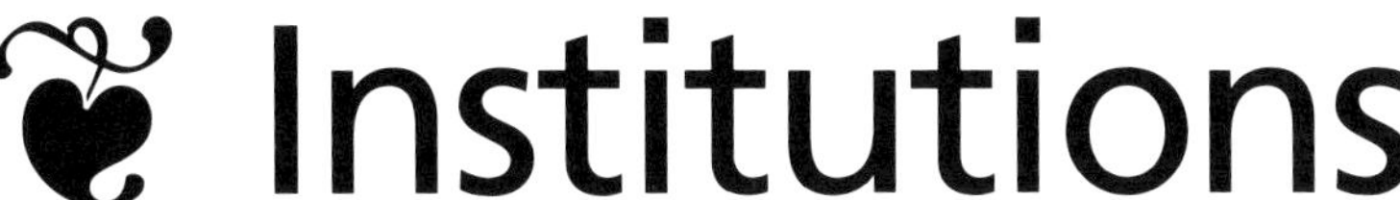 Institutions

The Osler-endowed Tudor and Stuart Club

 George T. Harrell, M.D.

The Tudor and Stuart Club was established by Sir William and Lady Osler at the Johns Hopkins University as a memorial to their only surviving son, Revere, who was killed in World War I.[1,2] Its purpose is to encourage in students a lifelong interest in literature.

William Osler had an intense lifelong interest in books, which began when he was a medical student. His interest was wide and emphasized the classics as well as the sciences and medicine. His collection now is at McGill University in Montreal, where the Bibliotheca Osleriana is housed in a separate beautiful setting, The Osler Library.

When Revere became an avid fisherman, his father gave him a first edition of Izaak Walton. He took the boy on his visits to bookstores and taught him how to examine catalogues critically for special items. He kept the books he purchased in the home.[3] From letters it is apparent Osler always intended that part of his collection eventually should go to Revere. The emphasis on the literature and especially poetry bore fruit in later years, as Revere began to buy books himself. At age eighteen, after he entered Christ Church College at Oxford, he drew a bookplate, which included a designation of himself as "Discip. IZ. WA."

Revere's first purchase, made in December 1913 at an auction at Sothebys, was for Landor's *Pericles and Aspasia,* for which he paid £1. No list of his purchases before 1916 was found. In a letter to Revere on his twenty-first birthday Sir William expresses pleasure "that of late years" Revere should have developed a taste for literature and fondness for old books.

In 1916, Revere began an acquisitions book, which appears to be handmade. He drew the title page in sepia ink. The first entry is for a 1640 first edition of a book of eighty sermons by John Donne, for which Revere paid £3. In all, he made forty-seven entries on six pages. Most titles are for books of the

Read at the annual meeting of the American Osler Society, May 3, 1983.

Reprinted with permission from *The Pharos of Alpha Omega Alpha, 47:23,* 1984

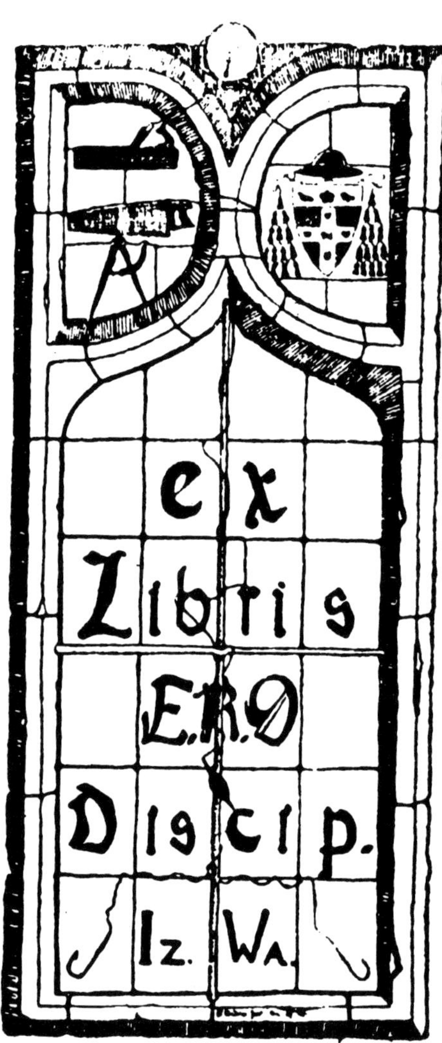

FIGURE 1 Bookplate of Revere Osler drawn when he was 18 years old.

sixteenth and seventeenth centuries, but many are of the nineteenth century. The last entry, dated May 12 (1917), was for a fourth edition of *Meditation upon Dobel.** On August 29, 1917, Revere was fatally wounded.

Endowment

On October 30, 1918, Osler wrote President Frank Goodnow of Johns Hopkins that, in recognition of his happy years in Baltimore and as a memorial to Revere, he had instructed the Toronto General Trust Company to hand over securities to the university. When sold they yielded $34,764, which was set up as the Edward Revere Osler Fund. The principal on September 30, 1982, had a value of $126,293.

*This entry, in Revere's handwriting, may actually refer to the book by T. Traherne titled *Centuries of Meditations* and edited by B. Dobell. The volume itself is missing from the collection.

The idea of access to a library for serious students was an old one of Osler's. In Baltimore and later in Oxford, he began to give keys to his home to a few selected students, who became known as "latch-keyers." In 1913, he gave a series of lectures at Yale, including one at the Elizabethan Club, which had been set up as a separate corporation for the study of literature.

Osler's letter to President Goodnow stated that in accordance with Revere's interests the fund was to encourage study of English literature in the Tudor and Stuart periods. He suggested that a literary club be formed with professors of English and undergraduate and graduate students of the department as members, with the university librarian ex officio. The books collected by Revere, with the later addition of special works from his own collection, were to be the nucleus of the club library, as a section of the departmental library. The income was to purchase books relating to the period and promote good fellowship and love of literature. The management of the club and expenditures of funds were to be in the hands of students, with qualifications for membership to be determined by the professors, the librarian, and William H. Welch of the medical school. Osler died December 29, 1919, before the club was organized.

On her death August 31, 1928, Lady Osler bequeathed £2000, with the note, "I give the following . . . to the Tudor and Stuart Club or Library of Johns Hopkins University." The remittance October 7, 1929, yielded $9700, which the university placed in a separate Lady Osler Fund. The principal September 30, 1982, had a value of $29,148.

Organization

Lady Osler was shattered by the deaths of her son and husband. Much of her communication was with the doctors she had known in Baltimore and Oxford. Though the club was to be located on the Homewood liberal arts campus, the medical school, some miles away in downtown Baltimore, was involved from the beginning through members of its faculty.

Lady Osler wrote April 3, 1922, that eight cases of books had been shipped. Her handwritten note was explicit "that the Library should be by itself and not in stacks of the General Library." She regretted she could not come herself, but hoped to later. She never did.

In May 1922 correspondence of Goodnow discussed whether the club was to have social or literary emphasis. At a meeting November 17 the location of the club was discussed. The choices were a new men's dormitory, which would have precluded women as members, the old Carroll mansion, which housed the Johns Hopkins Club, which did not permit women to enter, and Gilman Hall, where the English Department was located. The university decided in favor of Gilman which seemed to place more emphasis on the literary function favored by the librarian over the social function favored by some of Osler's friends.

In January 1923 two professors offered to give up their offices for conversion. Mrs. Robert Brewster, an original honorary member, thought the club room should be done in Tudor fashion and offered to pay for the work and the furnishings.

The minutes of the 1922 meeting in William S. Thayer's house end with a suggested committee to proceed with the organization of the club. The formal organization was completed January 16, 1923. Printed invitations were

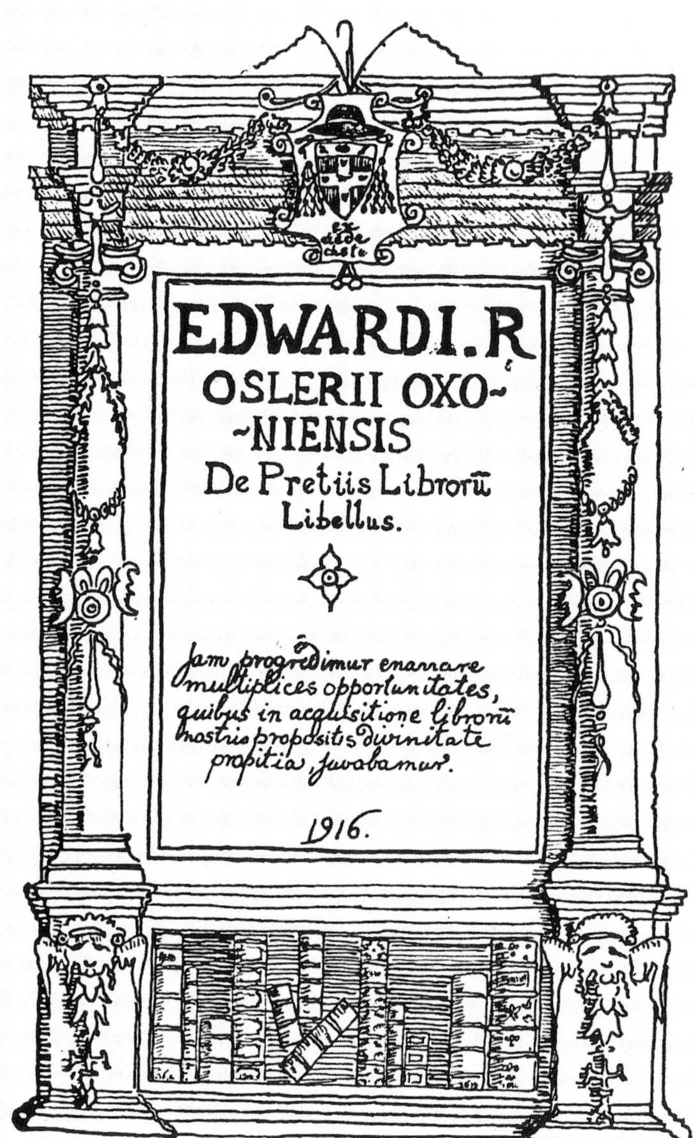

FIGURE 2   Title page of acquisitions book drawn by Revere Osler when he was 20 years old.

issued for the first public meeting, which was held 5 P.M., May 11, 1923, in the Civil Engineering Building. The formal opening of the club room was at 3 P.M., April 2, 1924. Letters during this period discussed whether only men would be members, a point never mentioned by the Oslers. Other letters questioned whether students or faculty in other departments could be invited to join if they had an interest in English literature. The president ruled they could.

In 1927, the club published the first small "Book" of the club with the text of Sir William's letter setting up the Edward Revere Osler Fund; the list of the charter members, honorary and active; the constitution and by-laws that had been adopted; and a poem to Revere Osler read by the author, Carol Wight, at the first formal meeting. Lady Osler had commissioned a portrait of Revere, which was unveiled in the club room January 27, 1926.[1]

Books

The books of the original shipment were individually wrapped in paper. A handlist of 857 titles alphabetically arranged by author, was mailed in March 1922. It is difficult to determine how many of the books actually were in Revere's collection, how many were added by his father or were later taken from Sir William's collection by Lady Osler and W. W. Francis. The original intention appears to have been to send Revere's books first. Some volumes contain his bookplate; his father never had a bookplate. A letter of Osler's indicates that the first editions of Milton, Shelley, Keats, and others are from his library.

By far the largest number of titles, ninety-eight, by or about an author are for Shelley (1792–1822). A letter of Osler's about Shelley's letters says, "Dear Izaak [Revere] was so interested in it and had become such a keen student of Shelley. The Everyman's library copy of poems he carried everywhere." It is a

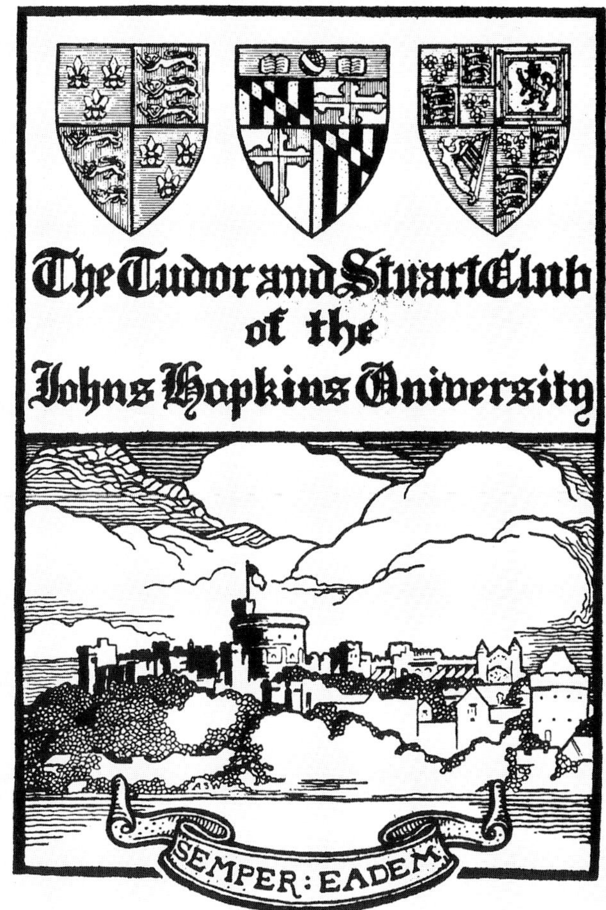

FIGURE 3   Bookplate of the Tudor and Stuart Club. The left crest is the Tudor, the central the University, the right the Stuart.

1910 pocket edition. The Montreal Library has a 4″ x 5″ book bound in red morocco that contains, in Sir William's handwriting, a list of forty-eight of Shelley's books. None of these now is in Montreal, but all appear in the handlist. Seven titles are by Keats (1795–1821) and seven about him. Revere clearly had a deep interest in nineteenth-century English poets.

From the notes by Francis on the Montreal list, it would appear the greatest number of books were from Osler's collection. Excluding duplicates, a count of the titles of original editions, reprints, or translations from or about the period shows thirty-five of the Tudor years with 153 titles of the Stuart period.

Books clearly about Revere's known interests include twenty-two by or about Walton, thirty-five about fishing, six on art, etching, or engraving, four on architecture, two on natural history and insects, one schoolboy algebra, but none on stamps or cabinet work. Of the books on fishing, thirty-four are by various authors published between 1531 and 1915. The list includes the 100,000th copy of Osler's textbook, the only publication of the father included, and Revere's Bible. The copy of Browne's *Religio Medici*, Boston, 1862, given by Sir William to Revere was noted as not to go since it was his father's favorite copy. It subsequently was used at Osler's funeral.

After Lady Osler's death in 1928, seventy-nine additional volumes were sent to Hopkins. No list of titles was found, and her will makes no mention of them. It is possible the books were kept in Revere's room by his mother and subsequently shipped by Sue Chapin or Francis.

When the original shipment arrived in Baltimore, no club room was available. It was university policy to have only departmental libraries. Accordingly, the books were placed in open stacks in Gilman Hall. The English professors' offices opened into the stacks, which also were available to students. Lady Osler had asked if a suitable room was available in Gilman Hall "so that men could take up books and enjoy them." The club bookplate designed by Mrs. Wight was printed in December 1923.

When the club room became available, some of the books were moved into that more secure situation. Lady Osler had recognized that there were "not a large number," but whether all could be placed behind the locked shelves is not known. Books began to disappear. A list of forty lost titles was prepared about 1936. The central climate-controlled Eisenhower Library on campus opened in 1964, and some part of the collection was moved into it.

The university had acquired Evergreen House, which is several miles from Homewood. It housed a collection of rare books in a climate-controlled environment and had a librarian, who, in January 1958, borrowed some books from the Tudor and Stuart collection for an exhibit. In July, 1969, the club asked permission to move "on deposit" to Evergreen books from Gilman, which was not air-conditioned. The Evergreen librarian moved 142 titles, which she found locked in a large safe located in a damp, airless closet off the club room. The books are now shelved behind locked grilles and arranged alphabetically with other volumes of English literature of the sixteenth and seventeenth centuries. One incunabulum is kept apart. All books have the club bookplate; some have Osler's name in his handwriting. A separate card file is maintained, but it is difficult to tell which books came from Osler's collection and which were bought by the club. Forty books contain Revere's bookplate. The books are used once or twice a month by graduate students or faculty in about equal numbers.

The books currently are housed in three places—the Club room in Gilman Hall, Eisenhower Library, and Evergreen House. All the books at all

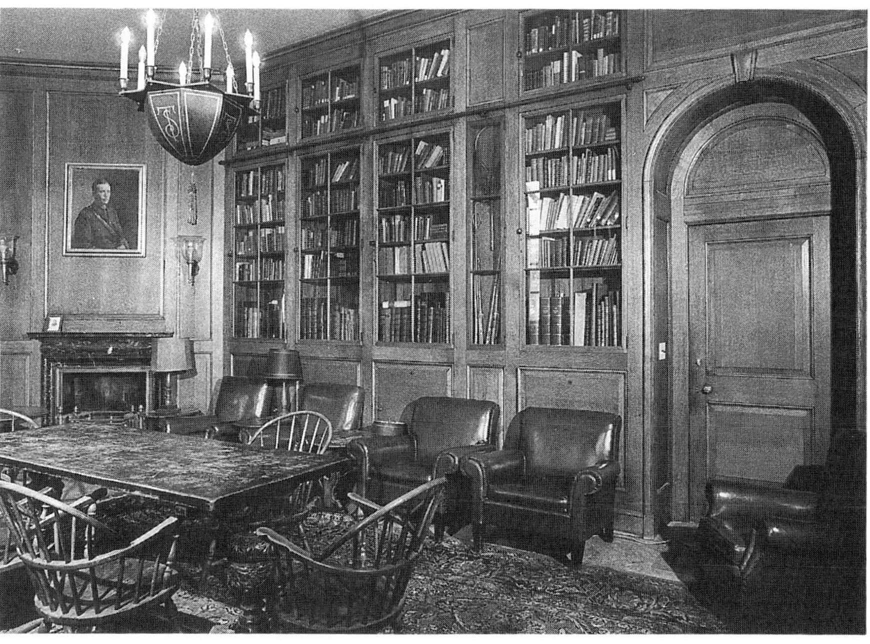

FIGURE 4   The Club room in 1983.

sites now are listed in the central catalog in Eisenhower. A university special collections librarian appointed in 1981 maintains the books presently in Eisenhower, but not as a distinct group.

Program

The early records of the club from 1918 to 1948 are fragmentary. Most minutes of meetings were handwritten in pencil. When the university archives were established in 1971, it was found most records covered only the period 1923–1943. The 1938 second and 1948 third small "Books" list the officers, members living and deceased, the lecturers and the titles of their talks. The only early summary of the club is that of John C. French in his 1946 history of the university.[4] The period from 1948 to the present is undocumented.

Members are elected by the board of governors. In the early years normally they included sixteen undergraduate men, eight from each of the upper two classes, and about the same number of male graduate students in English. An undated memorandum recommended that eight additional men could be elected by April of their sophomore year. "An undergraduate should be chosen partly for qualities of good fellowship and partly because of literary taste and ability, the latter qualities being of distinct importance." All male graduate students in English were elected "unless made undesirable by objectionable personal qualities." During the 1960s, women began to be admitted. All English graduate students now are elected, and 40 to 50 percent are women. The membership, including faculty, numbers about 200.

The board of governors always includes members from the medical school. The presidency alternates between faculty of the English department and the medical school. The secretary-treasurer, a student, remains responsible for the social functions. Some presidents elected from the medical faculty had been undergraduate members. Continuity in administration is achieved through the junior faculty member of the English Department serving as curator.

It was recognized from the start that the original collection was only a nucleus and not primarily of the Tudor and Stuart periods. The first board of governors decided to use the income accruing to concentrate on one author, Edmund Spenser (1552–99). By 1925, a distinguished collection of Spenser had been purchased, which helped in the recruitment of Edwin Greenlaw, who was named William Osler Professor of English Literature, a title that still is used.

It is not possible to determine how much of the cost of purchases in the early years came from income from the original endowment and how much from the later Lady Osler Fund. As late as 1940, occasional books were bought from the Edward Revere Osler Fund, but since then it has been used only for lectures and social activities. From at least 1933 on, the Lady Osler Fund has been used only for books. The librarians in the early years repeatedly recommended that more income be used for books and "less for cakes and ale." A faculty member recommended in 1970 that the operating budgets of the two funds be combined, but that has not been done.

The major scholarly activity has been the annual public lecture, which always is on a literary subject. The lecturers mostly have been professors of English. Some were literary critics, librarians, or authors. In the early years, most titles involved the literature of the Tudor and Stuart periods, but some had law, architecture, folklore, or the staging of plays as the subject. Almost all lectures have been published, those from 1923 to 1936 in the *Johns Hopkins Alumni Magazine* and those from 1937 to 1948 in *ELH,* the journal of English literary history sponsored by the club. The club also sponsors a lecture each January by a member of the medical faculty, but the subject is not always medical. Authors' readings and book talks for informal groups of thirty-five to forty members have been held in the club room. Some have been vividly remembered years later.

Social activities have included a formal dinner after the annual lecture for members and the lecturer. In the early years, afternoon teas in the English fashion were attempted in the club. A noon coffee hour with cigarettes was better attended. In the mid 1930s, up to three teas a year were given between 4 and 5 P.M., to introduce speakers to members. No teas are given now. During the thirties, five to six smokers with free distribution of cigars and cigarettes were given between 7:30 and 9:30 P.M. Now "smokers" follow the less formal evening lectures with free beer and a cold buffet served. When women were admitted, they objected to cigars. Smoking during meetings currently is discouraged.

The club has sponsored publication of work by faculty. Greenlaw embarked on a ten-volume edition of Spenser. Although he died in 1931, before it was completed, his colleagues finished the work. In 1933 Francis Johnson prepared a bibliography of Spenser's work printed before 1700. The club governors on April 11, 1934, appointed a standing committee on publications. Six faculty members wished to begin *ELH,* the journal of English literary history. They were to be the editors and assume full financial responsibility for a period of two years. The journal was successful from the start. On January 1, 1937, financial responsibility was assumed by the Hopkins Press. Editorial control remains in the club.

The club room is paneled in light oak. One wall has five locked, glass-front book cabinets, which extend to the ceiling. Interspersed is a small glass-front cabinet containing some of Revere's fishing rods and landing nets. At the far end of the room from the entrance door is an angled fireplace with Revere's portrait above the mantle.[1] On the other side is the closet holding the safe, which now contains only documents. A framed print of Revere's etching of Merton College in Oxford hangs on the wall. On the mat in pencil is written "With much love to the family and many apologies for the above Iz Wa Jr." A large oriental rug covers the floor. Six large leather overstuffed armchairs line one wall, and folding chairs to seat thirty-five are available. A large chest made by Revere stands against one wall.[1] A refectory table completes the furniture.

The club continues to encourage love of English literature. Osler believed that a lifelong interest in the classics as well as in medicine was essential for physicians and that study of the classics should begin in the student's preprofessional years and continue through medical school into their later careers. The involvement of the medical faculty from the inception of the club to the present day continues this tradition, but medical students rarely are reached. The annual public lecture, an ongoing feature, is now held in the Eisenhower Library. The number of informal lectures for members, including an annual lecture by medical faculty, held in the club room, seems to meet current needs. The founding and editorial responsibility for *ELH* has encouraged scholarship. Social activities throughout the year meet another of the Oslers' objectives. It has been physically impossible to house all the books in one room where members could sit and read. Acquisitions in recent years have been minimal. The income from the original endowment exceeds the requirements for the lectures and social activities. Some funds could be used for the purchase of books, as is being done with the later bequest.

References

1. Harrell, GT: The Oslers' son—Revere. Bull Hist Med 54:561–71, 1980.
2. Harrell, GT: The Osler family. JAMA 248:203–9, 1982.
3. Harrell, GT: Lady Osler. Bull Hist Med 53:81–99, 1979.
4. French, JC: The Tudor and Stuart Club. In French, JC: A History of the University Founded by Johns Hopkins. Baltimore, The Johns Hopkins Press, 1946, pp. 315–24.

Department of Retrospection
The Jefferson Medical College Connection:
A Letter From Sir William Osler

 Frederick B. Wagner, Jr., M.D.

On September 24, 1914, Sir William Osler was scheduled to deliver the introductory address to the ninetieth annual session of the Jefferson Medical College of Philadelphia. War conditions in England compelled him to cancel the engagement, but he sent a letter intended to be read to the students on that occasion. Unfortunately, it was delayed in transit and arrived a day late. Doctor J. Parsons Schaeffer, Professor of Anatomy, gave an address with apologies to the students for their disappointment.

Osler's letter was subsequently published by the students in *The Jeffersonian* (Vol. 15, October 1914). The original, a typed manuscript with handwritten corrections, was signed by Osler. It is reproduced in Figure 1.

This letter indicates that Osler had more than casual acquaintance with practically all of Jefferson's faculty of that era. This came about through his activities in the College of Physicians of Philadelphia, his consultations, and social life at the Rittenhouse Club and private homes. In his golden rule spirit he regarded Jefferson as a "sister institution" rather than a rival one.

Among the older set William W. Keen and Samuel W. Gross were his most intimate friends; among the younger were James Cornelius Wilson and Hobart A. Hare. Keen, Osler and S. Weir Mitchell cooperated in a driving force that obtained funds and books that greatly enlarged the library of the College of Physicians. Samuel W. Gross almost regularly invited Osler for Sunday dinners and tea at his home at 1112 Walnut Street, just two blocks from

Read at the annual meeting of the American Osler Society, April 12, 1986.

Reprinted with permission from *Transactions and Studies of the College of Physicians of Philadelphia,* 8:277, 1986

Dear Students.

I am, of course, sadly disappointed not to be able to address the students at Jefferson this year. I owe much to the men of this school - let me tell you in what way. The winter of 1869 -70 I had a bed-room above the office of my preceptor Dr. James Bovell, of whose library I had "the run". In the long winter evenings, instead of reading my text-books, 'Gray' and 'Fownes' and Kirkes, I spent hours browsing among folios and quartos, and all sorts of promiscuous literature with which his library was stocked. I date my mental downfall from that winter, upon which, however, I look back with unmixed delight. I became acquainted then with three old 'Jeff' men - Eberle, Dunglison and Samuel D. Gross. The name of the first I had already heard in my physiology lectures in connection with the discovery of cyanide of potassium in the saliva; but in his Treatise of the Materia Medica, and in his Treatise on the Practice of Medicine, (in the yellow brown calf skin that characterized Philadelphia medical books of the period) I found all sorts of useless information in therapeutics so dear to the heart of a second year medical student. Eberle was soon forgotten as the years passed by, but it was far otherwise with Robley Dunglison, a warm friend of three generations of American medical students. Thomas Jefferson did a good work when he imported him from London, as Dunglison had all the wisdom of his day and generation combined with a colossal industry. He brought

a great and well deserved reputation to Jefferson College. After all, there is no such literature as a Dictionary, and the twenty three editions through which Dunglison passed is a splendid testimony to its usefulness. It was one of my stand-bys, and I still have an affection for the old editions of it, which did such good service. (And by the way, if any one of you among your grandfather's old books find the 1st edition published in 1833 send it to me, please) But the book of Dunglison full of real joy to the student was the Physiology, not the knowledge, so that was all concentrated in 'Kirkes', but there were so many nice trimmings in the shape of good stories. One day we had returned from an interesting post mortem, and I asked my preceptor where to look for a good account of softening of the stomach, and he took from the shelf S. D. Gross's Pathological Anatomy, 2nd edition. I suppose there is not a man in this room who has opened the book - even great text-books die like their authors - and yet if any one of you wishes to read a good account of gastro-malacia, I cannot do better than in the book I have mentioned. And look, too, at the account of Typhoid Fever, written remember in 1845, five years before the differences between typhus and typhoid were recognized in England. Many and many a time I have had occasion to refer to this work, and always with advantage. Later I came to reverence the author as the Nestor of American surgeons. Not many years afterwards I got into mental touch with two more Jefferson men - Samuel Henry Dickson, one of the most brilliant teachers in medicine the school has ever had. His essays on life, sleep, pain etc. are full of good matter, and

especially let me commend to you his Study on Pneumonia. The other was John K. Mitchell, the great father of a still greater son, whom I learned to know in connection with his early studies on the germ theory of disease. I really came to Philadelphia through the good offices of Jefferson men. Early in the eighties I used to earn an honest penny by writing articles for the Medical News, of which Hays was the editor and Samuel Gross and Parvin his active collaborators. In 1884 when Professor Stillé resigned and Dr. William Pepper took the Chair of Medicine, there was a strong local field in for the Chair of Clinical Medicine. One day Samuel Gross said to Pepper "There's a young chap in the north who seems to dot his i's and cross his t's." You had better look him up". Well, the upshot was that the editorial committee I got the Chair. No small measure of the happiness of the five happy years I spent in Philadelphia came from my association with Jefferson men. Among the surgeons, Keen and Samuel Gross became intimate friends. They, with Brinton, Mears and Hearn, maintained the splendid surgical traditions of the school. With the seniors in medicine, Bartholow and Da Costa, I never got on quite so intimate terms, but they were always encouraging and friendly. The younger Jefferson set became my fast friends, particularly Wilson and Hare.

With best wishes for the progressive growth of the school, with which are associated many of the foremost names in the history of American medicine.

sincerely yours
W. Osler

FIGURE 1 Osler's letter to the students of Jefferson Medical College of Philadelphia.

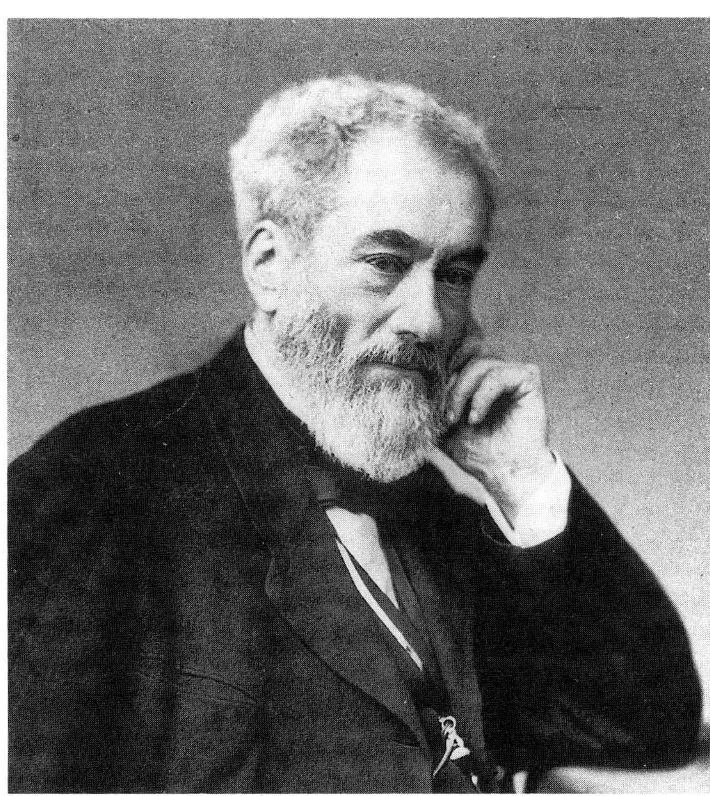

FIGURE 2   Robley Dunglison, M.D.

the Medical College. In the hospitality of the Gross household, Osler enjoyed the social graces of Mrs. Gross, who was destined later to become his wife.

Hobart A. Hare was initially a colleague of Osler at the University of Pennsylvania as Professor of Diseases of Children and succeeded Roberts Bartholow as Professor of Materia Medica and Therapeutics at Jefferson in 1891 for the next forty years. When Jacob Mendez DaCosta resigned as Chairman of Practice of Medicine in 1891, Osler was Jefferson's first choice for successor. On May 11 of that year Osler was propositioned by unanimous action of the Board of Trustees and of the Faculty with reference to the vacant Chair. A joint Committee consisting of Trustees, the Honorable Furman Sheppard and Ex-Mayor Fitler, with Dr. Hobart A. Hare requested the favor of a personal interview with Osler. The latter declined but strongly recommended his intimate friend J.C. Wilson for the post. Wilson carried the Chair with great distinction until 1911. He and Osler delighted in playing innocent jokes on each other. The most famous one on Osler's part is told by Harvey Cushing in his *Life of Sir William Osler*. Shortly before noon on May 7, 1892, Wilson stopped by Mrs. Gross's home, found her in the rear garden with Osler, and accepted a light luncheon. Mrs. Gross then excused herself with the statement that a hansom was waiting and she had to leave. Wilson promptly withdrew and a few hours later received a telegram from Osler: "It was awfully kind of you to come to the wedding breakfast."

Mr. William Potter Wear, a Trustee of Jefferson from 1941 to 1984, remembered as a little boy crossing the Atlantic with his grandfather, the

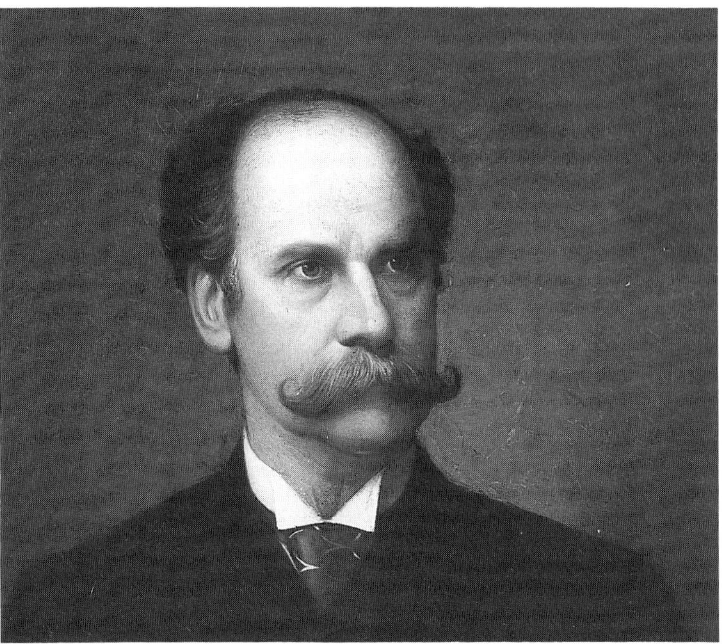

FIGURE 3   Dr. Samuel Gross, first husband of Lady Osler. Note resemblance to Osler himself.

Honorable William Potter, President of the Board. The latter was engaged in conversation with Osler at an adjacent deckchair. He overheard Osler remark: "The man you should have at Jefferson is Thomas McCrae." This was in September 1910 when J.C. Wilson was about to resign the Chair of Medicine, effective June 5, 1911. McCrae had married Osler's niece, Amy Gwyn, daughter of his sister Charlotte. He was a fellow Canadian who had been under Osler's instruction at Hopkins and was aiding in editing his former chief's *Principles and Practice of Medicine.* McCrae continued later editions after Osler's death, the ninth in 1922 to the twelfth in 1935. The McCraes were favorites of the Oslers and took occasional excursions together while visiting with them at Oxford. Through the revisions of his books, Osler for the rest of his life was in contact with McCrae, who kept him abreast of happenings at Jefferson. It was McCrae who had invited Osler to give the address in 1914, and Mrs. McCrae presented the manuscript to the Jefferson archives on May 21, 1936, the year after her husband's death.

Lady Osler never forgot her first love, Samuel W. Gross, and the first provision in her will of 1928 was a bequest of £5,000 to endow a lectureship in surgery at Jefferson in honor of her first husband's interest in tumors. This lectureship became a professorship in which the endowment increased more than tenfold. On September 25, 1984, at the Oslerfest in Oxford, a plaque was presented to Green College in honor of Lady Osler on behalf of Thomas Jefferson University and was hung in the main hall of the Osler mansion at 13 Norham Gardens, the so-called "Open Arms."

When the Philadelphia General Hospital was discontinued in 1977, the

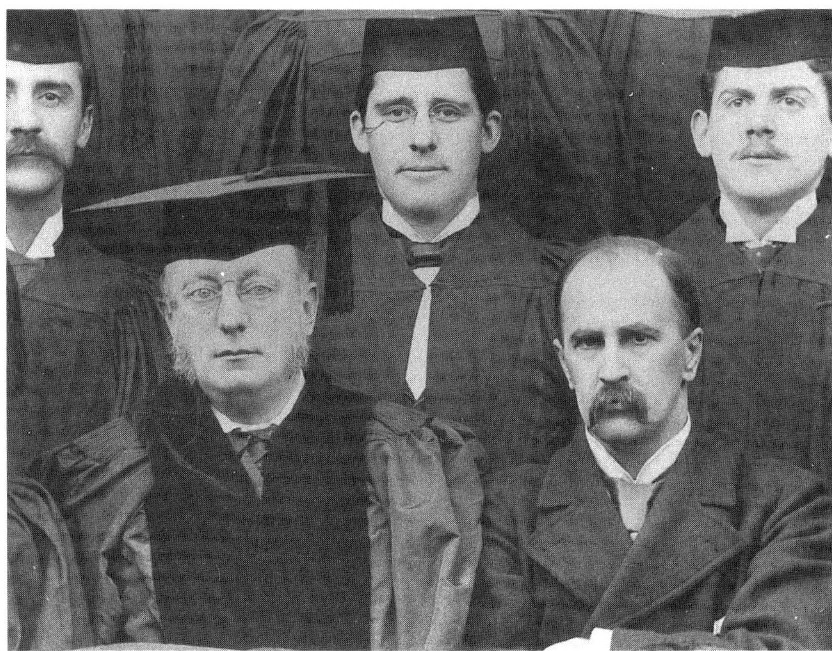

FIGURE 4   Osler with Dr. James C. Wilson at a meeting of the J.C. Wilson Medical Society at Jefferson Medical College in 1895.

Osler-Jefferson connection was strong enough to secure Dean Cornwell's painting of "Osler at Old Blockley." This portrait is prominently displayed in the main lobby of the Medical College. In defiance of those who speak of Osler in terms of myths and legends, his true spirit is much alive at Jefferson, where pride is taken in his various connections with this institution.

Sir William Osler and the Royal Society of Medicine, London

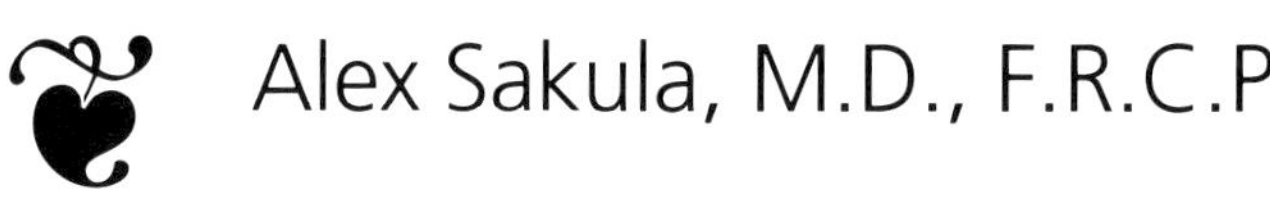

Alex Sakula, M.D., F.R.C.P.

Sir William Osler (1849–1919) (Figure 1) was the founder and first President of the Section of History of Medicine in the Royal Society of Medicine, London. This paper relates the story of the early years of the Royal Society of Medicine and Osler's association with the Society and the Section.

Origins of Royal Society of Medicine

The origins of the Royal Society of Medicine date back to the eighteenth century, when medical societies became fashionable as a means of facilitating scientific communication and professional and social contact among physicians and surgeons. The first British medical society was the Medical Society of London, founded in 1773 by the Quaker physician, John Coakley Lettsom (1744–1815).[1] The original membership of the Society comprised 30 physicians, 30 surgeons and 30 apothecaries. The personality of one of the early presidents, James Sims (1741–1820) gave rise to problems and in 1805 twenty-six members (among them such distinguished figures as Matthew Baillie (1761–1823) and Sir Astley Cooper (1768–1841)) decided to secede and establish a new society, the Medical and Chirurgical Society of London, which in 1834 received the Royal Charter from William IV.

The Royal Medical and Chirurgical Society flourished but, towards the end of the nineteenth century, many specialist societies were founded and the amalgamation of these with the Royal Medical and Chirurgical Society began to be mooted. Largely due to the initiative of its secretary-librarian, Sir John MacAlister (1856–1925) (Figure 2), the amalgamation was eventually achieved in 1907 when seventeen specialist societies (Figure 3) joined with the Royal Medical and Chirurgical Society to form the Royal Society of Medicine.[2] The Medical Society of London, however, stayed aloof and remains a separate society to this day.

Read at the annual meeting of the American Osler Society, April 27, 1989.

177

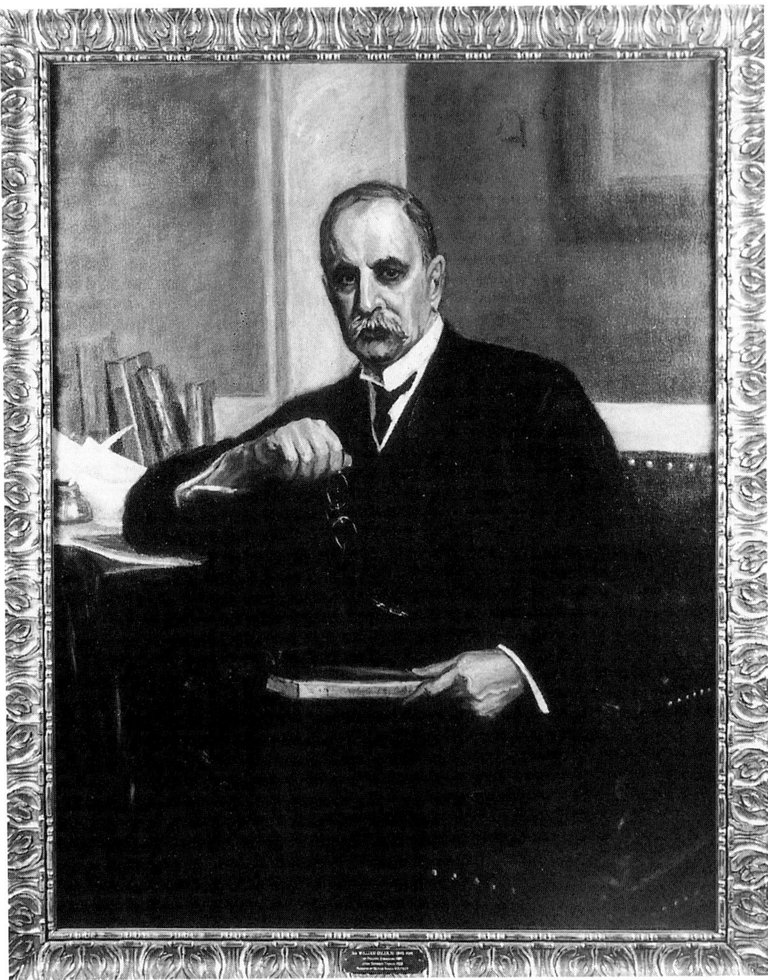

FIGURE 1 Sir William Osler. Portrait in oils by Seymour Thomas, 1908. Copy by Philippa Abrahams, 1989. (Courtesy of Royal Society of Medicine)

Osler's Role in the Early Years of the Royal Society of Medicine

Osler became Regius Professor of Medicine at Oxford in 1905. In London he sometimes visited the Royal Medical and Chirurgical Society in Hanover Square. When the amalgamation issue arose, he encouraged MacAlister and he was delighted when the Royal Society of Medicine came into existence. The first general meeting of the new Society was held on 14 June 1907 when Sir William Church FRCP (1837–1928) was elected President. Osler seconded his nomination and, in doing so, stated that money would have to be raised for the development of the library and for a new building, saying that "he who asketh much getteth much."[3] He later wrote:

> We baptised the Royal Medicine Society (*sic*) the other afternoon and had a most successful initial meeting[4]

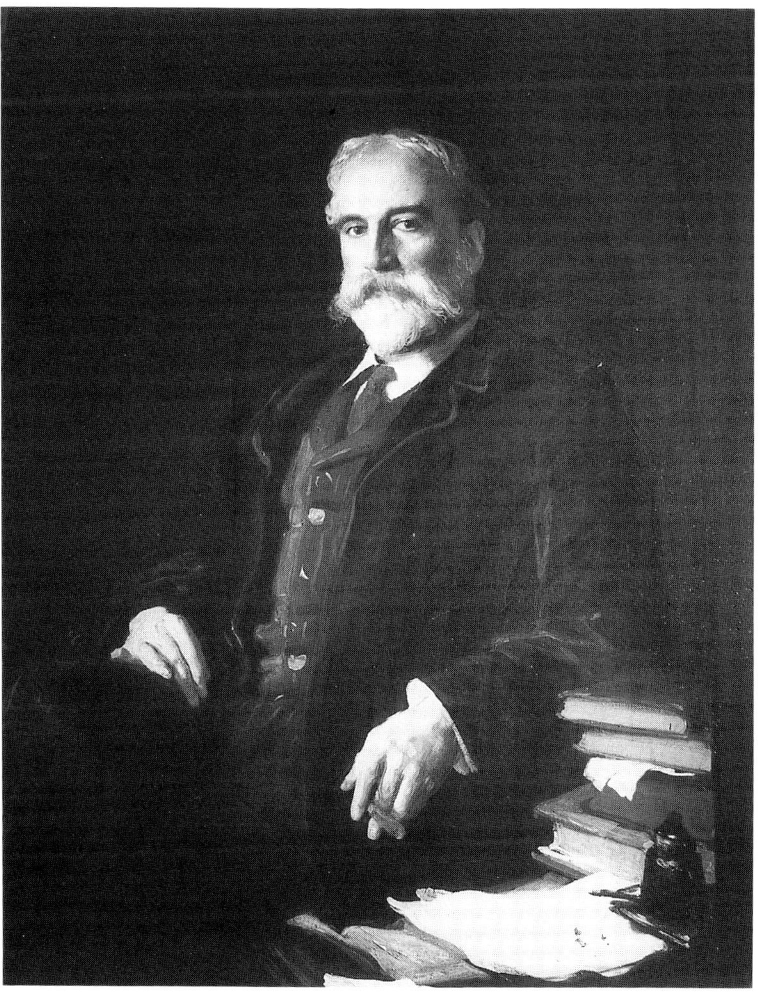

FIGURE 2 Sir John MacAlister. Portrait in oils by Eric Kennington, 1912. (Courtesy of Royal Society of Medicine)

Osler and his wife were present when the new building at 1 Wimpole Street (Figure 4) was formally opened by King George V and Queen Mary in 1912.

Osler was a member of Council during the first three years and was a member of the Library Committee until the end of his life. He took a special interest in the Clinical Section which he served as President in 1912. During World War I, he organized several meetings on matters of topical importance, viz, meningitis, paratyphoid, soldier's heart, and trench nephritis. When the war ended, he concerned himself with rehabilitation courses for the returning medical officers.

Osler and the Presidency of the Royal Society of Medicine

Osler was twice offered the Presidency of the Royal Society of Medicine, which he refused.

ROYAL SOCIETY OF MEDICINE

Date of Foundation

The Pathological Society	**1846**
The Epidemiological Society	**1850**
The Odontological Society of Great Britain	**1856**
The Obstetrical Society of London	**1858**
The Clinical Society of London	**1867**
The Dermatological Society of London	**1880**
The British Gynecological Society	**1884**
The Neurological Society	**1886**
The British Laryngological, Rhinological, and Otological Association	**1888**
The Laryngological Society of London	**1893**
The Society of Anesthetists	**1893**
The Dermatological Society of Great Britain and Ireland	**1894**
The British Balneological and Climatological Society	**1895**
The Otological Society of the United Kingdom	**1899**
The Society for the Study of Disease in Children	**1900**
The British Electro-Therapeutic Society	**1901**
The Therapeutical Society	**1902**

FIGURE 3   Specialist societies amalgamated with Royal Medical and Chirurgical Society, 1907. (From Calendar 1912–13, Royal Society of Medicine, p. 1)

The first occasion was in 1914 when he turned down his nomination with a telegram from Oxford (14 May 1914):

> Thank you so much but impossible to accept nomination. I have written. Osler.[5]

Sir John MacAlister responded with a letter (20 May 1914) so remarkable that it is reproduced here in full:

> My dear Mr. President-nominate,—Your telegram has given me a cruel shock, and I must earnestly beg—I should say implore—that you will reconsider your decision. You were nominated yesterday by the absolute unanimous vote of the whole Council of the society and, unless you prevent it, your election follows as a matter of course. It is not for me perhaps to say anything about the honour this is, for you have achieved such honours in your brilliant career that there is practically nothing left that will enhance them; but if you knew the traditions here you would understand what a special honour the election to the presidency of this society in your case means. It is for the first time in its history an entire departure from tradition, which demands that presidents of the society shall be the best of those *who have served it longest.* How strong this tradition is you will perhaps understand better if I tell you that some years ago a proposal to make Lord Lister President of the society had to be withdrawn. It is in some ways even a greater honour than the presidency of the College of Physicians, for the society is more broadly representative of the profession.

But I know that all that will count for nothing with you; but what I hope will count is the fact that many of the leading men of the society have been looking to you for some time as the future President, whose indomitable energy, progressiveness and large mindedness would help to place the society in the position that properly belongs to it, and it would be a bitter disappointment if now that the opportunity has come you hold back. The society wants a man who is above tradition and who will make precedents for himself, and there is none other who can fulfil that need as you can. In saying this I am not disparaging others, for your really unique position in the profession, and in the public estimation gives you opportunities of *doing things* which other men, however willing they might be, have not got.

I do not know if you have ever realized how much the Amalgamation owed to you. I remember, as vividly as if it were this morning, how at a time when I had practially given up hope, you came into my room at Hanover Square, and I told you of my dreams, and you urged me to "go right ahead, that the time was ripe, and I was not to worry about the old fogies." Your encouragement gave me just the stimulant that I needed at the time—for I was physically as well as mentally ill—and I went "right ahead," and even then hoped to see you President of the reformed society, and I cannot well express the bitter disappointment and discouragement it will be to me personally if you refuse this opportunity which may never come again.

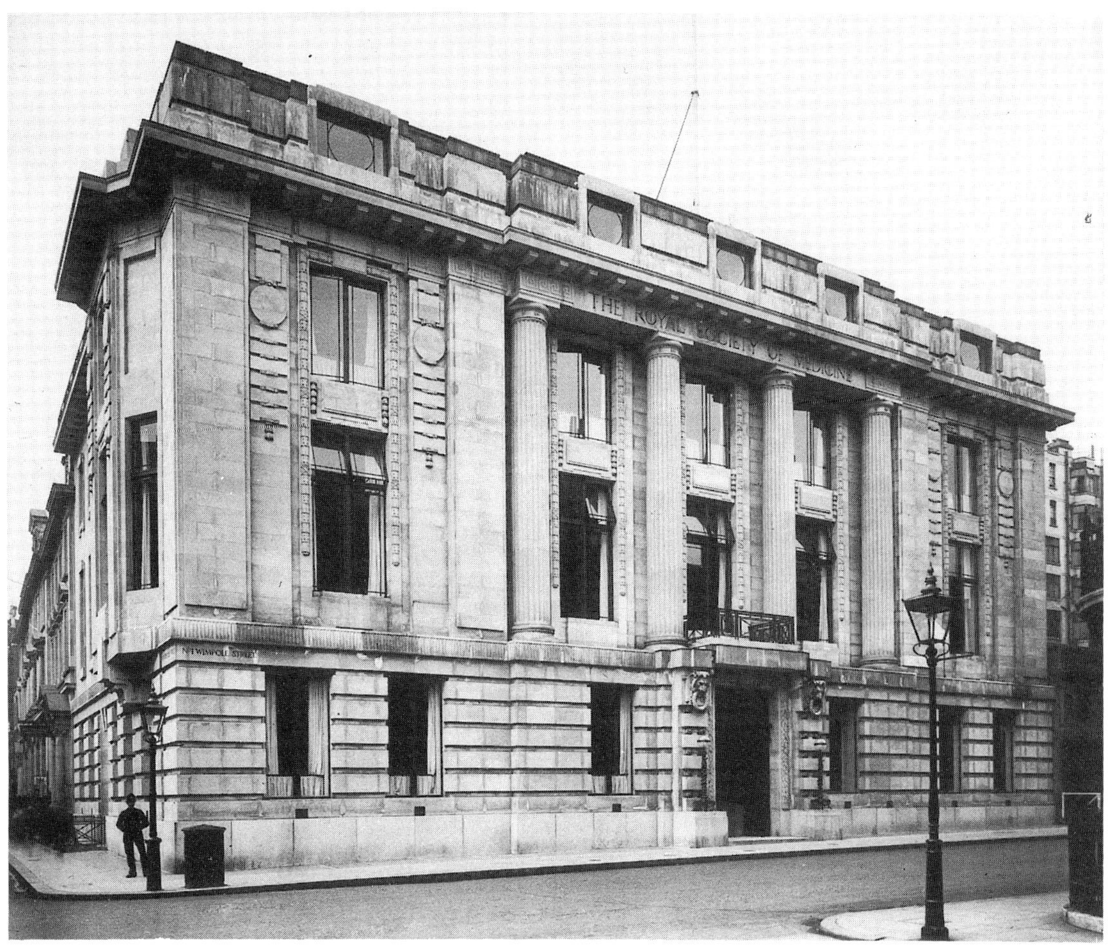

FIGURE 4   Royal Society of Medicine, 1 Wimpole Street, London W.1 (1912)

> Do not be afraid of the work, I will guarantee to save you all that; and you are
> so often in London that to preside at a monthly Council Meeting (the times
> for which can be fixed to suit you) should be no tax upon you. To parody the
> posters—"it is your inspiration we want." Up to now the presidencies have
> worked out in a perfectly rhythmical order, and this is the exact psychological
> moment for your presidency. Church was the necessary Amalgamating
> President, as he had presided at all the Amalgamation Meetings, and the
> Sections had to learn what amalgamation meant; then began the move and
> the new building, for which Morris was the best man and did yeoman service;
> settled in the new building the next thing that had to be done was to break the
> stupid old tradition, which prevented a specialist from occupying the chair,
> and Champneys as head of his specialty has done his duty well; and now,
> having amalgamated, built, and got rid of its fetters, what the society needs,
> and must have, is a new and inspiring energy to give it a good start on the
> great work that lies before it. It is your clear duty to accept, and for duty's sake
> you must not refuse. Yours sincerely and very anxiously. J.Y.W. MacAlister[6]

Osler replied in a letter (undated) from the Athenaeum:

> Dear MacAlister, Awfully sorry I cannot accept the nomination. It is not my
> job. I need not go into reasons. It is good of you to think of me. I see your
> hand in it. Sincerely yours, Wm. Osler.[7]

The second occasion that Osler refused the Presidency was in 1918. This time,
MacAlister wrote (8 May 1918):

> My dear Osler,—Once before you were offered and refused the Presidency of
> the Royal Society of Medicine—an unprecedented snub to the premier
> medical body of the Kingdom—and now I ask you unofficially and
> confidentially once more whether you will accept nomination, and I say to
> you quite seriously and solemnly that in the present crisis it is your duty to
> accept it, for from now on there are great things expected of, and to be done
> by the Society provided a man of light and leading is at its head, and you are
> the man to do it! It is the more important in view of the position you have
> taken with the Post-graduate Scheme. So please let me have a line or a
> telegram saying you accept. Yours sincerely, J.Y.W. MacAlister. I shall turn my
> face to the wall if you say 'No' for it is going to be my last lap. J.Y.W.
> MacAlister.[8]

Osler replied (10 May 1918) from the Victoria Hotel, Sidmouth:

> Dear MacAlister, I am more sorry than I can say; as I hate to refuse you
> anything; but it is impossible. On the previous occasion the *snub* as you call it,
> was certainly not meant as such. I regarded the offer as a great honour.
> Sincerely yours, Wm. Osler.[9]

It is of interest that in 1918, Osler was offered the Presidency of the Medical
Society of London which he also refused.

Osler and the Section of History of Medicine

There had been several previous attempts to form a Section of History of
Medicine but these had been unsuccessful. In 1912, Osler set about the task
with his usual vigour. In July 1912, he wrote to MacAlister:

> I have sent out 168 personal letters. . . . .

Sir Raymond Crawford (1865–1938), Registrar of the Royal College of Physicians of London later wrote:

> I saw a great deal of Osler in connection with the Section of History of Medicine at the Royal Society of Medicine. He was its father, and I doubt if it would ever have come into existence but for his quickening influence: he acted like a magnet in gathering together a company of original members. He was its first President; his own contributions were few and mainly biographical, and I do not think anyone could have discovered from them how fully he possessed the true historical sense, but his faculty of extracting contributions on every conceivable aspect of medicine from the most unproductive sources was invaluable to the Section; and that Osler was in the chair was a sure draw.[10]

On 20 November 1912, the first meeting of the Section of History of Medicine was held at 1 Wimpole Street. There were 160 members and Osler was elected the first President with many distinguished figures occupying the offices of Vice Presidents, Members of Council and Honorary Secretaries (Figure 5). The Transactions of that first meeting record Osler's inaugural remarks:

> In thanking the members of the Section for the honour of election as their first Chairman, Sir William Osler remarked that he had at least two qualifications—a keen interest in the subject and a certain academic leisure . . . . . . Physicians held very different views on the subject of the history of medicine. A majority were indifferent—too busy to pay any attention to it; a considerable number were interested to read articles or to listen to papers; then there were the amateur students, like himself, who dabbled in history as a pastime; and lastly there was a select group of real scholars. . . . . . It was to be hoped that this Section would form a meeting ground for the scholars, the students and for those who felt that the study of the history of medicine had a value in education.[11]

Osler then proceeded to deliver the first paper to the Section which was on Sir William Petty (1623–1687) and his letters written while he was Physician-General to the forces in Ireland. Petty had been Deputy Regius Professor of Medicine at Oxford in 1649 and was one of the founders of the Royal Society in 1662.

Regular meetings of the Section followed. Although Osler's personal contributions were few, he had the gift of extracting contributions from others. Osler was pleased with the progress of the Section and in 1913 wrote to both Silas Weir Mitchell and to Fielding Garrison that the History Section was doing well.[12,13]

In 1914, however, there must have been some criticism from a certain quarter since in a letter (17 November 1914) to MacAlister Osler wrote:

> It is not a good way, to pull up the turnips to watch their growth. We cannot make medical historians in a couple of years. If your friend will look over the material presented to the Section, while perhaps it does not indicate much research, I do not think there is much that could be called folk-lore or gossip. What is wanted in this country is not dilettante students like myself & some others but real scholars, & your friend will be interested to know that some of these are at work on serious medical research. . . . . . I think it is quite possible that we may gradually get associated with the history section a group of scholars capable of doing spade work. If your friend wants a job in the historical branches send him along. The harvest is plenteous but the labourers are few. Thank you all the same for his criticism, but if he looks over the papers he will come to my view that it is a bit bilious. Wm. Osler[14]

FIGURE 5   First Council of Section of History of Medicine (From Calendar 1912–13, Royal Society of Medicine, p. 32)

SECTION OF THE HISTORY OF MEDICINE

———

COUNCIL

President

Sir William Osler, Bart., M.D., F.R.S.

Vice-Presidents

Sir T. Clifford Allbutt, K.C.B., M.D., F.R.S.
Richard Caton, M.D.
Sir William S. Church, Bart., K.C.B., M.D.
Sir Henry Morris, Bart., F.R.C.S.
Sir Ronald Ross, K.C.B., F.R.S.

Hon. Secretaries

Raymond Crawfurd, M.D.	**D'Arcy Power, F.R.C.S.**

Other Members of Council

Sir Francis H. Champneys, Bart., M.D.	**R. O. Moon, M.D.**
S. D. Clippingdale, M.D.	**Sir Shirley F. Murphy, F.R.C.S.**
J. D. Comrie, M.D.	**J. A. Nixon, M.B.**
Alban Doran, F.R.C.S.	**Herbert S. Pendlebury, F.R.C.S.**
David Forsyth, M.D.	**H. D. Rolleston, M.D.**
James Galloway, M.D.	**F. M. Sandwith, M.D.**
Leonard G. Guthrie, M.D.	**A. F. Voelcker, M.D.**
E. Muirhead Little, F.R.C.S.	

On 28 May 1915, his tenth anniversary as Regius Professor, Osler noted in his account book:

> I have not done much in the profession here but have done the three useful things, or better, helped to 1. the Association of Brit. Phys. 2. The Quarterly Journal of Medicine 3. The Historical Section of the Roy. Soc. Med.[15]

Finale

During the past 77 years, the seed sown by Osler has taken root and the plant has been carefully tended by successive generations of medical historians. As current President of the Section of History of Medicine in the Royal Society of Medicine I am proud to report that Osler's plant continues to thrive.

Postscript

For many years it had been felt that it was a singular omission that the Royal Society of Medicine did not possess a portrait of Osler. In 1989, the author decided to commission Philippa Abrahams, a London Slade School diplomate, to paint a copy of the Seymour Thomas portrait of Osler and in January 1990 it was presented to the Royal Society of Medicine where it now hangs.[16,17]

References

1. Hunt, T. *The Medical Society of London,* 1773–1973 London; Heinemann, 1972
2. Sakula, A. *Royal Society of Medicine: Portraits, paintings and sculptures* London; Royal Society of Medicine, 1988
3. Cushing, H. *The Life of Sir William Osler* Oxford: University Press, 1940. p. 780
4. Ibid. p. 779
5. Ibid. p. 1094
6. Ibid. p. 1094–1096
7. Ibid. p. 1096
8. Ibid. p. 1289
9. Ibid. p. 1289–1290
10. Ibid. p. 1010
11. *Proceedings of Royal Society of Medicine,* 1913. 6. Transactions of Section of History of Medicine, p. 1
12. Cushing, H. Op. cit. p. 1061
13. Ibid. p. 1078
14. Ibid. p. 1130–1131
15. Ibid. p. 1164
16. Sakula, A. Sir William Osler's portrait by Seymour Thomas *Journal of Royal Society of Medicine.* 1990. *83.* 42–44
17. Sakula, A. *The Portraiture of Sir William Osler* London: Royal Society of Medicine, 1991

The 'Open Arms' Reviving: Can We Rekindle the Osler Flame?

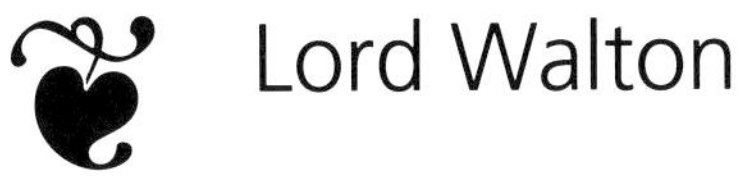 Lord Walton

However trite it may seem, I must begin by saying that it is a singular privilege to have been invited by the Society of which I am now deeply honoured to be an honorary member to give this annual lecture named after that most distinguished physician, founder member and past-President of this Society, Dr. Jack McGovern.

My own interest in medical history was first fuelled in my student days in the medical school of King's College, Newcastle, of the University of Durham, when early in the course I was introduced by an enthusiastic teacher to Osler's writings. Despite the constraints of wartime and of the student purse, I explored and searched whenever I could the bookshops of Tyneside; and when my colleagues sent me as a delegate to London meetings of the British Medical Students' Association, I scrutinised equally avidly those of Gower Street and the Charing Cross Road (especially the second-hand sections of H.K. Lewis and of Foyles) to collect whatever I could of Osler's writings. Having devoured Cushing's *Life of Osler,* which I believe to be one of the greatest; if not the greatest, medical biography ever written, I moved on to Fulton's *Life of Cushing* and many other biographies and autobiographies, both serious and popular, from pens as varied as those of Howard Haggard, Benjamin Ward Richardson, Johannes Freund, Oliver St. John Gogarty, Arturo Castiglioni and many more. I was, however, most affected by Osler's *Aequanimitas and Other Essays,* including particularly that on "The student life" which, despite the rather quaint, even archaic language, had a lasting impression upon me, engendering a reverence for Osler and his works which has lasted throughout my professional life. To find myself now, as Warden of Green College, responsible for the maintenance and upkeep of 'The Open Arms' at 13 Norham Gardens, where my wife Betty and I will soon take up residence, is a privilege and responsibility which I treasure greatly. As you are aware, we established some three years ago, with the support and active

Read at the annual meeting of the American Osler Society, April 26, 1989.

187

participation of this Society and of the Osler Club of London, the Friends of 13 Norham Gardens to help me and my colleagues in Green College to fulfil that task.

And before medical and scientific writing on topics like muscular dystrophy and neurological medicine became an abiding interest of mine and occupied most of my writing hours, I first put pen to paper for a medical student journal in 1944 and 1945 in two articles, the first on "Osler: a Great Physician" and the second on "Thomas Sydenham: the English Hippocrates." And later I was privileged in 1969 to deliver the Annual Osler Lecture to the Canadian Medical Association in Halifax, Nova Scotia. And when I handed over the Presidency of the British Medical Association (BMA) at its 150th anniversary meeting in 1982 to His Royal Highness the Prince of Wales, Stephen Lock, the editor of the British Medical Journal, independently invited myself and the other BMA chief officers to write articles on "The medical book I would most like to have written;" our articles were published in the Journal on 5 July 1982. I chose unhesitatingly Cushing's *Life of Osler* which, as I said at the time, gave a superb pen picture of the master, perhaps a trifle dated in its prose but nevertheless a truly great biography. How interesting is it to note that without any collusion Mr. Tony Grabham (now Sir Anthony), then chairman of the BMA Council, chose *Aequanimitas* for its lasting kindly message, as did Mr. David Bolt, Chairman of the Central Committee for Hospital Medical Services, who remarked that his ambition was perhaps less to have written this book than to be the kind of man who could have written it.

13 Norham Gardens: 'The Open Arms'

In his will, Sir William left his house to his wife, expressing the desire that on her death (or earlier if she so wished) the house be given to Christ Church College, of which he was a professorial fellow, "as the residence of the Regius Professor of Medicine." Sir William died in 1919. Lady Osler, who died in 1928, followed in her will Sir William's wishes and left the house to the Dean and Chapter of Christ Church to be "assigned by them as an official residence of the Regius Professor of Medicine in the University of Oxford for the time being, or to be otherwise applied by the said Dean and Chapter towards the endowment of the chair . . . in such manner as they might think fit." The contents of the house were left by Lady Osler to her brother, Mr. E.H.R. Revere, who in turn conveyed much of the furniture to Christ Church, and Mrs. Susan Chapin (Lady Osler's sister) attended to the arrangements. Some items of furniture were also offered to other members of the Revere family. But some of it which was still serviceable remained in 13 Norham Gardens. Sir Farquhar Buzzard on being appointed Regius Professor of Medicine in 1929 did not wish to occupy the house and it was let by Christ Church successively to two tenants, first Miss H.L. Hurlston and later a Miss Fairburn. And for a time during the Second World War the house was used to house part of the Mathematical Institute and as a hostel for the Society of Home Students which later became St. Anne's College. In 1953 Christ Church conveyed the property to the University to be held on trust, the trust being expressed in the same terms as in Lady Osler's will, and the University then became the Osler Trustees. Sir George and Lady Pickering took over the tenancy when Sir

George came to Oxford to become Regius Professor of Medicine in 1956 and remained there until 1968, when he was succeeded by Sir Richard Doll who, with Lady Doll, lived there until 1979. The new Regius Professor of Medicine, Henry Harris, then decided that he did not wish to take over the lease when appointed in 1979 and for some time the house remained vacant; some furniture was then stored and some was transferred to the country home of the Regius Professor in the almshouses at Ewelme. Some was distributed to other parts of the world including, for example, one of Osler's desks which went to the Osler Library at McGill University in Montreal. Another desk had previously been given to Dr. Palmer Howard in Iowa and other items of furniture had been handed down through the Revere family to Miss Revere of Boston who still lives on Beacon Hill.

In 1982 the University decided that as the house had been vacant for some time, it should "otherwise apply it towards the endowment of the Regius Professorship;" it therefore leased the house to Green College for 21 years from 1 August 1982, on condition that a quarter of the gross income received by the college from lettings of apartments and office accommodation therein would be paid to the Osler Trust, to bear part of the cost of the Regius Professor's stipend. Provision was made in the agreement that an apartment suitable for occupancy by a future Regius Professor of Medicine would be made available. At the same time it was agreed that the University Newcomers Club could occupy part of the premises on a sub-lease.

It is fascinating now to note the scale of the accommodation available in 13 Norham Gardens in 1929 just after Lady Osler's death. Apart from the large garden, garage, greenhouse and conservatory, there was a huge basement area with a kitchen, scullery, servants' hall, larder, wine cellar and other storage space, while on the ground floor, in addition to a very large hall, there were four reception rooms and a WC. The first floor (second in American terminology) had a boudoir, seven bedrooms, a dressing room, two bathrooms, two WCs and a housemaid's pantry, while on the second floor (or third, if you wish) were four bedrooms, a linen room, boxroom, sewing room, two bathrooms and again two WCs. When Green College took over the lease, funds were raised from Osler admirers both in the UK and overseas to carry out a programme of conversion through which four small apartments were created in the north end of the building, to be occupied by married students of the college. Three ground floor rooms and an area of the basement were allocated to the Newcomers Club, leaving the large entrance hall, the Osler library and the large adjacent office (formerly Lady Osler's drawing room) to be available for letting, as well as the spacious self-contained Regius Professor's apartment. From 1982 to 1989 that apartment was occupied by a Senior Visiting Research Fellow of Green College, Dr. Philippe Shubik, and he also rented the library and office in order to pursue his work in the field of toxicology and carcinogenesis.

Furniture and Memorabilia

As I have mentioned, one of Osler's desks from 13 Norham Gardens is now in the Osler Library at McGill and another is with Dr. Palmer Howard of Iowa. Some tables from the library remain in 13 Norham Gardens, as do the panelled walls and bookshelves, but some of the original chairs are now in the Regius Professor's apartment at Ewelme. However, the original terrace furniture is still available on the terrace at 13 Norham Gardens and was generously revarnished by Dr. and Mrs. Shubik.

The Acland Triptych

In about 1871, Sir Henry Acland, then Regius Professor of Medicine, commissioned Julian Drummond to make copies of portraits of Linacre, Sydenham and Harvey from the Royal College of Physicians and these were mounted in a triple frame and hung over the fireplace in Sir Henry Acland's library at 39 Broad Street, where the new Bodleian Library in Oxford now stands. When Osler paid his first visit to Oxford in 1894 to attend a meeting of the British Association for the Advancement of Science, he lunched with Sir Henry and was much attracted by the triptych. Mrs. Osler asked Sir Henry if she could have it copied to give to William for a birthday present; the copy went first to the Oslers' home in Baltimore, later being taken to Norham Gardens and installed in the library in 1907 after Sir William became Regius Professor. When Sir Farquhar Buzzard in 1929 decided that he did not intend to live there, Dr. Francis, then the Osler Librarian, with the permission of Lady Osler's executors, removed the portraits of Linacre, Harvey and Sydenham from their frames in the panelled library at 'The Open Arms' and took them to McGill where they now hang in a corner of the Osler Room in the McIntyre Building. The three frames remained empty until December 1986 when Dr. Alastair Robb-Smith, an Honorary Member of this Society and President of the Friends of 13 Norham Gardens, generously presented to the Osler Trustees (the University and Green College acting on their behalf) photographic facsimiles prepared by Mr. David Dickinson of the original portraits; these have been mounted into frames in the overmantel by Mr. Frank Samuels, so that the library fireplace in 13 Norham Gardens appears as it did in the illustration in Cushing's *Life of Osler*. Again through the energy and interest of Dr. Robb-Smith, the portrait of Sir Thomas Browne, author of *Religio Medici*, one of Osler's favourite works, which used to hang in the library of 13 Norham Gardens but which is now in Pembroke College, has been copied and suitably framed and now hangs in the library.

Other Memorabilia

While Osler's own collection of medical books and incunabula went, of course, to McGill University to establish the Osler Library, Green College is fortunate in having retained many of Osler's own publications including, for example, a first edition of his *System of Medicine* of 1910, two copies of the *Bibliotheca Osleriana,* and other notable works. We have also received from Mr. E.V. Quinn, former librarian of Balliol, many additional books and papers which he had purchased and which had previously been the property of Miss Mabel FitzGerald, a physiologist and friend of the Oslers who, being a woman, was not able to graduate in her youth from Oxford University but who was finally awarded an honorary MA at the age of 100. These are now housed in the Fellows' Room of Green College but are the property of the Friends and will be restored to the library of 13 Norham Gardens as the process of refurbishment continues. Some small items of china belonging to Sir William and Lady Osler are still in the library; a set of etchings by Revere Osler was generously donated by Dr. George Harrell, a head of Osler by Doris Appel by Dr. J.P. McGovern; a plaque commemorating the contributions of Lady Osler was given by Jefferson Medical College, Philadelphia, and another commemorating Osler's membership of the American Neurological Association by that association. Books have also been donated by Dr. Alec Cooke, Dr. Palmer Howard and Dr. Charles Roland, among others, while Dr. Glenn Knotts of Houston has given the Abram Belskie Medal of Osler created in 1972 to commemorate the foundation of the American Osler Society in Houston, Texas, in 1969. We were also amused to receive from Dr. W. M. Ramsden a silver cigarette case given by Sir William to his uncle, Dr. Walter Ramsden, with a card inscribed in Osler's handwriting saying: "Smoke and think of your good friend, William Osler!" And in May 1984 we received from Professor Michael Brain, son of the late Lord Brain, the D.Sc. gown worn by Sir William Osler when he received that honorary degree from Oxford University in 1904 when the BMA held its annual meeting there. That gown was later given by Lady Osler to Dr. Walter Morley Fletcher, first Secretary of the Medical Research Council, who in turn passed it on to his son, Charles Fletcher; he suggested to Lord Brain that the gown should be converted into a DM gown and given to the Royal College of Physicians of London, to be worn by College lecturers who hold an Oxford DM. However, the College already possessed such a gown and Sir Russell Brain, as he then was, said that he would prefer to give it, after conversion at his expense, to his son Michael, then a medical student, if and when he became an Oxford DM. In 1984 Michael Brain (now Professor of Medicine at McMaster University) decided to donate the gown to Green College for display in 13 Norham Gardens so that it would be available for wear by any future Regius Professor of Medicine or by any Warden of Green College holding a DM of Oxford. The gown is now suitably displayed in the hall. And I am sure that many members of the audience will have read with interest Michael Brain's account of his father's contacts with Osler in Oxford in 1919 published in the BMJ on 9 January 1988.

Repairs, Restoration and Vistors

I and the fellows and members of Green College are very conscious of the burden of responsibility that we have accepted in taking over the lease of *'The Open Arms.'* While the appeal of the early 1980s launched by my predecessor, Sir Richard Doll, raised substantial funds to assist in converting the house, it became clear soon after Green College took over the lease that as this was on a full repair and maintenance basis the college faced a major financial burden in simply maintaining its exterior fabric. In 1984 we learned that at least £50,000 would be required to carry out such a programme over a five to six year period. Hence in 1984 an appeal was launched to Osler admirers the world over, including members of the 19 Osler societies then in existence. We are very grateful to all of those, many present today, who have given substantial donations or have agreed to contribute by deed of covenant to assist us in fulfilling the task. I would like to pay a very warm tribute to the Osler Societies the world over which have supported us, including this Society, the Osler Club of London and the Japanese Osler Society vigorously led by Dr. Hinohara. Much invaluable support has also come from individuals in the UK but most notable have been the very generous contributions made by Dr. Jack McGovern in whose honour I am speaking today and who is now the Honorary Life President of the Friends. I must also say a very special thank you to Dr. Jeremiah Barondess and to his many colleagues in this Society for the successful approaches they made to colleagues and institutions in the United States, and to Dr. William Spaulding for his noble efforts in raising money for the Friends in Canada. A full list of contributions, both individual and institutional, was given in the 13 Norham Gardens newsletter No. 4 and is also displayed in the hallway at 13 Norham Gardens. These donations will make it possible for us now to complete this year the final programme of repairs involving much replacement of decaying stonework on the roof and gable ends of the building, on the entrance steps, on the terrace and above the bay windows, as well as repairs to the lead and slatework on the roof, pointing and restoration of brickwork and replacement of decaying wood.

Even during this programme of repair and refurbishment, it has been our great pleasure to welcome notable visitors from many countries who have come to see the Osler shrine. Among them have been physicians from the Netherlands, from Japan, from the Danish Osler Society, from the Osler Club of London, an international group who came on the *Osler Revisited* conference organised by Nicholas Dewey, a group of US physicians serving in Germany led by Bill Smith, a conference of UK postgraduate deans, Dr. and Mrs. R. McConnell of Liverpool, and many members of this Society including Jerry Barondess, Jim Warren, Nicholas Davies, Robert Kimbrough, Jim Reuler and David Mumford, and David Clarke (a Montreal student who was President of the McGill University Osler Society).

The Future

And what of the future? It is the intention of the Friends of 13 Norham Gardens during the next few years not only to see that Osler's former home is restored to a little approaching its former glory, but also to try to rekindle the Osler flame of international friendship between doctors, medical students and their families, and to make 'The Open Arms' a place which will be regarded by Osler's many disciples as being a fitting tribute to his memory and as helping to maintain the counsels and ideals which made him so famous. The University Newcomers Club, with its active programme for the wives and families of visitors to Oxford from other parts of the UK and from all over the world, is in one sense fulfilling this ideal. However, I am now happy to confirm that as the present Regius Professor does not wish to occupy the apartment at 13 Norham Gardens, the officers of Green College have invited my wife and myself to take over the lease of the apartment on relinquishing the Warden-ship of Green College this year; this we have gladly agreed to do. I have now raised the funds necessary to cover the costs of rental of the downstairs offices; and I intend to restore as best I can the library and office as a proper memorial to Osler, and to pursue a number of research projects in neurology and in the history of medicine from this exciting base.

Rekindling the Osler Flame

But rekindling the Osler flame does not only mean refurbishing his former Oxford home. At a time in medicine when resource constraints have beset medical care, medical education and medical research throughout the world, all of us working in these fields should surely do what we can, despite these difficulties, to recall and to instill in those whom we teach and to whom we offer our example in clinical practice the principles so clearly enunciated by Sir William in his writings. How interesting it is to speculate upon what might have happened had Osler taken the alternative path upon which he had set his heart when he first came to London in September 1872 at the age of 23. As a student, he was much impressed by R. Palmer Howard, Professor of Medicine at McGill in 1870–72, and it was Howard's ambition that William should train in ophthalmology with the ultimate objective of joining the teaching staff of

McGill and of Montreal General Hospital. When Canon Osler and William's brothers managed to raise the money needed to support him in his proposed programme of two years in the UK, he first found himself working in the Physiology Laboratory of University College, London, with John Burdon Sanderson. Nevertheless he was determined to emulate, if he could, William Bowman, England's best-known and most talented ophthalmologist. It was Bowman's advice that Osler should begin by working in physiology. While he was doing so the disturbing news came to him from Palmer Howard that a more senior candidate for the post of ophthalmologist in Montreal, Frank Buller, had emerged. It also turned out that Buller was an applicant for the house surgeon appointment at Moorfields upon which young William had set his heart. In the event, as Buller was appointed, Osler decided not to train in ophthalmology but, following in Howard's footsteps, to cultivate the whole field of medicine as it had never been cultivated before.

It is, of course, easy to pick out from Osler's writings many aphorisms as valid today as they were in his time. Neurologists like myself might perhaps question his comment that "Probability is the rule of life, especially under the skin. Never make a positive diagnosis." But in these days of AIDS and of the growing problem of alcoholism in our society, one can only reflect upon his opposite dictum: "Who serves the gods dies young—Venus, Bacchus and Vulcan send in no bills in the seventh decade." He repeated similar advice in a letter on "Rules for a sensible young fellow," written to A.L. Smith on 20 March 1907, recently resurrected by Giles Bullard in the 1986 Balliol Record and brought to my attention by Nicholas Dewey. His comment to the effect that "common sense nerve fibres are seldom medullated before forty—they are never even seen with the microscope before twenty" should perhaps be assessed along with the saying of Oliver Wendell Holmes the elder, whom he much admired, who wrote that "Science is a first-rate piece of furniture for a man's upper storey if he has common sense on the ground floor." I always enjoyed, too, his wry comment on one of the medical fashions of his age when he said that "the mental kidney more often than the abdominal is the one that floats." And how could one forget that "although one swallow does not make a summer, one tophus makes gout and one crescent malaria."

What a wonderful teacher Osler must have been. When one reads again his essay on "Teacher and student," in which he stressed the importance of acquiring a significant core of knowledge, based on the appreciation of principles rather than on the cramming of fact, he emphasised system and method, pointing out a lesson which all too many medical students found it difficult to learn, namely the importance of an orderly arrangement of one's work and the organisation of one's time. While the practice of medicine is indubitably an art, it must be firmly based upon science and scientific reasoning. How surprised I was, having played a major part in writing the General Medical Council's (GMC) Recommendations on Basic Medical Education in 1980, to turn back to Osler and to find that some of what I had fondly imagined might be personal gems were not at all new. Thus in relation to "Thoroughness" he confirmed that it was necessary to acquire a full and deep acquaintance of chemistry, anatomy and physiology and of the great principles based upon them. Students must also become familiar with methods by which knowledge is advanced (i.e. research) and must acquire such a knowledge of diseases and of life emergencies and of the means for their alleviation that they may become safe and trustworthy guides for their fellow men. Only through such an approach did he believe that the sloughs of charlatanism could be avoided. But he also roundly condemned cocksureness of opinion leading to a lively conceit in one's personal powers and stressed the vital importance of humility. I have long shared his admiration for Cowper, who said: "Knowledge and wisdom, far from being one, have oft times no connection. Knowledge dwells in heads replete with thoughts of other men, wisdom in minds attentive to their own. Knowledge is proud that he has learned so much, wisdom is humble that he knows no more." At the end of the day, as you all know, Osler saw as fundamental that master word in medicine which he suggested looms large in meaning. He regarded it, and I quote, as "the open sesame to every portal, the great equaliser in the world, the true philosopher's stone;" he thought that it would make the stupid man bright, the bright man brilliant and the brilliant student steady. "With it all things are possible and without it all study is vanity and vexation. To the youth it brings hope, to the middle-aged confidence, to the aged repose. It has been directly responsible for all advances in medicine during the past 25 centuries. Laying hold upon it, Hippocrates made observation and science the warp and woof of our art. Galen so read its meaning that 15 centuries stopped thinking and slept until awakened by Vesalius, the very incarnation of the master word. Harvey gave impulse with its inspiration to a larger circulation than he recognised, Hunter sounded all its heights and depths and stands out in our history as one of the great examples of its virtue. With it, Virchow smote the rock and the waters of progress gushed out, while in the hands of Pasteur it proved a very talisman to open to us a new heaven in medicine and a new earth in surgery." As you are all well aware, the master word was "work."

Osler the Philosopher

Not only, of course, was Osler a great physician and teacher, but it was clear from all that he wrote that he loved his profession and served it to the end of his days. The guild of doctors was one he regarded as being of noble ancestry, demonstrating solidarity without insularity, and a progressive character allowing the advance of knowledge and developments in medical science and in patient care, coupled with the all-pervasive benevolence and human understanding so fundamental to its practice. Among the sins which he saw in some colleagues were those of excessive nationalism, unalloyed provincialism and parochialism. When I re-read his comments on "Chauvinism in Medicine" I was reminded of the invitation which came to me in 1987 from the editor of the Oxford Medical School Gazette inviting me to comment upon the seven deadly sins as applied to medicine. This invitation prompted me to consider how these sins, namely lust, intemperance, ire, avarice, sloth, pride and envy, could be interpreted in a medical setting, and of course I concluded that all might at times be relevant, even if their respective importance in relation to medical practice may differ from the way that each is regarded by society as a whole.

Wearing one of my other hats as, until recently, President of the GMC, I confess that if one believed the salacious and sensational commentaries of the tabloid press upon the proceedings of its Conduct Committee, some doctors, driven by *lust,* appear to indulge in incredible, even unmentionable, sexual activities with patients of the opposite sex. But in fact the proportion of cases involving sexual misdemeanour is small in comparison with the whole (three out of the 53 cases handled by the committee last year)—a tiny problem when compared with the 24 doctors accused of serious neglect or disregard of their professional responsibilities to patients (also relatively few when derived from about 100,000 practising doctors in the UK).

Intemperance is, of course, a syndrome not unfamiliar (on occasion) in doctors and we cannot be proud of the fact that until about 1980 the incidence of cirrhosis of the liver was more than three times as great in doctors as in the general population. More recent figures suggest that its incidence in members of the profession is falling, but nevertheless addiction to alcohol or drugs is still by far the commonest cause of reference to the GMC's health procedures. Since 1980 over 150 doctors have been placed under supervision (a few have had their registration suspended) for this cause and about 10 doctors a month are now being referred to the National Counseling and Welfare Service for sick doctors.

Of less direct concern to the GMC but nevertheless worrying and troublesome is *ire*. The more I have seen of medicine in 42 years of clinical practice, the more I have recognised the crucial need for good communication between doctors and patients and the necessity of compassionate and humane management of sick people even when the doctor is weary and even when provoked or irritated by inconsiderate or irrational behaviour (patients, like doctors, sometimes lose their tempers and behave badly). But times out of number I received letters at the GMC from patients suggesting that doctors had been abominably rude, clumsy, arrogant, thoughtless or just simply unsympathetic, unfeeling or unkind. They said: "I don't want the doctor 'struck off'; please write and ask him (or her) to be nice to people in future"—but that, of course the Council couldn't do without involving the full panoply of quasi-legal procedures. *Avarice*, too, falls outside the GMC's statutory powers even though some letters complain about what, prima facie, looks like gross overcharging in private practice. Can we hope that the profession itself, with appropriate procedures at a local level, could satisfy public concern about some such matters?

Sloth, if I interpret the word literally, is I think pretty rare among doctors in clinical practice who are all too often, whether in junior resident posts or even when more senior, overworked and weary. And in family practice, too, the third night call during an epidemic or the stress of coping with an importuning patient in a crowded office can impose almost intolerable strains on a doctor's reserves of patience and understanding. But sick people are often frightened people and the diagnosis of acute meningococcal meningitis or of a perforated appendix in the middle of the night, followed by prompt action, can excuse several unnecessary calls which only an expert could judge with hindsight to have been unnecessary. No, sloth is not usually a problem with doctors—but perhaps the most difficult lesson of all for the young doctor to learn (as I said earlier) is how, in the face of competing demands and responsibilities, to be able to organise his or her time.

And so we are left with *pride* and *envy*. Relevant to medicine? Of course they are. If (with apologies to Rudyard Kipling) pride leads you to rely upon your own skill in diagnosis and management and to be so self-confident as to refuse the legitimate wish of a patient to seek a further (probably confirmatory) opinion, it comes before a fall. If intellectual and professional arrogance cloaks your opinions with an aura (to yourself) of infallibility, if that arrogance leads in turn to an inability or unwillingness to talk to a patient on equal terms with a full and frank discussion of pros and cons, if you are unable or unwilling to admit, on occasion, your uncertainties or even your mistakes, and if pride or envy leads you unjustifiably to criticise or disparage the views or advice given by a professional colleague, these are indeed deadly medical sins. For the days of "doctor's orders" are long past; the doctor/patient relationship is a partnership in which the doctor offers advice but it is up to the patient to decide whether or not to accept it.

Doctor/Patient Communication

May I now return to the question, so dear to Osler's heart, of communication between doctors and patients? Some of the greatest misunderstandings which arise between doctors and patients and their families occur when this is unsatisfactory. In the medical consultation, the keystone of clinical practice, the interview is the beginning. Interviewing skills can be examined, assessed and taught. It is salutary for a doctor to see a videotape recording of an interview conducted by himself. Even more important is the exposition or discussion in which the doctor must give clear and concise advice but must not strike an authoritarian role. Constraints of time in busy clinics or in overcrowded wards must be admitted. Equally important is the fact that patients often forget, misunderstand or misinterpret doctors' opinions and advice. Doctors themselves may be at fault by writing extremely complex prescriptions. For this reason, the profession should examine the possibility of producing more written advice to patients about the management of their illnesses. A working party which I chaired at the Nuffield Provincial Hospitals Trust produced a booklet for doctors and medical students ("Talking with Patients") which proved popular. Doctors should always remember that patients may be so distracted by anxiety that they cannot regularly remember what they are told. Sometimes, too, the patient's social and domestic circumstances may inflate or distort the significance of a trivial medical problem. Equally, too, there are patients who either find it impossible, or are unwilling, to comply with doctors' recommendations with regard to treatment.

Communication Between Doctors and Other Doctors and with Other Health Care Professionals

Just as doctor-patient communication is fundamental to good medical practice, communication between doctors in different specialties on the one hand and between doctors and other health care professionals on the other is equally important and often overlooked. The same working party of the Nuffield Provincial Hospitals Trust produced two further booklets highlighting some problems which had emerged as a result of our enquiries into intraprofessional communication. One social worker said to a doctor "I cannot hear what you say while what you are rings so loudly in my ears." But a hospital administrator also said wryly that it was his duty to serve the interests of 200 consultants, 195 of whom owed allegiance only to God and the other 5 did not even accept that limitation. I feel sure, too, that Osler would have felt just as concerned as did Dr. Alec Cooke in the talk he gave to the Oxford meeting of the Osler Club of London a few years ago in which he castigated the profession for its increasing use of acronyms, some of which he found increasingly unintelligible on studying hospital care records. Beginners, he felt sure, would have no difficulty in interpreting the meaning of WR for Wassermann reaction, PM for post-mortem, or D and C for dilatation and curettage. Even more advanced students would usually be quite happy in interpreting GFR, MCHC or DNA but might be compelled to hesitate a little in reading NCT for "not come through" or LSCS for "lower segment Caesarian section." But even honours students, he suggested, might be taken aback by EUAPS for "examination under anaesthetic of post-nasal space," DNSVI for "does not seem very ill," and especially when confronted by the final gem which he had found in a patient's notes as LASNULLLRSR, standing for "local anaesthesia, seventh nerve, upper lid, lower lid and retrobulbar space on the right." Surely, despite the temporal constraints which afflict us all in our clinical practice, we can do better?

Communication with the Media

Many doctors have also learned to their cost that communication with the media needs considerable skill and judgement. Charles Fletcher dealt admirably with this issue in his Rock Carling Lecture in 1972 and quoted with approbation Osler's warning in 1907 that the Delilah of the press may perhaps be courted with satisfaction but sooner or later was sure to play the harlot; it would thus "leave a man shorn of his strength, *viz.* the confidence of his professional brethren." How true that remains today when we all in medicine have been compelled to acknowledge increasing public interest in matters medical. This area, upon which I do not have time to dwell, requires exceptional expertise.

Epilogue

May I finally comment upon some of the fashionable but false antitheses which were so effectively demolished by Sir Douglas Black in his Rock Carling Lecture for 1984? Of his many verbal, philosophical and scientific gems I have time to select very few. When Faraday was asked by one sceptical of the value of science, "What use is electromagnetism?", his response was brief but compelling: "What use is a baby?" he said. All of us in clinical medicine know that there is no antithesis between the scientific and so-called holistic methods or between the scientific and the compassionate and caring, as all doctors, whatever their training and specialty, surely strive to practise whole-patient medicine. I am convinced that the good doctor is just as concerned with disease prevention as with cure. Nevertheless, Black did an invaluable service in stressing that those who feel that management and business skills may be used to buy results in the ever-changing and ever-challenging field of medical research must recognise that 'lavish finance can be impotent in the face of unripe time.' Parkinson in his 'laws of medical research' said much the same thing when indicating that research which does not define precisely a question to be asked, methods of answering it and a route to be followed may be as fruitless in medicine as is that which goes astray because of deficiencies in clinical knowledge, skills or experience.

As Osler so clearly indicated many years ago, clinical and laboratory science, combined with communication skills, must continue to be partners in our avowed aim of serving to the best of our ability our patients, future patients, knowledge itself and society. These may be truisms but it is upon their full recognition and application in our everyday contact with patients that a proper rekindling of the Osler flame depends.

Neurology

Osler and Neurology

 George C. Ebers, M.D.

William Osler's bibliography includes over 1400 papers, monographs, and notes touching on almost every subspecialty of medicine (Abbott 1939). He has been claimed by gastroenterologists (Cunha 1948), pediatricians (McGovern et al 1970; Robbins et al 1963), medical librarians, (Bett 1949), veterinarians (Giltner 1926–27) (Murphy 1960) obstetricians (Rucker 1952) and members of other disciplines as one of their own.

Osler published close to 200 papers, reviews, editorials and monographs dealing with neurology, but it is not widely recognized that his contributions to neurology exceed those to many of the other fields. For example, Osler's interest in neuropathology was entirely omitted from the recent excellent monograph "An Oslerian Pathology" (Rodin 1981). The purpose of this paper is to bring into focus his impressive neurological contributions and to document his substantial interest in the neurosciences.

Osler's activities in neurology constituted a microcosm of his overall medical contributions. His interests in the neurosciences began early. In 1884 he wrote on the comparative anatomy of the brain of the seal (Osler 1884a), having given a lecture on "the brain as a thinking organ" in the previous year (Osler 1883a).

The Mind-Brain Problem

Osler's early interest in what has been called the mind-brain problem very likely led him to carry out several studies on the brains of criminals, a subject of considerable controversy at that time. In 1879 Benedikt of Vienna (known eponymously by neurologists for Benedikt's syndrome) published a monograph on the abnormalities in the surface anatomy of the brains of criminals (Benedikt 1879). Benedikt had suggested that criminal brains showed the

Read at the annual meeting of the American Osler Society, April, 1984.

Reprinted with permission from *The Canadian Journal of Neurological Sciences*, 12:236, 1985 confluence of many primary fissures as well as an extra horizontal frontal gyrus. Osler was unable to confirm these findings. He studied the brains of two criminals and compared them to 34 brains obtained from autopsies at the Montreal General Hospital, noting that confluent fissures were found commonly in "normals" (Osler 1882a). He suggested that the appropriate controls for Benedikt's criminals would have been law-abiding individuals from the same race. Osler emphasized the dangers of attributing criminal behaviour to organic lesions and, in some moralizing uncharacteristic of his scientific papers, he expressed his belief in man's free will and responsibility for his own actions. One of the cases from this study illustrates Osler's tenacity in the pursuit of pathological material. Moreau, a man who had been convicted of axe-murdering his wife, was to be hanged at Rimouski, Quebec. Osler sent one of his residents to Rimouski in mid-winter to obtain this brain, not an easy task given the time of year and the transportation available (Cushing 1925). Despite his negative findings in criminal brains Osler went to the defense of Benedikt after a Lancet editorial noted the "collapse of Benedikt's attempt to furnish an anatomic basis for crime." In a letter to Lancet, Osler felt that more information was needed before firm conclusions could be reached (Osler 1882b). He kept up his interest in this question and the results of additional studies on criminal brains, which he called Series 2, constitute item 7666s in the Bibliotheca Osleriana.

Localization

It was an exciting time in the neurosciences when Osler came on the scene toward the end of the last century. The important studies of Hitzig and Ferrier and others had opened the way for clinical pathological study of focal cerebral lesions and localization of cerebral function was to preoccupy neurologists and neurophysiologists for several ensuing decades. Osler had a vivid interest in these developments and attended the International Medical Congress of 1881, sending back a report of the proceedings which was published. The discussion of localization by Ferrier, Brown-Sequard and others was the highlight (Osler 1881–82a). The level of sophistication in some of Osler's papers on localization is surprisingly high even when viewed in retrospect. He published a paper on sensory aphasia with word blindness in the same year as Dejerine's classical paper on this topic (Osler 1891; Dejerine 1891). He also wrote about the localization of sacral autonomic centres noting the difficulty in distinguishing conus from cauda lesions (Osler 1888a). He also described in the context of these cases a syphiloma of the sacral cord (Osler 1889a). Syphilis was indeed one of his major interests. He published on the inheritance of syphilis (congenital), on tabes dorsalis (Osler 1883b) and provided an excellent discussion of neurosyphilis in his classical text (Osler 1892a). The latter contribution has been emphasized (Harvey et al 1967). In Osler's time the relationship of tabes to syphilis was not certain even though the classical description of tabes by Romberg had occurred around the time of Osler's birth. However, in explaining the fact that some individuals developed tabes without a prior history of syphilis, Osler related a case of neurosyphilis in a physician whom he knew had had syphilis but who had subsequently denied it. Osler left little doubt that his sympathy lay with the view that tabes and general paresis of the insane were synonymous with syphilis.

Subdural Hematoma

Osler wrote an interesting paper on subdural hematoma while he was in Philadelphia (Osler 1888b). He recalled that in the 12 years in which he had been a pathologist at Montreal General Hospital he had not seen such a case. Of significance is the issue he took with the commonly prevailing notion that the disorder was an inflammatory one. Virchow appears to have been responsible for this notion, implicit in the term pachymeningitis hemorrhagica which he coined, (a term which is still used in a relatively recent text of neurology (Wilson 1940); but Osler in his microscopic analysis of subdural hematoma doubted an inflammatory etiology. Osler also made a relevant and accurate observation that many of these patients were found in hostels for the insane and that cerebral atrophy was often associated with this disorder. Although he denies ever seeing a case in Montreal, his original autopsy records include 2 cases which may well have been subdural hematoma, one acute and one chronic, in addition to an acute epidural hematoma. (Osler autopsy records-Osler Library, McGill University, Montreal). Osler was an early member of the American Neurological Association, presented papers at their meetings, and is seen in photographs of this organization taken in the 1890s. Osler wrote on encephalopathy and identified the toxic encephalopathy associated with pneumonia and uremia (Osler 1898; Osler 1882c).

Brain Tumors and Vascular Disease

He wrote several items on tumors of the brain both in the context of localization with clinico-pathological correlation and from the perspective of a working pathologist. He recorded a natural clinical remission in a cholesteatoma in a young physician in which he questioned whether or not the use of leeches had been responsible for the improvement (Osler 1887a). In another patient with Jacksonian epilepsy he invoked "Charcot's rule" with respect to localization (Osler 1884b). Charcot had noted that in cases of focal motor epilepsy, those with associated weakness had lesions involving the motor cortex whereas those without weakness had lesions adjacent to it.

Aneurysm was one of his favourite topics and he wrote numerous papers on aneurysms of the cerebral vessels. Osler thought embolism, endarteritis and atheroma were the chief causes and he supported an embolic mechanism by quoting a description of what may well have been a clot within an aneurysm rather than an embolus (Osler 1887b).

Separate from cerebral aneurysms, Osler had an interest in vascular disease in the nervous system and wrote numerous papers on this topic. In fact, Osler's first appearance in medical print concerned the case of an acute stroke in which Osler, then a young medical student, demonstrated a clot in the middle cerebral artery, perhaps one of the first times this had been documented (Reddy 1871–72) (see Figure 1). Osler attended Walt Whitman during the second of his strokes. He came to know Whitman through his relationship with Maurice Bucke, the former superintendent of the London (Ontario) Asylum for the Insane and a close friend of Whitman's (Cushing 1925).

Osler documented the occurrence of transient ischemic attacks (TIA's)

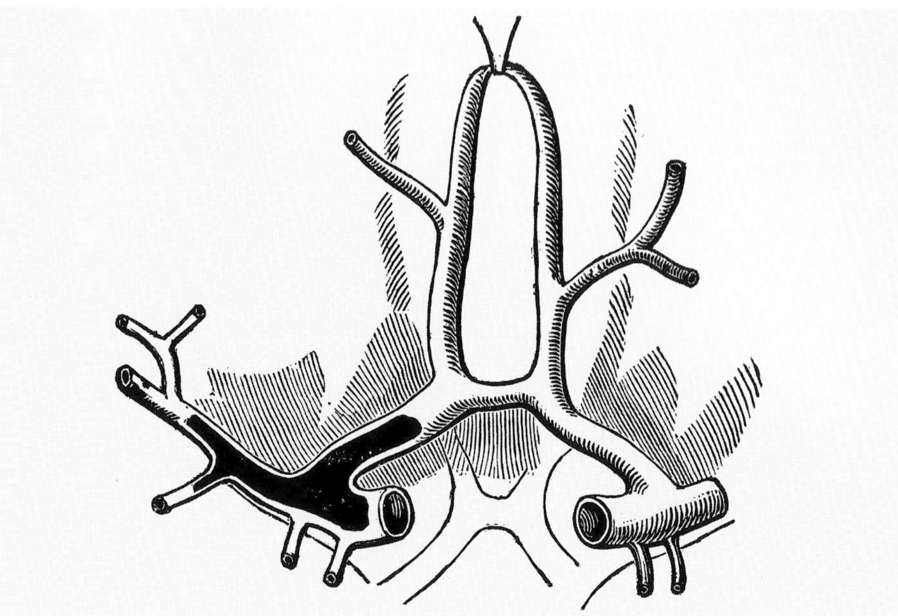

Figure 1 Diagram from paper by Reddy 1871–72 (autopsy by William Osler) showing clot in internal carotid-middle cerebral arteries.

in a 62 year old man shortly after Peabody's attribution of this phenomenon to arterial spasm (Peabody 1891). Osler had doubts about this mechanism in view of the sclerotic nature of the arteries. Osler's literary talents are nowhere more evident than in the description of another man "who had driven his engines at full steam" who also had episodes of transient cerebral ischemia. Referring to the case as "death at the top", he described the sufferer as a man devoted to Venus, Vulcan and Bacchus—a description surely more picturesque than our contemporary recording of cases of beer per week or pack-years of smoking (Osler 1911) (Osler 1911–12). It is interesting to note that Osler has been quoted as espousing spasm as a cause of TIA and also criticized for not embracing this concept by different authors in different generations (Russell 1912; Hachinski 1982). He was still alive to answer Russell's critique but tended not to commit himself completely (Osler 1912) on this issue, although he felt that spasm was the most plausible explanation. Contemporary thinking is that primary spasm is unlikely in the clinical setting he described. Also in the area of vascular disease, Osler reported a case of embolism of the anterior cerebral artery (Osler 1887c), cases of hemiplegia with typhoid fever (Osler 1900a), and a probable post-traumatic carotid cavernous fistula (Osler 1882–83). He wrote on the neurological complications of cases now strongly suggestive of lupus erythematosus (Osler 1895a; Osler 1900b; Osler 1903; Tumulty et al 1949). He also recorded the recurrent laryngeal palsy associated with mitral incompetence and its importance in the differential diagnosis of thoracic aneurysm (Osler 1909). In his autopsied case of this entity he documented the sclerosis of the nerve between the aorta and the left auricle. He also recorded the pupil sign of thoracic aneurysm, an observation which has at times been misquoted. The phenomenon of ipsilateral Horner's syndrome secondary to aneurysm is now well known and often attributed to Osler's description. In fact, going over the original paper, it appears that Osler described pupillary dilatation rather than constriction on the ipsilateral side (Osler 1910a). The reason for this was unclear although irritation of the sympathetic nerve was Osler's explanation. No less an authority than Fielding Garrison, summarizing Osler's contributions in his obituary notice, records that he was the first to relate mycotic aneurysms to bacterial endocarditis and to draw attention in his Gulstonian lectures on endocarditis to the cerebral presentations of this disorder including the complication of meningitis (Garrison 1920).

Movement Disorders and Psychiatric Disease

Osler maintained his early interest in psychiatric disease and wrote papers on post-febrile insanity (Osler 1890a), the Gilles de la Tourette syndrome which he likened to the Malay disease Latah (probably related to his interest in chorea) (Osler 1890b), and on the form of neurosis known as typhoid spine (Osler 1919a) thought by Pepper to be due to periostitis.

A number of publications addressed movement disorders. He doubted Charcot's view that Huntington's and Sydenham's chorea were similar and wrote an excellent monograph on chorea which is a model of a clinical epidemiologic study (Osler 1894a). The title page of this work is seen in Figure 2. Although Richard Bright had noted the association of heart disease with chorea it was Osler who solidly established it (Osler 1887d; Osler 1887e; Garrison 1920). He classified chorea and clearly separated hereditary chorea from the acquired form. This led to the adoption of rest as treatment for chorea because of the very frequent association with carditis which he helped establish. In his autopsied case of Huntington's chorea he noted the "well-recognized clinical trick" that such patients exhibit of raising their heel suddenly and standing on the balls of the toes. He overlooked the specific caudate nucleus atrophy of this disorder although he did notice that the ventricles were distended (Osler 1894b). He wrote on wry-neck with facial asymmetry contrasting the lack of progression in his two cases with its presence in Romberg's facial hemiatrophy (Osler 1892b).

Neuropathology

Osler's medical career was founded on solid pathological observation and his neurological contributions were usually backed up by careful neuropathological study. His interest in neuropathology was not casual—he wrote several papers on neuropathological methods, including an elegant study on the interstitial processes of the central nervous system which included detailed discussion on connective tissues in the nervous system and how they are involved in degenerative, inflammatory and developmental disorders. (Osler 1879; Osler 1892c). His studies on gliomas led him to doubt Klebs' contention that the nerve cells were involved in proliferation (Osler 1885–86). As a working neuropathologist he became aware of and learned many of the new German methods for study of the brain during his visits to Europe. Osler liked to indulge in "quinquennial brain dustings" and his visit to Europe in 1890 with Ramsey Wright of the University of Toronto was typical of this. Of special interest in the present context are the number of neurological figures he visited at that time. These included Strumpel, Weigert, Von Recklinghausen, Naunyn, Goltz, Edinger, Erb, Dejerine and Bouchard among others. He was impressed with Weidershein's use of different colours of chalk for teaching neuroanatomy and may have adopted this on his return (Osler 1890c). On one of his visits to Charcot's hospitals he was amused by Charcot's attempt to use hypnotism to cure a man with club feet of his inability to walk. He also observed hypnosis at the hands of Luys, a well known neurologist, who hynotized one of his nurses into giving a lecture on neuropathology, a feat which she performed but with which Osler was very much unimpressed, telling Ramsey Wright that this was "a circus".

Peripheral Nerve

Osler wrote about disorders of the peripheral nervous system including arsenical neuritis and post-typhoid neuropathy which in retrospect may well have been a form of what we now call the Guillain-Barré Syndrome (Osler 1895b). Cushing reports that while on a visit to Toronto Osler's nephew developed an acute paralysis with Osler discussing the differential diagnosis between polyneuritis and poliomyelitis, an issue he had dealt with in print (Osler 1886) noting the sensory changes and better prognosis in the former disorder. Still within the peripheral nervous system, Osler wrote about cervical rib and the neurovascular syndrome it produced. His two papers on the subject demonstrate his characteristic honesty in reporting and give some insight into the man himself. The first case was not correctly diagnosed but the clinical phenomena were clearly identified (Osler 1888c). Some years later when he came to the correct diagnosis he reported the case emphasizing how he had been mistaken previously (Osler 1910b). Osler also described the first case of facioscapulohumeral dystrophy in North America (Osler 1889b).

Meningitis

Osler had a special interest in the subject of meningitis and he wrote several papers and reviews in this area (Osler 1881–82b; Osler 1888d; Osler 1899a). A review of his writings on meningitis is particularly interesting as they document the evolution of general medical understanding of this disorder and the introduction of the lumbar puncture by Quincke which Osler advocated in the investigation of the problem. At the time of his first publications, there was no distinction among the various forms of meningitis. However, gradually specific forms of meningitis were identified—initially epidemic vs non-epidemic and subsequently pneumococcal vs meningococcal (Osler 1914–15; Osler 1919b).

Cushing's Disease

He made a "remarkable near miss" in the description of Cushing's Disease. He published a case of myxedema with glycosuria but in retrospect, on rereading the case reported, it is almost certain that this was a case of Cushing's Syndrome (Osler 1899b) as pointed out recently (Altschule 1980). The patient had abdominal striae and other typical features of the disorder. There is no evidence that Cushing (for whom this disease was eventually named) had ever discussed the condition with Osler. In Cushing's text on surgery of the head there is a sketch of a man with a bullet in his head which bears a distinct resemblance to Osler, perhaps the kind of literary joke one might have expected from Osler himself (Cushing 1908).

Neurological Associations

There is abundant other evidence of Osler's close association with neurologists. The neurologists Gowers and Bastian had written letters of support for Osler's application to the University of Pennsylvania. Osler wrote obituaries for Charcot, Mitchell and Horsley (Osler 1893a; Osler 1914; Osler 1916) and his review of Paget's biography of Horsley was Osler's last published work (Osler 1919c). In this review he described Horsley's removal of a spinal cord tumour as perhaps the most brilliant operation in the whole history of surgery. This latter work permits one to say that Osler began and ended his published medical career in the nervous system. He wrote two monographs of high quality on neurology dedicating the one on chorea to Gowers and that on cerebral palsy of children to Weir Mitchell (Osler 1889c) who had obtained his appointment to the Philadelphia Orthopedic Hospital and Infirmary for Nervous Diseases. The work for both these monographs originated at this institution.

Osler established a neurological journal club while at John Hopkins, the proceedings of which are to be found in the early issues of the Bulletin of the Johns Hopkins Medical School.

Osler made numerous contributions to textbooks and wrote the introduction for Hirt's Textbook (Osler 1889d). The three neurological chapters which he contributed to ''Pepper's System of Medicine'' comprised one half of the six chapters Osler wrote for this compendium (Osler 1893b; Osler 1893c; Osler 1893d). He wrote the chapter on ''Diseases the Direct or Indirect Result of Infection'' for ''A Textbook of Nervous Diseases by American Authors'', edited by Dercum (Osler 1895c).

Oslerian Reminiscences

Among Oslerian reminiscences was one written by neurologist Pierre Marie (Marie 1926) with whom Osler had visited on numerous occasions. Marie had also written a preface for an early French edition of Osler's textbook of medicine. Osler had numerous biographers and these included many medical and surgical neurologists such as Charles Mills, Dercum, Lewis, Penfield, Courville, Henry Viets, and of course Cushing.

Osler's Brain

Even after Osler's death his association with the nervous system continued, probably because of his interest in the mind-brain problem. Osler left his brain to the Wistar Institute in Philadelphia for study, an institution which Osler had helped to open years before. His brain, along with those of two other scholars,

Granville Hall and Edward Morse, were compared in intense detail (Donaldson et al 1928). The findings were also correlated with studies previously done by Myrtel Canavan (who is now eponymously remembered for Canavan's Disease) with the brains of the Southard family in Boston (Canavan 1926). Ernest Southard had been the Bullard professor of neuropathology at Harvard University in whose department Dr. Canavan had worked.

Following Archibald Garrod's seven year term, Osler's successor as Regius Professor of Medicine at Oxford was a neurologist, Sir Farquhar Buzzard, an additional Osler biographer (Buzzard 1928).

Oslerian Legacies

Osler's legacy to neurology is in part due to his great skills as a teacher. It is worth noting here that the accomplishments of his students are well known but, in particular, that the great English neurologist Sir Charles Symonds, as well as Lord Brain, were both influenced by Osler to pursue neurology. Symonds related that he decided on a career in neurology after seeing Osler diagnose a case of cervical rib (Brain 1960; Symonds 1969). It is certainly possible that Osler had an important influence on the development of 20th century neurosurgery through his relationship with Cushing. Osler was quick to identify, from his clinical pathological studies of the nervous system, the potential for surgical treatment of tumours of the brain localized by clinical findings. Did Osler push Cushing into neurosurgery? After Godlees' celebrated removal of a glioma, Osler wrote an editorial judging such an operation justifiable and possibly lifesaving (Osler 1885a). In a subsequent paper entitled "Conditions of the brain suitable for operative interference", Osler noted that ganglionic hemorrhage was not appropriate. He stated that tuberculomas, gliomas, sarcomas and carcinomas occurred in decreasing order of frequency and that tumours of the dura looked very promising (for surgery) (Osler 1889e). He also mentioned the possibility of treating epilepsy with this new modality. It would seem quite possible that Osler conveyed his enthusiasm for this nascent field to Cushing, a close friend and protégé

Osler the Neurological Clinician

Although it has recently been suggested that Osler possibly "did not have the feel for clinical neurology" (Matthews 1982) the observations in the present review give reason to think otherwise. Riese has published a case detailing the autopsy findings of a patient with symptoms of Parkinson's disease. It was subsequently found that Sir William Osler had made the diagnosis of multiple sclerosis some 50 years previously and this in fact was confirmed at autopsy (Riese 1952). Osler did recognize Parkinson's disease. Thomas McCrae related the story of a patient with a slowly developing neurological disorder who had had opinions from a remarkable list of American, British, French and German physicians and Osler had been the first to suggest the correct diagnosis—Parkinson's disease (McCrae 1926).

In Osler's writings he relates how he tested for 2–point discrimination and used the rim of the stethoscope to elicit tendon reflexes (Osler 1883b). Osler diagnosed one of the first cases of acromegaly in North America and in

ON

CHOREA

AND

CHOREIFORM AFFECTIONS

BY

WILLIAM OSLER, M.D.

FELLOW OF THE ROYAL COLLEGE OF PHYSICIANS, LONDON ; PRESIDENT OF THE ASSOCIATION
OF AMERICAN PHYSICIANS ; PROFESSOR OF MEDICINE JOHNS HOPKINS UNIVERSITY,
AND PHYSICIAN-IN-CHIEF JOHNS HOPKINS HOSPITAL, BALTIMORE.
FORMERLY PHYSICIAN TO THE INFIRMARY FOR DISEASES OF THE NERVOUS SYSTEM,
PHILADELPHIA

LONDON

H. K. LEWIS, 136 GOWER STREET, W.C.

1894

Figure 2 Title page of Osler's monograph "On Chorea" dedicated to Gowers.

his letters to house staff it was clear he was on the lookout for such a case even prior to seeing one because he had read Pierre Marie's classic description in the journal Brain or perhaps had discussed it with him (Osler 1890c; Tigertt 1971). Osler wrote on the neurological examination including discussions of brain murmurs in children (Osler 1880) and variations of the normal knee jerk (Osler 1887f).

In reviewing Osler's published writings it is extraordinary how often he was on the correct side of what seemed to have been controversial issues. Examples of these include the subdural hematoma, and tabes dorsalis. Although in retrospect it is possible to find Osler occasionally in error, such as in his early views on the spontaneous generation of blood platelets (influenced by Bastian), it is indeed uncommon. Osler's papers and chapters make entertaining reading today, replete as they are with literary references, aphorisms and medical wisdom, occasional social commentary, and above all, accurate observation. It is fair to state that a few of his papers were not memorable. Oslerian encounters in neurology brought the well known therapeutic nihilist to a discipline spare in practical treatments. Osler's view that nitroglycerin was helpful for epilepsy has not been substantiated (Osler 1888e). Osler's failure in the use of acupuncture analgesia has been recorded (Cushing 1925; Anonymous 1974). He did not find success in treating patients with locomotor ataxia by hanging them upside down for three minutes at a time as suggested by Charcot (Osler 1889f). Nevertheless, Osler's papers usually stand in striking contrast to those adjacent to his in the journals in which he published.

Osler played an important role as a general medical critic for his ability to determine flaws in others' works no doubt added to his general reputation and the esteem in which he was held. In the neurological area we can credit him with "debunking" the gross changes said to be characteristic of the brains of criminals, and the denial of "typhoid spine" as a specific disease entity. He formally reviewed many neurological works for the general medical literature, including Gowers on the spinal cord (Osler 1885b), Bramwell on the same (Osler 1885c) and Mitchell on diseases of women (Osler 1885d).

My interest in Osler was kindled by curiosity as to whether multiple sclerosis is increasing in prevalence. Osler's records and writings have proved to be most interesting in this context. Osler described the first case of multiple sclerosis in Canada at autopsy (Osler 1880–81a) shortly after the description of the first North American case (Seguin et al 1878).

He identified a number of cases premortem and postmortem (Osler 1880–81a; Osler 1880–81b). In some 786 patients autopsied over eight years in the Montreal General Hospital, Osler identified one definite case and two possible cases of this disorder (G. Ebers 1982; Osler autopsy records, Osler Library McGill University, Montreal). Although these data are obviously severely limited they may represent the best evidence concerning the prevalence of multiple sclerosis 100 years ago in Osler's time.

In summary it can be stated that Osler's neurological contributions were numerous, and many were first rate. His autopsy records provide a remarkable account of contemporary neurological disease through the eyes of an accurate and careful observer. Both these and his clinical studies of the nervous system have been under-appreciated. Osler belonged as much to Neurology as to any other field of medicine.

Acknowledgements

I would like to acknowledge the help of Marilyn Franciszyn of the Osler Library, Mrs. Sheila Swanson of the Toronto Academy of Medicine Library and Professor C. G. Roland of McMaster University for helpful discussions and to Drs. William Gibson and C. A. McDowell of the University of British Columbia for reviewing the manuscript. This paper was presented in part at the Osler Society meeting in Atlanta, April 1984 and at the American Academy of Neurology (Ebers 1982).

References

Abbott M (1939) Classified and Annotated Bibliography of Sir William Osler's Publications. Montreal, The Medical Museum, McGill University.

Altschule MD (1980) A near miss—Osler's early description of Cushing's syndrome. N Eng J Med 302:1153–55.

Anonymous (1974) Osler, Peter Redpath and acupuncture. Osler Library Newsletter 16.

Benedikt M (1879) On the Brains of Criminals (translated by Dr. Fowler). W. Wood and Co. New York.

Bett WR (1949) Osler the medical historian. Med Press, 222:35–37.

Brain R (1960) Osler and medicine today. Can Med Assoc J 83:349–354.

Buzzard F (1928) The pain, penalty, and prohibitions of old age—can they be prevented. Bull N Y Acad Med 4:1068–1077.

Canavan MM (1926) Ernest Elmer Southard and his Parents: A Brain Study. University Press, Cambridge, Massachusetts.

Cunha F (1948) Osler as a gastroenterologist. Almeda California Times—Star Press.

Cushing H (1908) Surgery of the head. *In:* Surgery: Its Principles and Practices. Edited by W. W. Keen, 3:248.

Cushing H (1925) The Life of Sir William Osler. Oxford, Clarendon Press.

Dejerine J (1891) Sur un cas de celite verbale avec agraphie, Suivi D'Autopsie Mem Soc Biol 3:197–2

Donaldson HH and Canavan MM (1928) A study of brains of three scholars: Granville Stanley Hall, Sir William Osler, Edward Sylvester Morse. J Comp Neurol 46:1–95.

Ebers GC (1982) Osler and Neurology. Neurol 32(2):A229.

Garrison FH (1920) Sir William Osler, 1849–1919. Science, li:55–58.

Giltner W (1926–7) Osler and veterinary medicine. J Am Vet Med Assoc 69:422–432.

Hachinski V (1982) Transient cerebral ischemia: A historical sketch. *In:* Historical Aspects of the Neurosciences. Edited by F. C. Rose and W. F. Bynum, Raven Press, New York.

Harvey AM, McKusick VA (1967) Osler's Textbook Revisited. New York, Appleton-Century-Crofts.

Marie P (1926) Osler—educateur. Int Assoc Med Mus Bull 9:9

Matthews WB (1982) Osler oration. J Royal Soc Med 25:307–314.

McCrae T (1926) The influence of pathology on the clinical medicine of William Osler. Int Assoc Med Mus Bull 9:37–41.

McGovern JP, Davison WC (1970) Osler and pediatrics. Am J Dis Child 119:5.

Murphy DA (1960) Osler now a veterinarian. Can Med Assoc J 83:32–35.

Osler W (1879) On Giacomoni's method of preserving the brain. Can Med Surg J viii:16–17.

Osler W (1880) On the systolic brain murmur of children. Bost Med Surg J ciii:29–30.

Osler W (1880–81a) Cases of insular-sclerosis. Can Med Surg J ix:1–11.

Osler W (1880–81b) A contribution to the question of spastic spinal paralysis. Can Med Surg J ix:100.

Osler W (1881–82a) The VII international medical congress London. Can Med Surg J, Montreal, x:121–125.

Osler W (1881–82b) Case of tubercular meningitis. Can Med Surg J x;603–606.

Osler W (1882a) The brains of criminals. Can Med Surg J x:385–398.

Osler W (1882b) The brains of criminals. Lancet II:38.

Osler W (1882c) Uremic delirium at a very early stage of interstitial nephritis. Arch Med, New York, vii:213–215.

Osler W (1882–83) Cerebral aneurism and hemorrhage: Erosion of internal carotid into cavernous sinus six weeks after a blow on the head. Can Med Surg J xi:335–358.

Osler W (1883a) On the brain as a thinking organ. Can Nat x:109.

Osler W (1883b) Pre-ataxic tabes dorsalis. Med News, Philadelphia, xliii:197–199.

Osler W (1884a) The brain of the seal. Can Rec Nat Sci i:64.

Osler W (1884b) Fibroglioma of upper end of ascending frontal gyrus. J Nerv Ment Dis xliv:82–83.

Osler W (1885a) Removal of a brain tumor (unsigned editorial). Med News, Philadelphia, xlvi:75.

Osler W (1885b) The Diagnosis of Diseases of the Spinal Cord by W. R. Gowers (initialled book review). Am J Med Sci, Philadelphia, lxxix:218–219.

Osler W (1885c) Diseases of the spinal cord by Byron Bramwell. The Second Edition, Edinburgh: Young J., Pentland, 1884. (Initialled book review). Am J Med Sci, Philadelphia, xc:504.

Osler W (1885d) Lectures on Diseases of the Nervous System, Especially in Women, by S. Weir-Mitchell. Second Edition, Phila. Lea Bros. & Co. (unsigned book review). Med News, Philadelphia, xlvii:162.

Osler W (1885–86) The structure of certain gliomata. Med Times, Philadelphia, xvi:394–395.

Osler W (1886) Multiple neuritis. Med News, Philadelphia, xlix:10–11.

Osler W (1887a) Case of cholesteatoma of the floor of the third ventricle and infundibulum. J Nerv Ment Dis xiv:657–73.

Osler W (1887b) Aneurism of the larger cerebral arteries. Trans Path Soc Phil xiii:87–93.

Osler W (1887c) Embolism of the left anterior cerebral artery - softening of the left frontal lobe. Trans Path Society Phil, 202–203.

Osler W (1887d) Chorea and heart disease. Med News, Philadelphia, li:509.

Osler W (1887e) The cardiac relations of chorea. Am J Med Sci, Philadelphia, civ:371–386.

Osler W (1887f) The variations of the normal knee jerk (editorial). Med News, Philadelphia, li:601.

Osler W (1888a) On lesions of the conus medullaris and cauda equina and the situation of the ano-vesical centre in man. Med News, Philadelphia, lii:669–671.

Osler W (1888b) Note on pachymeningitis hemorrhagica. J Nerv Ment Dis, New York, xiii:608–612.

Osler W (1888c) Enlargement and congestion of the right arm following exercise of the muscles. J Nerv Ment Dis, New York, xiii:246–248.

Osler W (1888d) Epidemic cerebral spinal meningitis (unsigned editorial). Med News, Philadelphia, lii:269.

Osler W (1888e) Note on nitroglycerin in epilepsy. J Nerv Ment Dis, New York, xiii:38–39.

Osler W (1889a) Case of syphiloma of the cord of the cauda equina—death from diffuse central myelitis. J Nerve Ment Dis xiv:499–507.

Osler W (1889b) On a case of simple idiopathic muscular atrophy involving the face and scapulo-humeral muscles. Am J Med Sci xcviii:261–265.

Osler W (1889c) The Cerebral Palsies of Children. K. R. Lewis, London.

Osler W (1889d) Introduction in: Hirt, Ludwig. Diseases of the nervous system translated by A. Hoch, Appleton and Co., New York.

Osler W (1889e) On conditions of the brain suitable for operative interference. Can Pract 14:165–67.

Osler W (1889f) Treatment of locomotor ataxia by suspension. Med News, Philadelphia, liv:323.

Osler W (1890a) Cases of post-febrile insanity, Johns Hopkins Hospital Reports, Baltimore, ii:46–50.

Osler W (1890b) On the form of convulsive tic associated with coprolalia, etc. Med News, Philadelphia, lvii:645–647.

Osler W (1890c) Letters to my house physicians. N Y Med J lii:81;163;191;-274:333.

Osler W (1891) A case of sensory aphasia: word-blindness with hemianopsia. Am J Sci ci:219–224.

Osler W (1892a) The Principles and Practice of Medicine. D. Appleton and Co. New York.

Osler W (1892b) On the association of congenital wry-neck with marked facial asymmetry. Arch Ped, New York, ix:81–85.

Osler W (1892c) Interstitial processes in the central nervous system. Trans Cong Am Phys Surg 1891, New Haven, ii:144–146.

Osler W (1892–93) Note on arsenical neuritis following the use of Fowler's solution. Mont Med J xxi:721–724.

Osler W (1893a) Jean Martin Charcot, memorial notice. Johns Hopkins Hospital Bulletin, Baltimore, ix:87–88.

Osler W (1893b) Organic Disease of the Brain in: A System of Practical Medicine by American Authors. Edited by W. Pepper, Philadelphia, i:669–725.

Osler W (1893c) Diseases of the Nerves in: A System of Practical Medicine by American Authors. Edited by W. Pepper, Philadelphia, i:805–849.

Osler W (1893d) Disease of the Muscles in: A System of Practical Medicine by American Authors. Edited by W. Pepper, Philadelphia, i:850–858.

Osler W (1894a) On Chorea and Choreiform Affections. P. Blakiston Son & Co., Philadelphia.

Osler W (1894b) A case of hereditary chorea. Johns Hopkins Hospital Bulletin, Baltimore, v:119–120.

Osler W (1895a) On the visceral complications of Erythema Exudativum Multiforme. Am J Med Sci 110:629–646.

Osler W (1895b) Neuritis during and after typhoid fever. Johns Hopkins Hospital Reports, Baltimore, v:397–416.

Osler W (1895c) Diseases the direct or indirect result of infection: *In:* A Textbook of Nervous Diseases by American Authors, Edited by F. X. Dercum, Philadelphia, 203–226.

Osler W (1898) Cerebral features of pneumonia. Maryland Med J, Baltimore, xxxviii:381–383.

Osler W (1899a) On the etiology and diagnosis of cerebral spinal fever. Br Med J i:1517–1529.

Osler W (1899b) An acute myxoedematous condition with tachycardia, glycosuria, melaena, mania and death. J Nerv Ment Dis, New York, xxvi:65–71.

Osler W (1900a) Hemiplegia in typhoid fever. Johns Hopkins Hospital Reports, Baltimore, viii:363–371.

Osler W (1900b) The visceral lesions of the erythema group. Br J Derm 12:227–245.

Osler W (1903) On the visceral manifestations of the erythema group of skin diseases. Trans Assoc Am Phys 18:599–624.

Osler W (1909) Paralysis of the left recurrent laryngeal nerve in mitral valve disease. Mont Med J xxvii:79–83.

Osler W (1910a) The pupil symptom in thoracic aneurysm. Practitioner, London, lxxiv:417–422.

Osler W (1910b) Certain vaso-motor sensory and muscular phenomena associated with cervical rib. Am J Med Sci, Philadelphia, New York, cxxix:469–472.

Osler W (1911) Transient attacks of aphasia and paralysis in the states of high blood pressure and arteriosclerosis. Can Med Assoc J i:919–926.

Osler W (1911–12) A case of recurrent aphasia with high blood pressure (discussion). Proc Royal Soc Med, London, v. Clinic Section, 113.

Osler W (1912) Cerebral angiospasm. Lancet ii:1463.

Osler W (1914) Silas Weir Mitchell MD, LLD. Br Med J i:120–121.

Osler W (1914–15) The epidemiology of cerebral spinal meningitis (remarks and discussion). Proc Royal Soc Med, London, ix, Therapeutics and & Pharmacology, sect. 1–5.

Osler W (1916) Sir Victor Horsley (unsigned obituary). Br Med J ii:165.

Osler W (1919a) Typhoid spine. Can Med Assoc J ix:490–496.

Osler W (1919b) Influenza pneumonia: bilateral rigidity, spinal meningitis with hemorrhage into the theca vertebralis and nerve roots. Lancet, i:501.

Osler W (1919c) Book review. Oxford Magazine xxxviii:175.

Peabody G (1891) A contribution to the symptoms and pathology of endarteritis obliterans. Address to The Practitioners Society, New York.

Reddy J (1871–2) On paralysis with aphasia. Can Med J viii:407–408.

Riese W, Jones GL, East IE, Beamer-Maxwell E, Davis HE (1952) Disseminating demyelinating process of over 50 years duration first seen by Dr. William Osler. Confinia Neurologia 12:113–120.

Robbins BH, Christie A (1963) Sir William Osler the pediatrician. Am J Dis Child 106:124–129.

Rodin AE (1981) Oslerian pathology: an assessment and annotated atlas of museum specimens. Coronado Press, Lawrence, Kansas.

Rucker MP (1952) Sir William Osler's obstetric interests. Bull Hist Med 26:153–160.

Russell W (1912) Motor and speech paralysis due to cerebral angiospasm. Lancet ii:1351.

Seguin EC, Shaw JC, van Derveer A (1878) A contribution to the pathological anatomy of disseminated cerebrospinal sclerosis. J Nerv Ment Dis 5:284.

Symonds C (1968) Letter to Charles G. Roland, M.D. February 24, 1968. JAMA, 210:2239.

Tigertt WD (1971) Osler on acromegaly. Can Med Assoc J 105:1336.

Tumulty P, Harvey AM (1949) Disseminated lupus erythematosus. Bulletin of the Johns Hopkins Hosp. 85:47–73.

Wilson SAK (1940) Neurology. Edited by A N Bruce: E. Arnold Co. London.

William Osler and "the special field of neurological surgery"

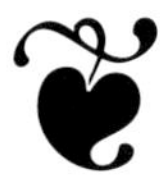 Dee James Canale, M.D.

√ Harvey Cushing's paper, "The special field of neurological surgery," published in the *Bulletin of The Johns Hopkins Hospital* in 1905, constitutes a recognized milestone in the establishment of neurological surgery as a separate surgical specialty in the United States. The main point the author wishes to make here is that the very special friendship of Sir William Osler, influencing, encouraging, stimulating Cushing at the particular time that it did (1901 to 1905), was probably the primary positive influence that made it possible for Cushing to achieve specialization in neurological surgery and to make his considerable contribution in this field.

KEY WORDS • William Osler • Harvey Cushing • neurological surgery • specialization • history of neurosurgery

Neurological surgery began as a special branch of surgery in the latter part of the 19th century as a result of a number of discoveries in medicine, especially the adoption of Lister's principles of aseptic surgery and the development of clinical neurology associated with the rise of the great schools of neurology. Cushing himself recognized that the foundation of neurological surgery rests on the work of Victor Horsley in England and Sir William MacEwen in Scotland.

In the United States, Harvey Cushing was the pre-eminent figure in the development of neurological surgery, along with Charles Frazier and Charles Elsberg. Moreover, Cushing went further than the earlier great British and continental neurosurgeons in that he was the first to limit his practice to neurological surgery. Of perhaps greater significance is his development of a school of neurological surgery which eventually would attract surgeons from abroad to work in his clinic,[44] making him, according to Cairns, "the father of modern brain surgery."[4]

When neurological surgery actually began in America is difficult to pinpoint. The specialty was probably established with Cushing's paper, "The

Read at the annual meeting of the American Osler Society, May 4, 1988.

Reprinted with permission from *Journal of Neurosurgery, 70*:759, 1989 special field of neurological surgery,'' published in March, 1905[17] (Fig 1). Indeed, this subject was significant enough that Cushing revisited the ''special field'' with addresses ''. . . five years later'' in 1910[19] and ''. . . after another interval'' in 1921.[15] Some observers stated that Cushing established neurosurgery as a specialty in the United States in 1908 with the publication of ''Surgery of the head''[20] in *Surgery, Its Principles and Practice,* edited by Keen, who coincidentally proposed the subject to Cushing in 1905. Cushing later stated that the original 1905 paper was written shortly after his decision to limit his surgical work to the nervous system.[18] In this paper, Cushing described the pitfalls of the then common practice of the neurologist calling in an ''operator,'' a surgeon who had little knowledge and perhaps less interest in the problem at hand. Cushing felt that those who focused their studies in this particular field of neurology should do their own operating. In spite of strong opposition to operative specialization from many of his surgical friends, he believed that this was important.

The 1905 paper serves more as a reference point in time than as a medical landmark. Thus, in a brief period of only 4 years following his year abroad, Cushing had established the specialty of neurological surgery in the United States with its beginning in Baltimore. William Osler played a very significant role in influencing and aiding Cushing in this endeavor. Osler certainly advocated specialization.[41]

Harvey Cushing served as William Halsted's resident from 1896 to 1900. Learning Halsted's meticulous surgical techniques uniquely prepared him to adapt these techniques and others to the new field of neurological surgery.[22,35,52] He was able to take advantage of the Professor's increasing absence from the clinic and the operating room to develop his own surgical skills to a very high degree.[31] Halsted gave his resident a good deal of freedom, and Cushing made the most of it with a high degree of scientific curiosity and almost limitless energy. Cushing also had a giant ego to go along with these other qualities. Finishing his training under Halsted undoubtedly would have led to a number of promising opportunities for a career in general surgery; indeed, an offer was made to him to join the staff at Western Reserve in June,

THE SPECIAL FIELD OF NEUROLOGICAL SURGERY.[1]

BY HARVEY CUSHING, M. D.,

Associate Professor of Surgery, The Johns Hopkins University.

Gentlemen:—In response to the friendly request of Dr. Crile, your presiding officer, I shall attempt to formulate some personal views concerning a branch of surgery, which, in this country at least, largely owing to the allurement of other and more immediately promising fields of operative endeavor, has hardly received the attention it deserves.

Through the generosity of Dr. Halsted, his junior associates have been given, in a measure, the privilege of directing the work in some of the subdivisions of his large surgical clinic, in order that they may concentrate their efforts toward advancement along particular lines. It has thus fallen to my lot, temporarily and under his guidance, to control the group of cases which present features chiefly of neurological interest; and it is upon the present possibilities and limitations, as well as upon the future outlook for this department of surgery, that I shall briefly dwell tonight.

To many of us as students, neurology was the *pons asinorum* of the medical curriculum. Nor can I recall any very earnest efforts to cross the bridge, particularly by those of us whose ability to visualize lesions, that probably had never been seen under the microscope nor handled in the gross, was—to say the least—not abnormally developed; and who, for the stimulation of their interest, needed certainties of diagnosis and assurances of therapeutic results. Even for a student, whose inclinations from the beginning may tend in this direction, a steady prosecution of the subject is beset with great discouragements. Special training is necessary before one can obtain a working knowledge of the underlying pathological processes, without which the clinical superstructure is built upon sand. The morbid anatomy of the lesions is greatly obscured by the imperfections of our methods of examination, but still more because they are but rarely seen except at the autopsy table and then only in their terminal stages. Furthermore, owing to the technical difficulties of our present laboratory methods, so long a time often elapses before the histological alterations in the tissues are demonstrable, that, in the interim, our recollection of the clinical picture has become dimmed and interest has fled elsewhere. That the morbid physiology of the subject—its experimental side—when compared with the researches that have been made in other directions, has hardly been touched, may be a matter of

[1] An Address delivered before the Academy of Medicine of Cleveland, November 18, 1904. Reprinted from the *Cleveland Medical Journal*, January, 1905.

FIGURE 1 Title page of Harvey Cushing's landmark paper ''The special field of neurological surgery,'' published in *The Bulletin of The Johns Hopkins Hospital,* in March, 1905.[17]

1900. Halsted actually did nothing to encourage Cushing to embark on a surgical specialty, although he eventually did allow Cushing, albeit somewhat reluctantly, to devote his energies to surgery of the nervous system. Elliott Cutler tells us that Roy McClure, another of Halsted's residents, recalled what took place when Cushing asked Halsted's permission to specialize. The Professor's reply was, "Why, Dr. Cushing, we had only two cases of brain tumor last year!" Cushing persisted, however, and Halsted subsequently said, "All right, the field is yours."[23]

In contrast, William Osler played an all-important role in shaping Cushing's early career as the foremost neurosurgeon of his time. This remarkable friendship has been clearly described in the splendid Presidential Address to the American Osler Society by Jeremiah Barondess in 1984.[2] This friendship has traditionally been credited by Fulton[29–31] and Penfield[43] for shaping Cushing's interest in the human and cultural aspects of medicine, including medical history, book collecting, and medical institutions, rather than the strictly professional side of medicine. Ebers[26] raised the question, "Did Osler push Cushing into neurosurgery?" The evidence suggests not, but that Cushing made his own decision to specialize in neurosurgery, with Osler supplying many of the key ingredients which paved the way for Cushing's success.

Unfortunately, the most likely source from which one would expect to learn of this connection (namely, the Osler biography[11]) is silent on the subject. As Fulton[29] noted, Cushing left himself out of the book completely. This unnecessary anonymity regrettably leaves a void in the records for the years 1900 to 1905, when Cushing was most closely associated with Sir William Osler. William Welch[53] noted that this was almost unparalleled in a biographer. Dr. William Feindel (personal communication, 1987) noted that this circumstance was similar to the apostle John's veiled references to himself in the "Gospel according to St. John" in the New Testament.

One of the curious aspects of Cushing's career was that his development of neurosurgery at The Johns Hopkins Hospital was not associated with a dominant school of clinical neurology, as was the case in Great Britain, on the continent, and even in Philadelphia, where William Spiller and Charles K. Mills were coworkers and were responsible with Charles Frazier for much of the latter's early neurosurgical endeavors. The development of neurosurgery in New York likewise was dominated by a group of prominent neurologists, who invited Charles Elsberg to join them at the New York Neurological Institute in 1909. It was apparent that even as a resident Cushing felt that a surgeon should have the responsibility of acting largely on his own diagnosis, and that he should be impelled seriously to study his own cases before they came to the operating table.[14] This environment was in sharp contrast to that in Philadelphia, where Charles K. Mills considered that ". . . one of the functions of the neurologist is to superintend and direct operative procedures upon the brain and spinal cord by the surgeon."[27]

It was precisely the unique milieu of clinical neurology at The Johns Hopkins Hospital, with William Osler as the dominant figure, that nurtured the aggressive Cushing in his quest for the new subspecialty. George Ebers[26] has clearly demonstrated Osler's place in neurology; moreover, Russell DeJong[25] has stated that the history of American neurology in the latter part of the 19th century would not be complete without William Osler. It was not Osler's position as head of the traditionally prominent clinical neurology service that provided the foundation for Cushing's neurosurgical growth, but rather his counsel and friendship during Cushing's last 2 years as a resident, his year abroad, and those intimate years from 1901 to 1905 when Cushing was a "latchkeyer." Osler is said to have been a spiritual father to Cushing, and to have had a keener understanding of Cushing's own restless nature than almost anyone.[29] Indeed, in their stimulating influence over others to accomplish some good piece of work, Osler and Weir Mitchell had no rivals.[36]

Before discussing neurology in the early days at The Johns Hopkins Hospital, I will make a brief digression for a look at Osler's Philadelphia days which will reveal connections that later played a role in Cushing's development. A favorite photograph from the Osler biography is the picture of Osler at the Orthopedic Hospital and Infirmary for Nervous Diseases, which illustrates in a sense "the complete Osler." He is shown here with attending staff, nurses, and patients—two children possibly with cerebral palsy or chorea, who may have become the subjects of two monographs he wrote during this period.[37,38] Also shown are open atlases on the table, a skull, and what appear to be fixed specimens of brain (Fig. 2). Osler's appointment to the hospital was secured by Weir Mitchell.[3] Osler was to become intimate friends with Mitchell and with others, including W.W. Keen—the most important 19th century American surgeon to operate with success on the brain. These lasting friendships made in Philadelphia, which will be referred to again later, had special significance for Harvey Cushing.[24]

When The Johns Hopkins Hospital opened in 1889, Osler was appointed Physician and Chief of the Hospital. He was in charge of three departments in the outpatient dispensary, one of which was the "Department of Nervous Disease." Working with Osler in this Department was Dr. Henry Thomas, who was appointed Assistant in Nervous Diseases, and who soon began to give weekly clinical lectures. Thomas, the son of a trustee of Johns Hopkins University, was a graduate of the University of Maryland School of Medicine, where his interest in neurology was awakened by Professor Miles. Thomas spent a year in Europe studying in Vienna and working under Wilhelm Erb in Heidelberg; however, he probably learned more neurology from Osler.[1] Thomas admitted that Osler was looked upon as a guiding star of the younger clinicians, and stated that: "What good there is in me as a teacher and physician I owe to him."[48] After The Johns Hopkins Medical School opened in the autumn of 1893, Osler gave Thomas charge of neurological training, and Thomas was appointed Clinical Professor of Nervous Diseases in 1896.

Reviewing case reports in the *Bulletin of The Johns Hopkins Hospital*, the reader gets the feeling that Osler had the final word on the Neurology Service. An example is a case report of a neurological disorder presented to the hospital medical society in February, 1894, which concludes with the statement: "In Dr. Osler's unavoidable absence, I am unwilling to make any definite statement as to the diagnosis in this case."[45] Another example is a brain-tumor patient of Dr. Thomas.[50] Osler saw the patient on April 10, 1896, "confirmed the diagnosis" of a brain tumor, and advised "pushing the iodide and mercury." The patient, failing to improve, was again seen by Osler with Thomas 3 weeks later, and Osler "urged the operation." Dr. Keen, who was asked to perform the surgery, successfully removed a large left frontal meningioma. Osler and Thomas were present during the surgery, and examined the tumor carefully, "while waiting for the hemorrhage to be arrested." This report illustrates Osler's active participation in neurological cases and, in addition, his appreciation for surgery for certain disorders of the brain.

Osler's recognition of the place of surgery in treating certain disorders of the nervous system becomes clear through his association with Sir William

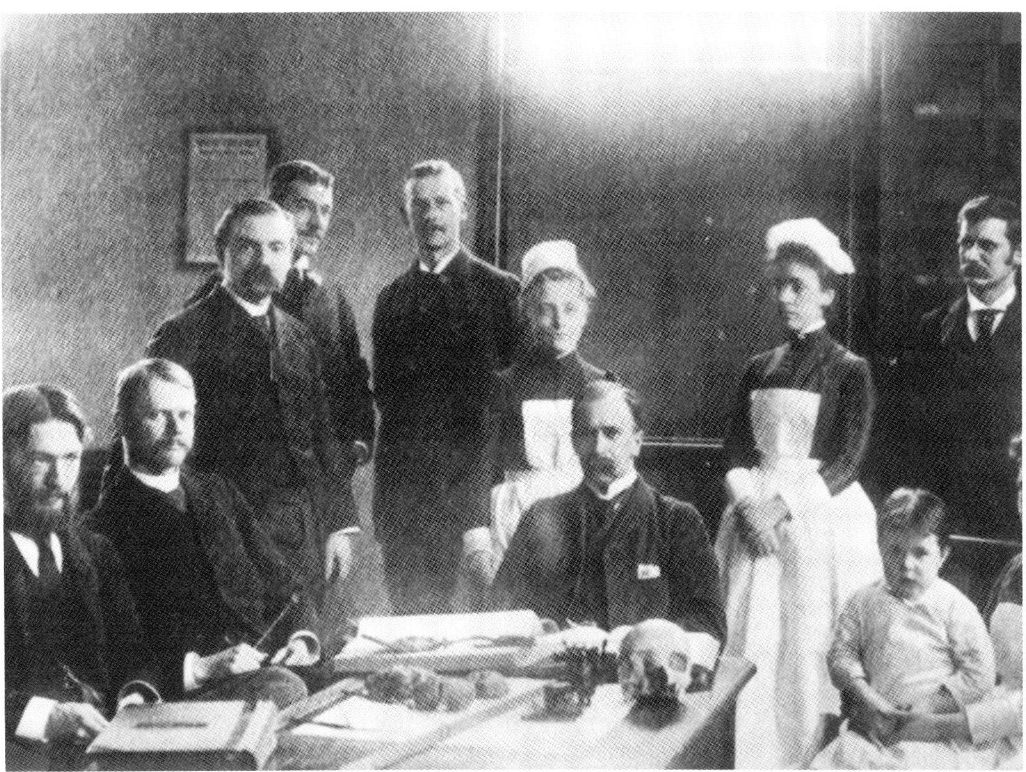

FIGURE 2   Photograph of William Osler surrounded by (from left to right) J.M. Catell, Guy Hinsdale, J.P. Willitts, J.K. Mitchell, G.E. de Schweinitz, Miss C. Dalziel, Mrs. Green, Joseph Otto, Miss J. Dalziel, and two young patients. The picture was taken at the Orthopedic Hospital and Infirmary for Nervous Diseases. (Reproduced from Cushing H: *The Life of Sir William Osler*. Oxford: Clarendon Press, 1925.)

Gowers and Victor Horsley and their work in London. Theirs was probably the leading center of neurology at this time. In August, 1894, Osler spent a few days with Gowers in London.[11] He had been a friend of Gowers since 1878. It is interesting that Osler's monograph, *On Chorea and Choreiform Affections*,[38] published that same year (1894) is dedicated to Gowers. During this same visit with Gowers, Osler observed Victor Horsley remove a meningioma. Osler had first met Horsley one summer evening in 1878 while Horsley was a student at University College. Probably no other American neurologist had a closer insight into the pioneering work of Horsley than Osler, who followed Horsley's career closely as he became the greatest Hunterian surgeon of his day.[42] It is easy to understand why Osler advocated surgical treatment of certain brain and spinal cord tumors, brain abscesses, and subdural hematomas, citing primarily the work of Horsley in the first edition of his book *The Principles and Practice of Medicine*.[39]

This was the setting when Cushing arrived in Baltimore in 1896, the same year that Keen operated on the patient mentioned above. Cushing's first formal piece of writing was "Haematomyelia from gunshot wounds of the spine. A report of two cases, with recovery following symptoms of hemilesion of the cord."[9] One of the cases had been presented previously to The Johns Hopkins Hospital Medical Society on May 3, 1897. Discussing the case, Dr. Thomas stated: "I know of no case in the hospital records that has been worked up so carefully as this."[47] Recalling this experience 25 years later in his

Presidential Address to the American Neurological Association, Cushing stated: "The opportunity personally to study for the first time a neurological case, which though a nonoperative one had drifted into and was permitted to remain in a surgical ward, made a great impression on me, and, spurred on by H.M. Thomas and L.F. Barker, with the report of this case I started on my inky way."[13] It is significant that, through 1905, Cushing coauthored only one neurological paper with Henry Thomas, and that was on the subject of lesions of the brachial plexus."[49] This probably represents his desire to make his own neurological diagnosis. Cushing also had a tendency to omit credit to coworkers, a concern Osler would address later.

In all likelihood, Osler acted increasingly as Cushing's chief stimulus and mentor during the last 2 years of his residency. Osler counseled Cushing regarding an offer from the Department of Surgery at Western Reserve University in 1899 and, along with Welch, encouraged his "young friend" to go abroad for a year of study.[29] One incident in particular stands out during this period. In April, 1900, Cushing was requested by W.W. Keen to read a paper on gasserian ganglion resection at a meeting of the College of Physicians of Philadelphia.[12] Cushing reported on his surgical technique, illustrated with drawings from four cases of gasserian ganglion resection for trigeminal neuralgia. He had operated on his first case in 1899, barely a year before. As William German noted, "Here we find the young H.C. [Harvey Cushing], not yet five years out of medical school, speaking in the Temple to the Elders in neurology and surgery."[32] In addition to Keen, participants included William Spiller, Frances Dercum, Robert Abbe, and Charles Dana. Cushing's paper was brilliant, though a year later Spiller and Frazier would demonstrate that retrogasserian section of the trigeminal root was a superior procedure.[46] It is doubtful that Cushing had met or had any direct association with Keen prior to that meeting. How was it then that Cushing was invited to give this important paper by the then dean of the American surgeons and America's greatest pioneer brain surgeon? The invitation may well have been initiated by William Osler, whose very warm personal friendship with Keen would have brought Cushing's work to Keen's attention.[28]

Encouraged by Osler and Welch to go abroad for a year of study, Cushing sailed for England in June, 1900.[51] It was his intention to give priority to study with men whose interests were neurological, especially Kocher, Horsley, and Sherrington. It was during his first month in England that Cushing first came into intimate contact with Osler. Osler was spending the summer in England "brain dusting." According to Fulton, Osler must have gone out of his way to include Cushing in many social and senior scientific gatherings he would not otherwise have been included in.[29,31] Osler's interest in Cushing is illustrated in his response, in the spring of 1900, to an inquiry about Cushing by one of his Yale classmates. Osler replied: "Your friend Cushing has opened the book of surgery to a new place."[51]

Initially, after arriving in London, Cushing spent only a brief time with Horsley. During this period, he watched Horsley perform several operations on brain and spinal cases. His year abroad was highlighted, however, by his work in Berne under Theodore Kocher. Cushing's brilliant experiments demonstrating the effect of intracranial pressure on systemic blood pressure had been suggested by Kocher.[5,29] This was to be one of the most important fundamental neurophysiological discoveries. Cushing had become interested in Kocher through his original study of his case of hematomyelia of the spinal cord. Kocher was greatly admired by Halsted, with whom he had much in common.[22] Cushing then spent a month in Turin in northern Italy in the laboratory of the Italian physiologist, Angelo Mosso, repeating his Berne experiments.[51]

Cushing returned to England in early July. He had written to Horsley about working with him, but Horsley advised him to visit Sherrington in Liverpool. After spending 3 days with Osler, whose friendship with Sherrington dated from 1894, Cushing went up to Liverpool."[33] Here he found valuable experience operating on primates in Sherrington's laboratory. Cushing impressed Sherrington with the surgical technique he used on these animals, as well as with his illustrations of his experiments. Later Cushing stated that he had no idea during his year abroad that he would specialize in neurological surgery.

Cushing returned to the United States and Baltimore in August, 1901, largely due, as he later said, to pressure brought to bear by Welch and Osler. Halsted delayed Cushing's appointment until October of that year. It was finally agreed, however, that, in addition to "other duties," Cushing would get the neurological cases.

It was at this time that Cushing, along with Thomas Futcher and Henry Barton Jacobs, moved into 3 West Franklin Street next door to the Oslers, and became one of the "latchkeyers" for the next 4 important years. Settling in at The Johns Hopkins Hospital, he began to undertake some private work and took over the course in operative surgery for 3rd-year students. Referrals were infrequent, especially of neurological cases.[13] In the decade ending in 1899, only two brain-tumor cases had been operated on at The Johns Hopkins Hospital, and both patients had died. Because of their uncertainties and fears, physicians were reluctant to refer patients for cranial surgery during this period.

A few months after returning to Baltimore, Cushing was invited by W.W. Keen to give the Mütter lecture in Philadelphia in December, 1901.[51] Cushing described the work he had done in Hugo Kroneckor's laboratory in Berne. The problem of "Hirndruck" and the relationship between intracranial pressure and blood pressure had been suggested by Professor Theodore Kocher.[16]

A year later in November, 1902, Cushing returned to Philadelphia at the request of Charles Mills to discuss his paper on brain tumors. Cushing stated: "Little could I have known about the subject. I had had perhaps a case or two at the Church Home and Infirmary, but could scarcely have had any successful cases at the time in question."[29] Following the talk, he was invited by Weir Mitchell, whom he met now for the first time, to come to his home. Cushing spent the evening and into the early morning hours with Mitchell, his son Jack, and W.W. Keen, talking about books and sampling some old Madeira wine. Osler's Philadelphia connection can be seen again in this professional and social encounter.

Osler assisted Cushing perhaps indirectly in his early endeavors in neurosurgery, but he helped him directly and in a substantive manner by referral of patients. In the Mütter lecture, Cushing described, in addition to his experimental studies, clinical observations of three cases of increased intracranial pressure with medullary failure resulting in death. Two of the cases, including one of a cerebellar cyst, were referred by Dr. Osler.[16]

In March, 1902, Cushing presented a ninth case of gasserian ganglion extirpation to The Johns Hopkins Hospital Medical Society.[8] In discussing the patient, Osler stated: "It is really a difficult thing to get physicians to appreciate the extraordinary benefit of this operation. The doctor under whose care the patient was, consulted me several times about it and it was with

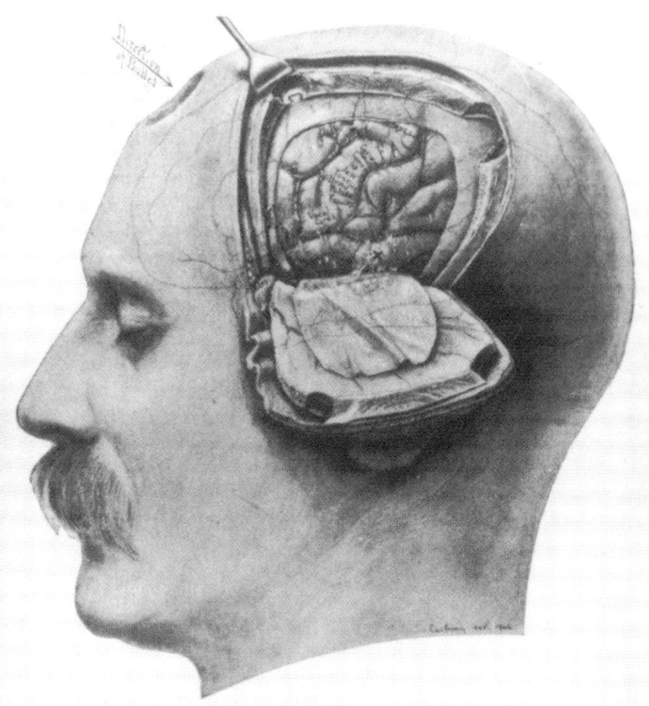

FIGURE 3 Drawing by Cushing used to illustrate his chapter "Surgery of the head" in Keen WW (ed): *Surgery, Its Principles and Practice*. Philadelphia: WB Saunders, 1908, Vol 3, pp 17–276. The patient shows the unmistakable likeness of William Osler.

some difficulty that I persuaded him to have the operation performed." In 1903 and 1904, two additional cases of trigeminal neuralgia were referred by Osler to Cushing for surgery. The latter case was operated on by Cushing in Montreal, apparently the first operation of its kind done there.[29] The first brain-tumor case that Cushing operated on was one of a tumor in the pituitary region. Referred by Osler in 1902, the patient underwent three operations without the tumor being located, and eventually died.[15]

One of Cushing's most important early contributions to neurosurgery was his method of subtemporal or occipital decompression for inaccessible brain tumor. This procedure, devised by Cushing, afforded rather dramatic relief for those patients with increased intracranial pressure and failing vision. This method allowed decompression with opening of the dura, and permitted closure such that the wound did not break down with resulting cerebral fungus. Cushing reported 15 cases in 1905.[7] In two of the three examples described in this report, the referring physician was William Osler.

Cushing's first operation for removal of a benign intradural spinal tumor was performed in November, 1903.[10] Osler's note of the case indicating his confidence in Cushing is worth quoting: "When the patient first consulted me I suspected cervical caries or pachymeningitis. It was not until after his admission to the hospital, and more careful study of the case with Dr. H.M. Thomas, that tumor was suspected. I urged early operation, feeling sure that the condition would not be made worse." This tumor, probably a meningioma, was quite rare in those days, and was similar to Horsley's famous case. This was Cushing's first intradural spinal cord tumor, and he considered it as perhaps a "once in a lifetime case." Cushing stated: "Due to the early and unequivocal diagnosis made after the patient's admission to Dr. Osler's service, and his prompt transference for operation without the customary period temporizing with antiluetic treatment, the case seems in many respects the most satisfactory of any heretofore recorded."[10] What better source of referral than from the most eminent and widely influential physician of his time.

Early in 1904, W.W. Keen offered Cushing the Chair in Surgery at Jefferson Medical College. Cushing eventually declined the offer after consultation with Osler.[34] Perhaps more important, however, was the fact that Keen would ask him, in August, 1905, to write the "Surgery of the head" section for *Surgery, Its Principles and Practice*,[20] which he edited and which was finally published in 1908 (Fig. 3). This represented Cushing's first systematic treatise on brain surgery, and established him as the leader of the new specialty. By this time, Cushing's growing reputation was bringing him both students and increasing numbers of patients.[51]

As indicated earlier, Cushing established neurosurgery as a specialty with his paper, "The special field of neurological surgery." The paper was originally presented to the Academy of Medicine in Cleveland in November, 1904, and was subsequently published in the *Bulletin of The Johns Hopkins Hospital* in March, 1905. A photograph of Cushing taken at about that time with Halsted and his "All-Star" team is presented in Fig. 4. The theme of the paper, after a review of the status of surgery for various disorders of the nervous system, was the necessity for specialization in surgery of the nervous system. Cushing emphasized that the surgeon should work closely with the neurologist and, moreover, be familiar with all aspects of neurology, and not simply act as a technician to be called in at the last moment by the neurologist. The importance of the 1905 paper is even more obvious in his paper on the same subject 5 years later.[19] In the 1905 paper, Cushing's discussion of surgery on brain tumors was largely confined to the decompression procedure for

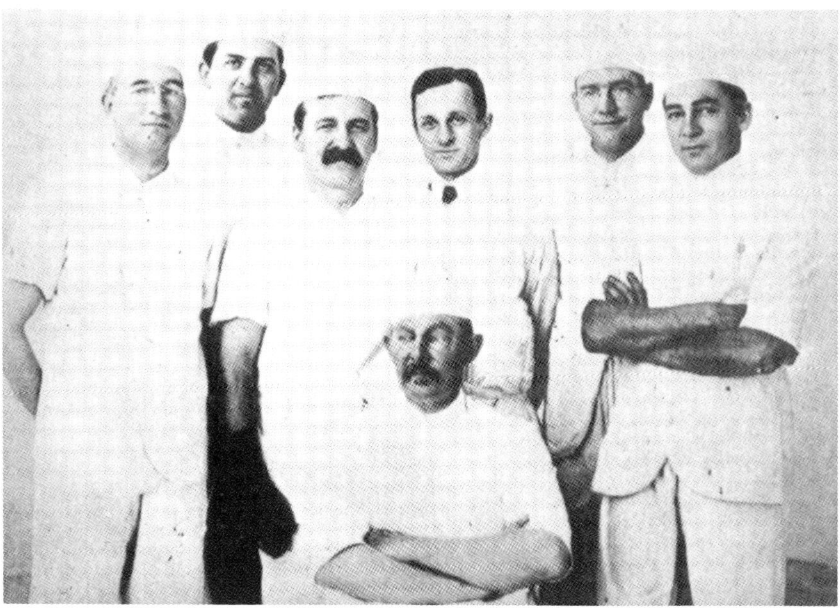

FIGURE 4 Photograph of the young Harvey Cushing 1 month preceding presentation of his paper "The special field of neurological surgery." The legend reads: "Halsted's 'All-Star' Team. Standing: Young, Follis, Finney, Cushing, Bloodgood, Mitchell. Seated: Halsted. 5 October, 1904." (Original photograph is in the Yale Medical Library, New Haven, Connecticut.)

temporary relief of symptoms in cases of brain tumor, which were "few and far between." By 1910, however, he had performed some 250 operative procedures on 180 patients with brain tumors. Cushing also noted that other young men were preparing to specialize in neurological surgery.

The sixth edition of Osler's *The Principles and Practice of Medicine* was published in 1905.[40] In the preface, dated May, 1905, just when he was leaving Baltimore and The Johns Hopkins Hospital, Osler thanked Harvey Cushing of the Surgical Clinic along with H.M. Thomas of the Neurological Department for revision of the section on the nervous system.[6] What an acknowledgment of Cushing and of the new specialty for him to be able to contribute his experience to the newest edition of the "most used and useful book in medicine."[21]

In summary, William Osler was, by his counsel, encouragement, association with influential figures in neurology, and (most importantly) his referral of neurological cases, of paramount importance in Harvey Cushing's development of the then new "special field of neurological surgery." The specialty was established by Cushing at the end of his closest and most intimate association with William Osler during the Baltimore period prior to Osler's departure in May of 1905 to become Regius Professor of Medicine at Oxford.

Finally, Cushing spoke of a particular quality of Osler that to him was especially significant: ". . . perhaps because of his unusual powers of visualizing disease gained in the post-mortem room, he was far more tolerant than most of his contemporaries in the so-called surgical invasion of the traditional province of internal medicine . . . ; and it has been said of him that few physicians have ever shown better surgical judgement or had a more instinctive and certain knowledge of the proper moment for surgical intervention."[11]

Acknowledgment

The author is grateful to Ms. Florence M. Bruce for her assistance with the writing and overall preparation of the manuscript.

References

1. Barker LF: Henry M. Thomas, M.D., 1861–1925. *Arch Neurol Psychiatry* 16:78–81, 1926
2. Barondess JA: Cushing and Osler: the evolution of a friendship. *Trans Stud Coll Physicians Phila* 7:79–111, 1985
3. Burr AR: *Weir Mitchell: His Life and Letters.* New York: Duffield, 1929
4. Cairns H: Harvey Cushing: a surgeon's tribute. *Lancet* 2: 857–858, 1939 (Letter)
5. Cushing H: Concerning a definite regulatory mechanism of the vasomotor centre which controls blood pressure during cerebral compression. *Bull Johns Hopkins Hosp* 12:290–292, 1901
6. Cushing H: Diseases of the nervous system, in Osler W (ed): *The Principles and Practice of Medicine, ed 6.* New York/London: D Appleton, 1905, pp 867–1110
7. Cushing H: The establishment of cerebral hernia as a decompressive measure for inaccessible brain tumors: with the description of intermus-

cular methods of making the bone defect in temporal and occipital regions. *Surg Gynecol Obstet 1*:297–314, 1905

8. Cushing H: Exhibition of surgical cases. A ninth case of Gasserian ganglion extirpation. *Bull Johns Hopkins Hosp 13*:248–249, 1902

9. Cushing H: Haematomyelia from gunshot wounds of the spine. A report of two cases, with recovery following symptoms of hemilesion of the cord. *Am J Med Sci 115:* 654–683, 1898

10. Cushing H: Intradural tumor of the cervical meninges. With early restoration of function in the cord after removal of the tumor. *Am Surg 39*:934–955, 1904

11. Cushing H: *The Life of Sir William Osler.* Oxford: Clarendon Press, 1925

12. Cushing H: A method of total extirpation of the Gasserian ganglion for trigeminal neuralgia. By a route through the temporal fossa and beneath the middle meningeal artery. *JAMA 34*:1035–1041, 1900

13. Cushing H: Neurological surgeons: with the report of one case. *Arch Neurol Psychiatry 10*:381–390, 1923

14. Cushing H: The physician and the surgeon. *Boston Med Surg J 187*:623–630, 1922

15. Cushing H: *The Pituitary Body and Its Disorders. Clinical States Produced by Disorders of the Hypophysis Cerebri. An Amplification of the Harvey Lecture for December 1910.* Philadelphia/London: JB Lippincott, 1912

16. Cushing H: Some experimental and clinical observations concerning states of increased intracranial tension. *Am J Med Sci 124*:375–400, 1902

17. Cushing H: The special field of neurological surgery. *Bull Johns Hopkins Hosp 16*:77–87, 1905

18. Cushing H: The special field of neurological surgery after another interval. *Ohio State Med J 17*:293–302, 373–380, 1921

19. Cushing H: The special field of neurological surgery: five years later. *Bull Johns Hopkins Hosp 21*:325–339, 1910

20. Cushing H: Surgery of the head, in Keen WW (ed): *Surgery, Its Principles and Practice.* Philadelphia: WB Saunders, 1908, Vol 3, pp 17–276

21. Cushing H: William Osler, the man. *Ann Med Hist 2*:157–167, 1920

22. Cushing H: William Stewart Halsted, 1852–1922. *Science 56*:461–464, 1922

23. Cutler E: Memoir: Harvey (Williams) Cushing 1869–1939. *Ann Surg 111*:663–672, 1940

24. Davidson GA: Men of Osler's time. *Bull Vancouver Med Assoc 26*:183–192, 1950

25. DeJong RN: *A History of American Neurology.* New York: Raven Press, 1982

26. Ebers GC: Osler and neurology. *Can J Neurol Sci 12*:236–242, 1985

27. Elsberg CA: The development of neurological surgery in New York during the past twenty-five years. *J Mt Sinai Hosp 9*:413–418, 1942

28. Erikson GE: Sir William Osler and William Williams Keen. *Osler Library Newsletter, Vol II,* 1972

29. Fulton JF: *Harvey Cushing. A Biography.* Springfield, Ill: Charles C Thomas, 1946

30. Fulton JF: Harvey Cushing: in appreciation. *Sci Mon 49*:477–479, 1939

31. Fulton JF: Harvey Cushing's early training. *Bull NY Acad Med 23*:545–563, 1947

32. German WJ: Trigeminal neuralgia, in Matson DD, German WJ (eds): *Harvey Cushing 1869–1939. Selected Papers on Neurosurgery.* New Haven: Yale University Press, 1969, pp 41–42

33. Gibson WC: The friendship of Osler and Sherrington, in Barondess JA, McGovern JP, Roland CG (eds): *The Persisting Osler*. Baltimore: University Park Press, 1985, pp 181–186

34. Green JR: William Williams Keen, M.D., pioneer American neurological surgeon. *BNI Quart I(4):* 15–28, 1985

35. Horrax G: Harvey Cushing, '95. *Harvard Medical Alumni Bulletin 14:*15, 1939

36. Keen WW: *The Surgical Operation on President Cleveland in 1893 Together with Six Additional Papers of Reminiscences*. Philadelphia/London: JB Lippincott, 1928

37. Osler W: *The Cerebral Palsies of Children*. Philadelphia: Blakiston, 1889

38. Osler W: *On Chorea and Choreiform Affections*. Philadelphia: Blakiston, 1894

39. Osler W: *The Principles and Practice of Medicine*. New York: D Appleton, 1892

40. Osler W: *The Principles and Practice of Medicine, ed 6*. New York/London: D Appleton, 1905

41. Osler W: Remarks on specialism. *Boston Med Surg J 126:*457–459, 1892

42. Osler W: Sir Victor Horsley (unsigned obituary). *Br Med J ii:*165, 1916

43. Penfield W: The passing of Harvey Cushing. *Yale J Biol Med 12:*323–326, 1940

44. Sachs E: The most important steps in the development of neurological surgery. *Yale J Biol Med 28:*444–450, 1955

45. Smith FR: A case presenting the group of symptoms termed astasia-abasia. *Bull Johns Hopkins Hosp 5:*13–16, 1894

46. Spiller WB, Frazier CH: The division of the sensory root of the trigeminus for the relief of tic douloureux: an experimental, pathological, and clinical study, with the preliminary report of one surgically successful case. *Univ Penn Med Bull 14:*341–352, 1901

47. Thomas HM: The Johns Hopkins Hospital Medical Society (unsigned). *Bull Johns Hopkins Hosp 8:*195–197, 1897

48. Thomas HM: Some memories of the development of the medical school and of Osler's advent. *Bull Johns Hopkins Hosp 30:*185–189, 1919

49. Thomas HM, Cushing H: Exhibition of two cases of radicular paralysis of the brachial plexus. One from the pressure of a cervical rib, with operation. The other of uncertain origin. *Bull Johns Hopkins Hosp 14:*315–319, 1903

50. Thomas HM, Keen WW: A successful case of removal of a large brain-tumor from the left frontal region. Opening and packing of the lateral ventricle with iodoform-gauze. *Am J Med Sci 112:*503–522, 1896

51. Thomson EH: *Harvey Cushing: Surgeon, Author, Artist*. New York: Henry Schuman, 1950

52. Tilney NL: Harvey Cushing and the Oxford connection. *Surg Gynecol Obstet 155:*89–94, 1982

53. Welch WH: A great physician and medical humanist. *Sat Rev Lit 2:*309–310, 1925

Harvey Cushing and Pediatric Neurosurgery

 Dee James Canale, M.D., and
Lawrence D. Longo, M.D.

Harvey Cushing made fundamental and seminal contributions to pediatric neurosurgery. Early in his surgical career, he described the diagnosis and treatment of subdural hematomas in newborn infants. Important investigations on the cerebrospinal fluid and the nature of hydrocephalus were carried out under his direction, first by Walter Dandy and Kenneth Blackfan in the Hunterian Laboratory at the Johns Hopkins School of Medicine, and shortly afterward by Lewis Weed at the Laboratory of Surgical Research at Harvard. Cushing's principal interest throughout his professional career was the surgical treatment of brain tumors. By his careful clinical examination of patients, Cushing described for the first time a typical and composite picture of the more common tumors of the posterior fossa in children, particularly the cerebellar astrocytomas and medulloblastomas. Percival Bailey, working under Cushing's supervision at Harvard, studied and classified the glioma group of brain tumors. This contribution by Bailey was a major factor in the understanding of the characteristics and natural history of these tumors. In the closing years of Cushing's surgical practice, he published three major papers summarizing the characteristics, clinical picture, and treatment of the more common brain tumors in the pediatric age group. As a result of his exceptional surgical skill and innovations, he was able to achieve a surgical mortality of only 4% in operations on brain tumors in children. These landmark papers secured Cushing's place as a pioneer in pediatric neurosurgery. (*Neurosurgery* 27:602–611, 1990)

Key words: Harvey Cushing, Percival Bailey, Cerebellar tumors, Glioma classification, Pediatric neurosurgery.

Probably the chief architect and builder of the specialty of neurosurgery was Harvey Williams Cushing (1869–1939).[7] Among Cushing's major accomplishments were his contributions to neurosurgery of children and adolescents.[28,37] To quote John Farquhar Fulton (1899–1960),

Read at the annual meeting of the American Osler Society, May 9, 1990.

Reprinted with permission from *Neurosurgery, 27:*602, 1990

> Harvey Cushing was widely known in three distinct capacities—as a great physician, as the founder of a school of neurosurgery, and as a humanist of unusual literary attainment. ([27] pp 477).

Perhaps Cushing's greatest neurosurgical contribution was in the field of intracranial tumors, which became the main focus of his professional life. His meticulous surgical technique, learned from the "Professor," William S. Halsted (1852–1922), was especially important in his development of this "special" field of neurosurgery. Additionally, he developed technical aids that greatly enhanced the ability to remove tumors. These included the silver clip for occlusion of blood vessels and the use of the electrosurgical instrument for tumor removal, which he introduced with William T. Bovie (1882–1958).[12,18,19]

Cushing's special interest in intracranial tumors is evident in his writings. Three of his principal monographs deal with pituitary tumors, acoustic tumors, and meningiomas.[13,15,22,23] His interest in tumors, as will be shown later, also culminated in three classic reports in which he described, for the first time, the clinical features, classification, natural history, and successful surgical treatment of the more common brain tumors of childhood.

Cushing's first paper relating to pediatric neurosurgery, "Concerning Surgical Intervention for Intracranial Hemorrhages of the New-born," was published in 1905.[9] He reported on four infants who, after either prolonged labor and spontaneous delivery or a difficult delivery, were depressed and developed seizures and other neurological signs. Cushing operated a few days after birth, finding massive subdural hematomas. Two of these newborns survived, one with apparently minimal sequelae. Cushing thus demonstrated that surgery on such newborns could be successful.

Cushing's "Surgery of the Head," published in 1908 in *Surgery, Its Principles and Practice,* edited by William W. Keen (1837–1932)[10], was the first definitive American work on neurosurgery.[31] In this work, Cushing further discussed treatment of neonatal injuries to the skull and nervous system. He described the recognition and treatment of hydrocephalus, including congenital hydrocephalus in the newborn associated with spina bifida (meningomyelocele).

Cushing reported 12 cases in which he used a new technique in operating on patients in whom the ventricles communicated with the lumbar subarachnoid space. He trephined the L5 vertebra through a laparotomy and transperitoneal approach, combining this with a laminectomy, and placed a silver cannula that connected and drained the subarachnoid space into the peritoneal cavity. Although he reported a "considerable measure of success" in these 12 cases, long-term follow-up was wanting. Later, however, he noted that none of the surgical procedures gave uniform results.[11] A lumbar subarachnoid-peritoneal shunt had not previously been reported. This principle of treating hydrocephalus, long abandoned, would eventually be rediscovered, improved upon, and adapted to the modern treatment of hydrocephalic infants.

The first attempt at shunting the cerebrospinal fluid into the jugular vein was done by Roy McClure, a resident of Halsted's working in the Hunterian Laboratory. The experiments were done "on the suggestion of Dr. Alexis Carrel and with the encouragement of Dr. Cushing."[14,36]

McClure conducted six experiments on normal dogs. He anastomosed a segment of external jugular vein, taken from the contralateral neck, from the subdural space to the external jugular vein on the ipsilateral side, placed so the valves would prevent retrograde flow of blood toward the subdural space.

The end-to-end anastomosis of the veins was done by the Carrel method. The procedure was performed on one patient of Dr. Cushing's, a 10-month-old baby who had had progressive hydrocephalus since a premature birth. Numerous ventricular and lumbar punctures had been made, affording only temporary relief. The condition was felt to be a case of unilateral external hydrocephalus with fluid in the subdural space. A subdural external jugular shunt was performed under cocaine anesthesia using a cephalic vein from the father's arm. The baby tolerated the surgical procedure well, but a few hours after surgery, developed sudden elevation of temperature and died.[36] This was the first use of an operation that, years later, would be refined into a useful procedure for shunt placement in hydrocephalic patients.

In the Hunterian laboratory of Surgical Research at the Johns Hopkins Medical School, Cushing initiated various studies on the cerebrospinal fluid that profoundly influenced other investigators, such as Walter E. Dandy (1886–1946), Lewis H. Weed (1886–1952), and Kenneth D. Blackfan (1883–1941).[29] Cushing's first paper on this topic was published in 1914.[14] In this paper, Cushing reviewed the current knowledge of the formation, absorption, and characteristics of the cerebrospinal fluid. Going beyond the suggestion of Key and Retzius[33] that the cerebrospinal fluid was absorbed by the Pacchionian granulations, Cushing held that the arachnoid villi along the major longitudinal sinuses, the dural sinuses in the middle cranial fossa, and the larger convexity veins were the major sites for absorption of cerebrospinal fluid. He noted that after Weed's studies, he (Cushing) abandoned his "preconceived idea" of a valvular action in the arachnoid villi. The function of the arachnoid villi was the "chief emphasis" of his studies at this time.[14]

Weed concluded that "the chief method of return of cerebrospinal fluid to the general circulation is by a process of filtration through the arachnoid villi into the great sinuses." Weed also believed that absorption from the cranial subarachnoid space was much more rapid and in a much greater amount than that from the spinal portion.[38]

Cushing also noted the acceleration of the development of hydrocephalus after surgical repair of one of the major forms of spinal or cranial meningoceles in infants. He was of the opinion that the hydrocephalus was the result of failure of absorption in the arachnoid villi and not always due to blockage of the foramen of Magendie.[14]

Cushing's interest in cerebrospinal fluid studies and hydrocephalus unfortunately was associated with one of the regrettable schisms in American neurosurgery. Cushing selected Walter Dandy to be his assistant resident and appointee in the Hunterian Laboratory for the academic year 1911–1912. During that year, as Fulton noted, a conflict of personalities arose relating to Dandy's investigations, ([28] p. 316). Dandy and Blackfan had begun their classic studies on experimental hydrocephalus in 1911. As Cushing was leaving Baltimore to take up his new appointment at Harvard and the Brigham Hospital, he placed Dandy's papers in a box of materials from the Hunterian Laboratory he was taking with him to Boston. As Fox later recounted, Dandy removed his records, stating that it was his work, and that it would remain in Baltimore. For Cushing, this apparently was the "final straw," and shortly afterwards, he informed Dandy that he would not be taking him to Boston.[26] What part, if any, Cushing had in initiating these experiments other than allowing them to be performed in his laboratory, is unknown. Cushing certainly had a strong interest in hydrocephalus in children. This landmark experimental work by Dandy and Blackfan proved for the first time that cerebrospinal fluid was secreted by the choriod plexus and absorbed diffusely by the pia-arachnoid veins.[24,25] These classic experiments formed the basis of our understanding of the nature and treatment of obstructive and communicating hydrocephalus.

Because of his rigid temperament and precipitous decision over this affair, Cushing's Laboratory of Surgical Research at Harvard lost credit that it surely otherwise would have gained for this outstanding work. A great opportunity to find a solution to the problem of hydrocephalus was lost.[29] It is a pity that Cushing did not recall that he had been in exactly the same situation as Dandy when he was working under Kocher's direction in Berne just a few years earlier.[28]

Lewis Weed, who also had begun experimental studies on cerebrospinal fluid and the pituitary gland in the Hunterian Laboratory, was invited by Cushing to go to Boston. Weed continued his important studies on cerebrospinal fluid as a fellow in charge of the Laboratory of Surgical Research in 1912.[37,38] Weed added to Dandy's work by demonstrating that cerebrospinal fluid is principally absorbed in microscopic arachnoid villi found in the major cerebral veins and resembling Pacchionian granulations. This in itself was an important contribution to the understanding of hydrocephalus, a condition relatively more frequent in infants and children, for which satisfactory surgical treatment lay in the future.[38,39]

Cushing's most important contributions to pediatric neurology and neurosurgery were made over a period of 4 years, from 1927 to 1931.[29] This work actually began in the summer of 1922, when Cushing asked Percival Bailey (1892–1973), his assistant resident and the Arthur Tracy Cabot fellow in the surgical research laboratory, to create a histological laboratory for the study of his collection of brain tumors. Bailey began first to classify the gliomas, working on this intermittently for the next 3 years. Virtually all the work was done by Bailey, who later held some natural resentment toward Cushing for the latter's failure to acknowledge his contributions properly. Nevertheless, in Cushing's later years, Bailey generously expressed his affection for Cushing.[4,30]

The results of the glioma studies were first reported by Cushing in the Cameron Prize Lectures given at the University of Edinburgh in October 1925.[16] The completed monograph by Bailey and Cushing, "A Classification of Tumors of the Glioma Group on a Histogenic Basis with a Correlated Study of Prognosis," appeared in 1926.[6] Here, for the first time, was an orderly classification of gliomas with their natural history and clinical course. This study included a total of 414 cases of glioma in Cushing's series, of which Bailey did histological tissues studies on 254. Based on the predominant cellular configuration, Bailey classified these tumors into 13 categories. This histological categorization was the first ever, and formed the basis for all subsequent classifications. From this study, it was determined that approximately 40% of gliomas had a relatively favorable prognosis if correctly diagnosed and operated on.[6,16,32] The study also showed that certain of these tumors—for example, the ependymoblastomas, the unipolar spongioblastomas, and the medulloblastomas—were predominantly tumors of the pediatric age group.

Studying these cases further and adding another 159 cases, Bailey reduced and simplified the glioma classification to 10 groups. Cushing carefully reviewed the survival figures. The new classification of 1927 correlated the tumor types with survival.[1] Bailey also published a valuable histological atlas of these gliomas.[2]

THE INTRACRANIAL TUMORS OF PREADOLESCENCE

REPORT OF A CLINIC FOR THE COMBINED MEETING OF THE PEDIATRIC
SECTION OF THE NEW YORK ACADEMY OF MEDICINE, THE
PHILADELPHIA PEDIATRIC SOCIETY, AND THE NEW
ENGLAND PEDIATRIC SOCIETY, HELD AT THE
PETER BENT BRIGHAM HOSPITAL,
BOSTON, OCT. 16, 1926

HARVEY CUSHING, M.D.
BOSTON

Gentlemen: I was the more ready to accept Dr. Sisson's invitation to address you because of a letter recently received from a distinguished neurologist in a distant city. Relative to a chapter on nervous diseases he is preparing for a general textbook of pediatrics, he wrote to ask if we had ever seen any recoveries after the removal of tumors of the brain in children, adding that in his personal experience the operations were either fatal or gave bad results.

It is fair to say that the operations on children are in the long run less favorable than those on adults, for reasons that will be pointed out. Nevertheless, the results are excellent, as I think you will come to admit. Otherwise, one would hardly be willing to devote his life to such a business. Moreover, the results improve year by year as our diagnostic acumen is sharpened and as our knowledge of the life history of the lesions increases.

My accredited title, "Neurological Surgery in Childhood," is far too broad to think of compassing in a single clinic. Even the tumors of the central nervous system, to which I shall confine my remarks (for these are the most commonly overlooked lesions and for that reason the ones that should most interest you), would be beyond the possibilities of an hour's exercise.

What I plan to do is to parade for you all the patients under 15 years of age that happen at this time to be in the hospital, either awaiting operation or convalescing after operations for tumor. This will give you an idea of the conditions with which we deal and of the immediate results.

I will subsequently show a few patients from the neighborhood who have been good enough to report for the purposes of this exercise, so that we may learn something of the more favorable end-results.

INCIDENCE OF TUMORS OF THE BRAIN IN CHILDHOOD

As a point of departure, Dr. Louise Eisenhardt, who for the past several years has kept personal track of our tumor series, has put on the

FIGURE 1 Title page of Cushing's paper, "The Intracranial Tumors of Preadolescence." [From *American Journal of Diseases in Children* 33:551–584, 1927. Reproduced with permission.]

In 1923, Paul Martin (1861–1937) and Cushing reported seven cases of glioma of the optic nerve. Four of the seven cases occurred in children. The authors emphasized the frequent finding of optic atrophy, a common finding of erosion of the anterior clinoid process on x-ray, and the association of the tumor with von Recklinghausen's neurofibromatosis.[34]

Cushing's first report on his series of pediatric brain tumors in 1927 was "The Intracranial Tumors of Preadolescence"[17] (Fig. 1). Of 1,108 verified tumors, 154 had occurred in patients under 15 years of age. In this paper, Cushing noted that 40% of adult tumors—namely, meningiomas, acoustic tumors, and pituitary tumors—are "practically excluded from the children's list." The gliomas were found to make up 75% of childhood brain tumors, with cerebellar or infratentorial tumors being twice as common as those

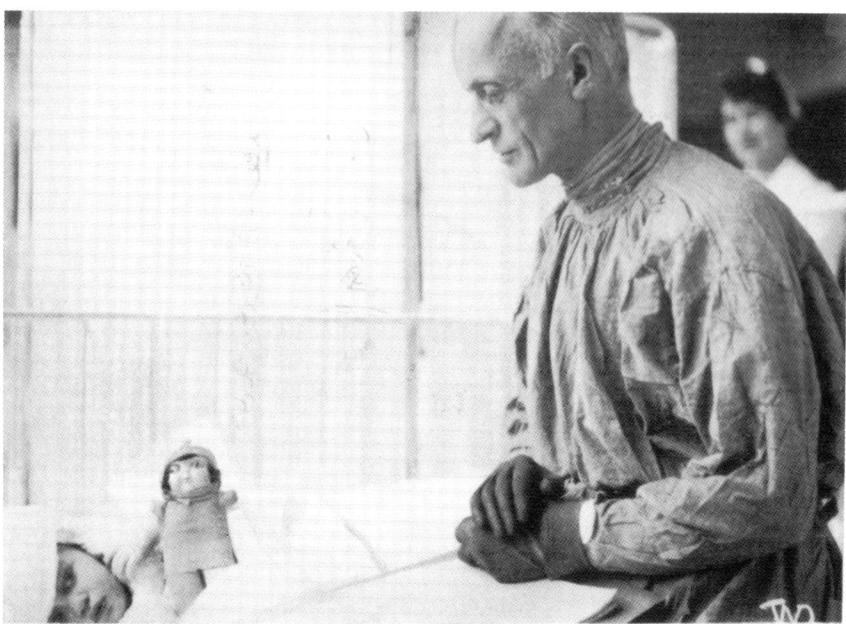

FIGURE 2 Harvey Cushing examining a young patient a few days after removal of a cerebellar tumor. [Courtesy of the Yale Medical School Library, New Haven, Connecticut.]

occurring above the tentorium. The other tumors included a small group of congenital tumors, such as craniopharyngiomas, tuberculomas, and blood vessel tumors.

Cushing stressed the diagnostic vicissitudes that confront the physician who examines the child with a brain tumor, and urged careful and repeated examination of the optic fundi, as most children with tumors of the posterior fossa developed increased intracranial pressure with papilledema. In this report, Cushing cited a recent letter from a distinguished neurologist in "another city" whose experiences with operations on brain tumors in children had either been fatal or produced poor results. In contrast, the results in Cushing's clinic were hopeful, in that cerebellar astrocytomas were twice as common as the more malignant medulloblastoma, and patients with these tumors had an average postoperative survival of more than 6 years. Moreover, the operative mortality had steadily dropped in the years preceding these reports.

Within the next 2 years, two additional seminal papers on brain tumors in children appeared. The first of these described Cushing's experiences with cerebellar medulloblastomas,[20] and the next, his experiences with cerebellar astrocytomas.[21] Cushing is shown examining a young patient a few days after removal of a cerebellar tumor in 1928 in a photograph by Thomas W. Dixon (Fig. 2). The essay on medulloblastomas, a term coined by Percival Bailey,[5] was a classic that can hardly be improved upon today (Fig. 3). The series of 61 cases includes 6 early cases operated on at the Johns Hopkins Hospital in which the true nature and behavior of the tumors were not recognized. Also, these 6 operations were performed before the introduction of the suction apparatus and electrosurgical instrument[19] (Fig.4).

Cushing described a "composite" of symptoms typical of these tumors:

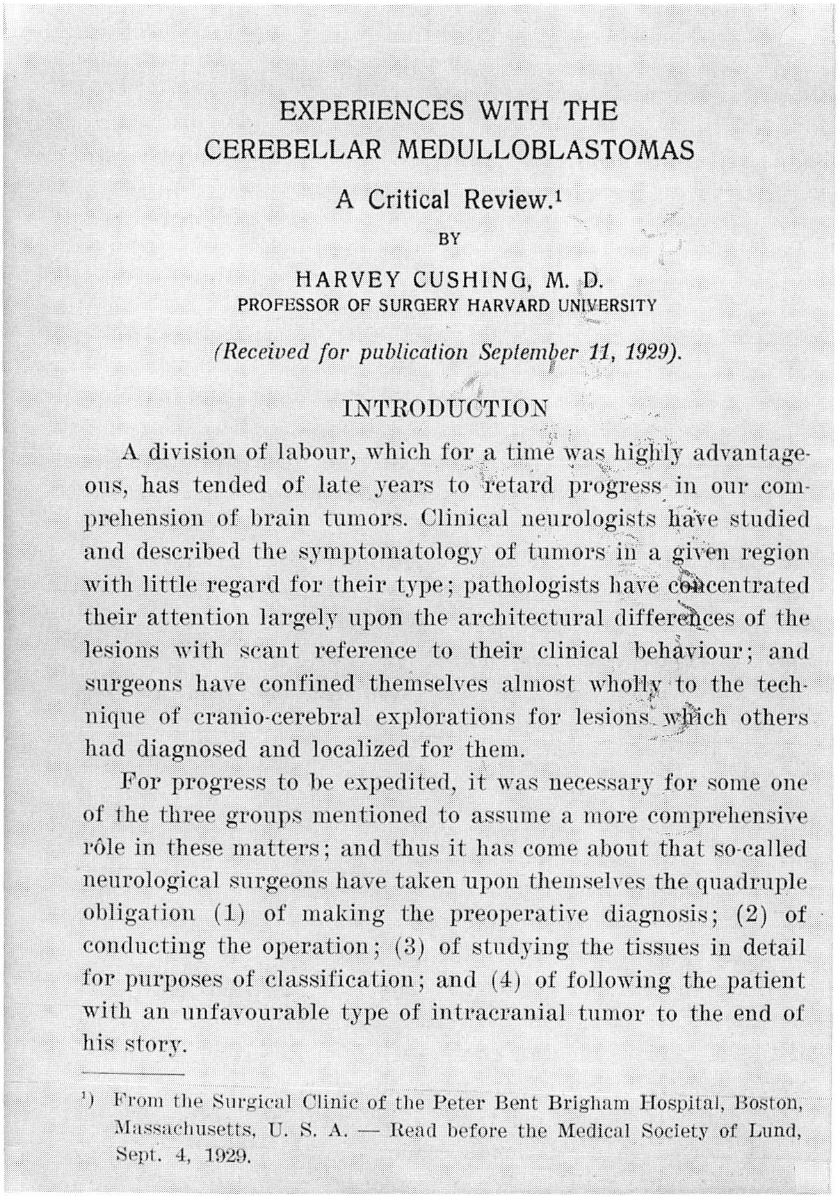

EXPERIENCES WITH THE CEREBELLAR MEDULLOBLASTOMAS

A Critical Review.[1]

BY

HARVEY CUSHING, M. D.
PROFESSOR OF SURGERY HARVARD UNIVERSITY

(Received for publication September 11, 1929).

INTRODUCTION

A division of labour, which for a time was highly advantageous, has tended of late years to retard progress in our comprehension of brain tumors. Clinical neurologists have studied and described the symptomatology of tumors in a given region with little regard for their type; pathologists have concentrated their attention largely upon the architectural differences of the lesions with scant reference to their clinical behaviour; and surgeons have confined themselves almost wholly to the technique of cranio-cerebral explorations for lesions which others had diagnosed and localized for them.

For progress to be expedited, it was necessary for some one of the three groups mentioned to assume a more comprehensive rôle in these matters; and thus it has come about that so-called neurological surgeons have taken upon themselves the quadruple obligation (1) of making the preoperative diagnosis; (2) of conducting the operation; (3) of studying the tissues in detail for purposes of classification; and (4) of following the patient with an unfavourable type of intracranial tumor to the end of his story.

[1] From the Surgical Clinic of the Peter Bent Brigham Hospital, Boston, Massachusetts, U. S. A. — Read before the Medical Society of Lund, Sept. 4, 1929.

FIGURE 3   Title page of Cushing's paper, "Experiences with the Cerebellar Medulloblastomas" [From *Acta Pathologica, Microbiologica et Immunologica Scandinavica* 7:1–86, 1930. Reproduced with permission.]

A preadolescent child previously in good health begins to complain of headaches or of suboccipital discomfort and to have occasional attacks of vomiting without preliminary nausea, usually on first arising in the morning. Attendance at school meanwhile may continue but the teacher soon notices that the child is listless or inattentive and the character of its work noticeably falls off. Ere long it is apparent that there is some unwonted clumsiness of movement and awkwardness in gait. The mother may find that the child quickly outgrows its caps and she thinks the head enlarges unduly fast. In course of time it is noticed, at home or at school, that the child's sight is

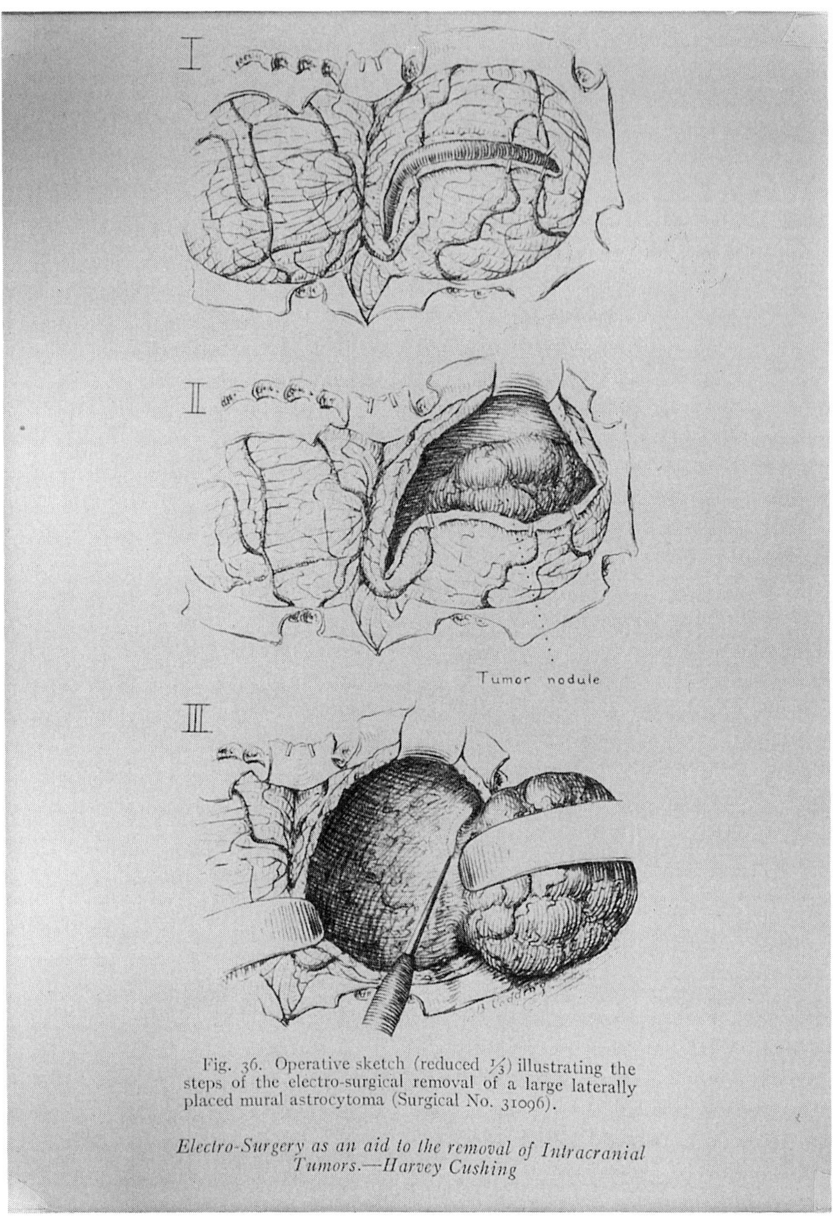

Fig. 36. Operative sketch (reduced ⅓) illustrating the steps of the electro-surgical removal of a large laterally placed mural astrocytoma (Surgical No. 31096).

Electro-Surgery as an aid to the removal of Intracranial Tumors.—Harvey Cushing

FIGURE 4   Operative sketch by Mildred Codding showing Cushing using the electrosurgical instrument to remove a laterally placed mural astrocytoma [From Cushing H: Electro-surgery as an aid to the removal of intracranial tumors. With a preliminary note on a new surgical-current generator by W.T. Bovie. Ph.D. *Surgery, Gynecology & Obstetrics* 47:751–784. 1928. Reproduced with permission.]

impaired; or a beginning squint of one eye may be detected, even in the absence of any complaint of double vision. The family doctor, who has previously suspected some gastro-intestinal disorder, may then have the eyegrounds examined and to the surprise of everyone a choked disk is found. Three or four months on the average have elapsed, and at about this stage of the malady many cases first come under hospital care.

Should the condition not be recognized so soon, the symptoms relentlessly progress. The clumsiness increases until the gait gradually

SURGERY, GYNECOLOGY AND OBSTETRICS

AN INTERNATIONAL MAGAZINE, PUBLISHED MONTHLY

Volume LII   FEBRUARY, 1931   Number 2

EXPERIENCES WITH THE CEREBELLAR ASTROCYTOMAS[1]

A Critical Review of Seventy-Six Cases

HARVEY CUSHING, M.D., Boston

I. INTRODUCTION

WHAT has been chiefly contributory in recent years to the success of operations for intracranial tumors has been the tendency of those interested in the subject to concentrate upon the behaviour and traits of special tumors in special situations. This was hardly possible when these operations were few and far between, but now that they are of daily occurrence it becomes increasingly evident that tumors of each particular kind occupy favoured sites and evoke a similar and therefore recognizable set of symptoms. This being so, it becomes possible with some degree of assurance to foretell in a large percentage of cases what particular type of lesion will be encountered, what it will look like when brought to view, and what surgical procedure offers the best prospect not only of the immediate amelioration of symptoms, but, in an ever enlarging percentage of cases, of permanent cure.

As an outcome of this change in attitude and with the growing conviction that the point of origin of tumors of different kinds is not purely accidental, it is no longer highly profitable to discuss the effects of brain tumors in general, to describe the symptomatology of tumors in a given region irrespective of their specific nature, or to deal with tumors of comparable histology irrespective of their location.

For this reason, those of us who have been at this business longer than others begin to feel the obligation of handing on from time to time the results of our surgical experience with tumors of particular kinds in particular situations. This sort of information, however, is admittedly difficult to transmit, for though the general principles may be more or less the same, no two of these operations are precisely alike, and in the process of carrying out what at the best is a complicated and often hazardous procedure, unforeseen circumstances may arise which wholly modify its intended course. When to take great risks; when to withdraw in the face of unexpected difficulties; whether to force an attempted enucleation of a pathologically favourable tumor to its completion with the prospect of an operative fatality, or to abandon the procedure short of completeness with the certainty that after months or years even greater risks may have to be faced at a subsequent session—all this takes surgical judgment which is a matter of long experience and which can scarcely be transmitted by the written word.

Surgical judgment, indeed, is a more or less inspirational quality which is variable and elusive, all surgeons being conscious of having it in hand on some occasions, of losing it on others. It is a good deal like a game which even the best and most consistent player foozles for some unaccountable reason at

[1] Being the basis of the second Arthur Dean Bevan Lecture of the Chicago Surgical Society delivered October 3, 1930, before the joint meeting of the Chicago Surgical Society, the Institute of Medicine of Chicago, Chicago Neurological Society, the Society of Internal Medicine, the Chicago Pediatric Society, and the Chicago Society of Medical History.

129

FIGURE 5 Title page of Cushing's paper "Experiences with the Cerebellar Astrocytomas." [From *Surgery, Gynecology, & Obstetrics* 52:129–204, 1931. Reproduced with permission.]

becomes so ataxic walking without support is difficult; vomiting grows more frequent, the child begins to lose weight; the muscles become wasted and atonic; there may be a slight facial palsy; the internal squint may become bilateral and finally 'fainting spells' occur, characterized by extensor rigidities that may be precipitated by slight changes in position. Ere this the child will have become bedridden. The whole story if uninterrupted by operation may cover a period from eight to nine months ([20], pp 43–44).

Diagnosis of such tumors at this time was largely clinical, as today's sophisticated neuroimaging tests were unknown. Despite improvement in surgical techniques, survival was still measured in months. The problem of

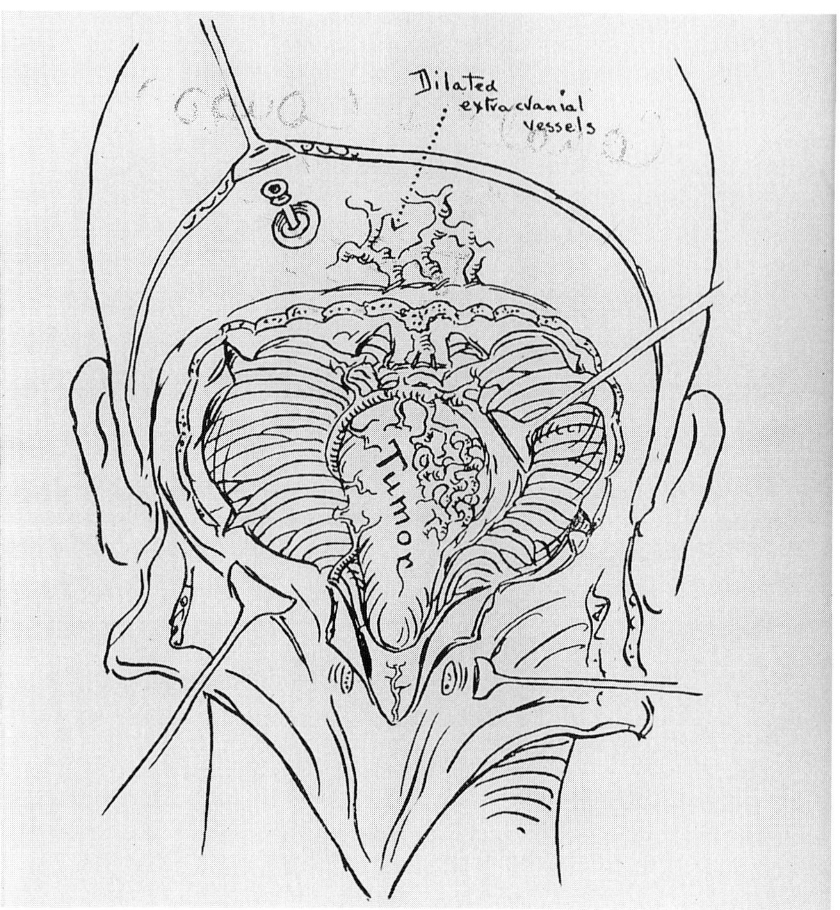

FIGURE 6   Cushing's rough postoperative sketch to indicate the approximate situation and appearance of the field and operative findings of a medulloblastoma. [From Cushing H: The intracranial tumors of preadolescence. *American Journal of Diseases in Children* 33:551–584. 1927. Reproduced with permission.]

spinal seeding and the beneficial effects of radiation therapy were noted, however.

Further studies of Cushing's cases led to the conclusion that it was advisable to radiate the entire cerebrospinal axis after an operation for medulloblastoma, since a fatal outcome was inevitable once the patient developed symptoms from seeding.[3]

The 1931 article, "Experiences with the Cerebellar Astrocytomas," summarized Cushing's experience with these more favorable tumors[21] (Fig. 5). Here he acknowledged Bailey's "highly important contributory role." Again, though differing in some aspects from the medulloblastomas, a composite clinical progression was given:

> A child apparently normal in all respects begins toward the end of the first
> decade, possibly after a fall of an attack of whooping cough, to have early

morning headaches with vomiting. Nothing much is made of this by the family doctor, should he be called in, for the child subsequently feels perfectly well, has had breakfast and wants to go out and play. This daily performance may continue for a considerable time, the child even going to school meanwhile. There may then be a remission of weeks or perhaps months and the episode be forgotten. On their recurrence, the symptoms are likely to be more pronounced and are apt to be ascribed to some gastro-intestinal disturbance. This appears the more probable since the child finds that straining at stool brings on a headache and there is a tendency to become constipated. What is more, a mild daily laxative usually serves completely to mask the symptoms.

This sort of thing continues off and on until it becomes evident that the child is a little clumsy at play and gets knocked over easily. Very possibly, ere this, the periodic headache and vomiting will have ceased completely or at least have occurred at much longer intervals; and if parents are observant they may notice that the child's head in the interim has increased in size more rapidly than it should. This, however, is usually discounted for the child meanwhile has become free from complaints and in all respects appears alert and well.

Matters may run on in this way for an indefinite time, possibly with some increase in clumsiness of movement or in some instances with no noticeable change whatever until it suddenly becomes apparent, perhaps at school, that the child's sight is poor. To counteract this glasses are usually prescribed: but even should an ophthalmoscope be resorted to, a child's retina is less easily examined than that of an adult and because of the decompressive effects of the enlarging head, the optic papillae often show no measurable swelling and the fact of their being pale and with margins blurred may easily pass unrecognized.

Due to the insidious nature of the symptomatic onset, it is in this pre-amaurotic stage of the process that even today the victims of these mid-cerebellar astrocytomas, unfortunately continue to be admitted to hospital, ([21] pp 147–148).

This series included 76 cerebellar astrocytomas. The children tended to become asymptomatic at an older age, and to have symptoms of longer duration and a greater loss of vision than those who had medulloblastomas. Of perhaps greater importance was Cushing's discovery that removing the mural nodule in the cystic cerebellar astrocytomas would commonly lead to a long remission or cure. The importance of this surgical characteristic of the cystic cerebellar astrocytomas had not previously been recognized or reported.

These papers on brain tumors in children, illustrating the classic clinical picture and detailing the surgical aspects of the cases, including the beautiful illustrations drawn by Mildred Codding from Cushing's operative sketches, give some idea of the principles that made Cushing a great neurosurgeon[35] (Figs. 6 and 7). Cushing firmly believed that a surgeon should be familiar with all aspects of his cases; hence he did his own careful examination of each patient and did not rely on a neurologist or someone else.[8] He carefully recorded his cases, a habit he probably learned from William Osler (1849–1919).[7] As Cushing pointed out in the cerebellar astrocytoma article,

What has been chiefly contributory in recent years to the success of operations for intracranial tumors has been the tendency of those interested in the subject to concentrate upon the behavior and traits of special tumors in special situations ([21] p. 129).

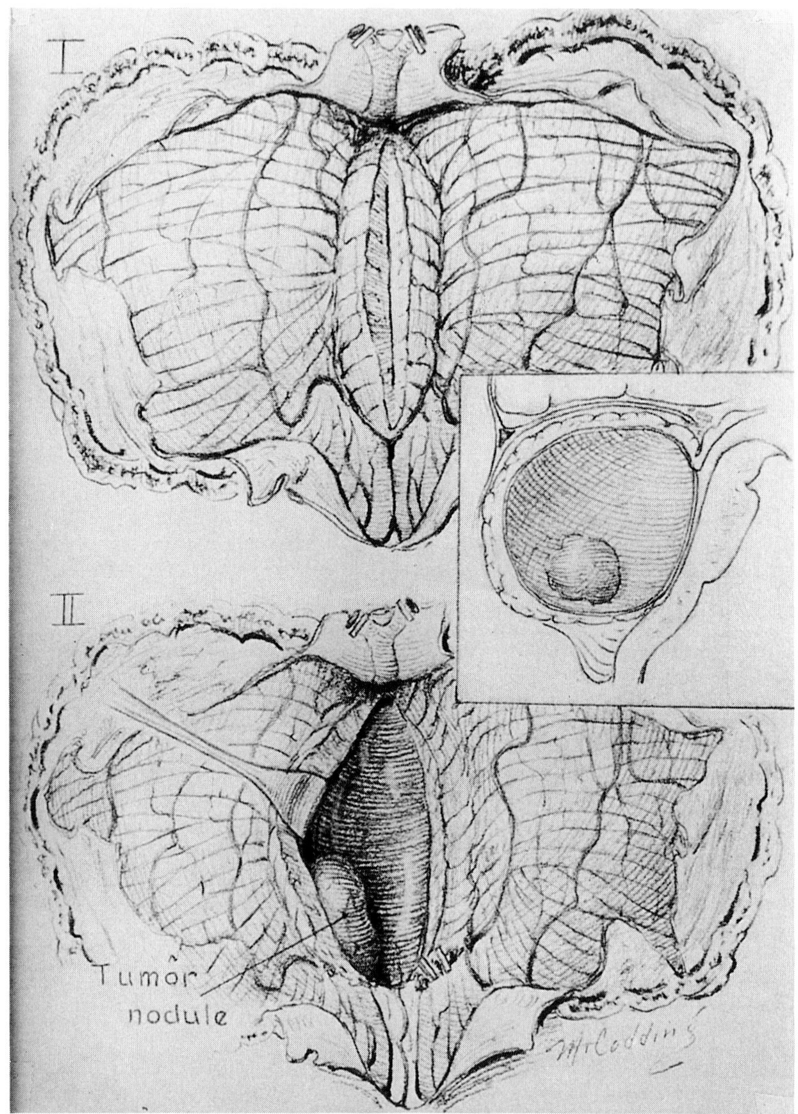

FIGURE 7 Illustration by Mildred Codding of case of astrocytoma showing a central cyst with a small, laterally placed mural nodule. [From Cushing H: Experiences with the cerebellar astrocytomas. A critical review of seventy-six cases. *Surgery, Gynecology & Obstetrics* 52:129–204, 1931. Reproduced with permission.]

This is best illustrated by a case mortality of only 4% in the last 25 consecutive operations on these cerebellar tumors, a remarkable accomplishment in view of the prolonged and radical nature of the operations.[21]

This was Cushing's last major paper on brain tumors before his retirement in 1933. He undoubtedly had the largest operative experience in brain tumors in children, despite operating in the Brigham Hospital, which was not a children's hospital. Nevertheless, Cushing's reputation and skill brought him a wide referral of such patients.

In his Cameron Prize Lectures at the University of Edinburgh, Cushing included an assessment of the contributions from his students and fellow surgical investigators:

> I do not know that I personally am to be credited with anything more than the introduction of a few trifling technical procedures which in time are almost certain to be superseded. However . . . a teacher's influence . . . should be centrifugal, his own ideas being far less important than the ideas which radiate from his pupils and theirs in turn. One of the greatest satisfactions of my professional life . . . has been my privilege to appoint annually some younger man who has been put in independent charge of a laboratory of experimental surgery . . . , ([16] p. xii).

Harvey Cushing, through his many contributions to the field of neurosurgery, made fundamental contributions to child neurology. As noted by several biographers[28,37] he set an example in the application of the scientific method to clinical problems, especially those involving tumors of the brain. He trained and influenced most of the neurosurgeons of his era in America and many from abroad. His landmark papers secured his place as the pioneer surgeon dealing with brain tumors in children. Cushing's singular dedication to his major life's work can be understood in his statement:

> The surgery of brain tumors may be likened without being trivial to a form of major sport which is played against an invisible but utterly relentless antagonist quick to take advantage of every misplay and faulty move. And when the time comes to make public one's score, it is done somewhat apologetically, but with the expectation that others may profit by it and with the assurance they will come to improve upon it ([21], p. 130).

Acknowledgments

The authors express thanks and appreciation to Ms. Florence M. Bruce and Mrs. Brenda J. Kreutzer for their editorial assistance and word-processing skills.

Received for publication, November 28, 1989; accepted, final form, April 25, 1990.

Reprint requests: Dee James Canale, M.D., 1314 Peabody Avenue, P.O. Box 41619, Memphis, TN 38174–1619.

References

1. Bailey P: Further remarks concerning tumors of the glioma group. Bull Johns Hopkins Hosp 40:354–389, 1927.
2. Bailey P: Histologic atlas of gliomas. Arch Pathol Lab Med 4:871–921, 1927.
3. Bailey P: Further notes on the cerebellar medulloblastomas. The effects of roentgen radiation. Am J Pathol 6:125–135, 1930.
4. Bailey P: Pepperpot, in Bucy, PC (ed): *Neurosurgical Giants. Feet of Clay and Iron.* New York, Elsevier, 1985, pp 73–89.
5. Bailey P, Cushing H: Medulloblastoma cerebelli: A common type of midcerebellar glioma of childhood. Arch Neurol Phychiatry 14:192–224, 1925.
6. Bailey P, Cushing H: *A Classification of the Tumors of the Glioma Group on a Histogenetic Basis with a Correlated Study of Prognosis.* Springfield, IL, Charles C Thomas, 1926.

7. Canale DJ: William Osler and "The Special Field of Neurological Surgery." J Neurosurg 70:759–766, 1989.

8. Cushing H: The special field of neurological surgery. Bull Johns Hopkins Hosp 16:77–87, 1905.

9. Cushing H: Concerning surgical intervention for the intracranial hemorrhages of the new-born. Am J Med Sci 130:563–581, 1905.

10. Cushing H: Surgery of the head, in Keen WW (ed): *Surgery, Its Principles and Practice.* Philadelphia, WB Saunders, 1908, pp 17–276.

11. Cushing H: Hydrocephalus, in Osler W (ed): *Modern Medicine.* Philadelphia, Lea & Febiger, 1910, vol 7, pp 459–466.

12. Cushing H: The control of bleeding in operations for brain tumors. With the description of silver "clips" for the occlusion of vessels inaccessible to the ligature. Ann Surg 54:119, 1911.

13. Cushing H: *The Pituitary Body and Its Disorders. Clinical States Produced by Disorder of the Hypophysis Cerebri. An Amplification of the Harvey Lecture for December, 1910.* Philadelphia, JB Lippincott, 1912.

14. Cushing H: Studies on the cerebro-spinal fluid and its pathway. J Med Res 26:1–19, 1914.

15. Cushing H: *Tumors of the Nervus Acousticus and the Syndrome of the Cerebello pontine Angle.* Philadelphia, WB Saunders, 1917.

16. Cushing H: *Studies in Intracranial Physiology and Surgery. The Third Circulation. The Hypophysis. The Gliomas.* London, Oxford University Press, 1926.

17. Cushing H: The intracranial tumors of preadolescence. Am J Dis Child 33:551–584, 1927.

18. Cushing H: *MacEwen Memorial Lecture: The Meningiomas Arising from the Olfactory Groove and Their Removal by the Aid of Electro-Surgery.* Glasgow, Jackson, Wylie & Co (Publishers to the University), 1927.

19. Cushing H: Electro-surgery as an aid to the removal of intracranial tumors. With a preliminary note on a new surgical-current generator by W.T. Bovie, Ph.D. Surg Gynecol Obstet 47:751–784, 1928.

20. Cushing H: Experiences with the cerebellar medulloblastomas. A critical review. Acta Pathol Microbiol Scand 7:1–86, 1930.

21. Cushing H: Experiences with the cerebellar astrocytomas. A critical review of seventy-six cases. Surg Gynecol Obstet 52:129–204, 1931.

22. Cushing H: The basophil adenomas of the pituitary body and their clinical manifestations (pituitary basophilism). Bull Johns Hopkins Hosp 50:137–195, 1932.

23. Cushing H, Eisenhardt L: *Meningiomas. Their Classification, Regional Behavior, Life History, and Surgical End Results.* Springfield, IL, Charles C Thomas, 1938.

24. Dandy WE, Blackfan KD: An experimental and clinical study of internal hydrocephalus. JAMA 61:2216–2217, 1913.

25. Dandy WE, Blackfan KD: Internal hydrocephalus, an experimental, clinical and pathological study. Am J Dis Child 8:406–482, 1914.

26. Fox WL: The Cushing-Dandy controversy. Surg Neurol 3:661–666, 1975.

27. Fulton JF: Harvey Cushing: An appreciation. Sci Monthly 49:477–479, 1939.

28. Fulton JF: *Harvey Cushing, A Biography.* Springfield, IL, Charles C Thomas, 1946.

29. German WJ: Cerebral spinal fluid, in Matson DD, German WJ, and a committee of the American Association of Neurological Surgeons (eds): *Harvey Cushing. Selected Papers on Neurosurgery.* New Haven, Yale University Press, 1969, p 274.

30.   Harvey Cushing Society: *Harvey Cushing's Seventieth Birthday Party, April 8, 1939.* Springfield, IL, Charles C Thomas, 1939.
31.   Horrax G: Harvey Cushing, 1869–1939. Surg Gynecol Obstet 69:828–834 1939.
32.   Horrax G: Some of Harvey Cushing's contributions to neurological surgery. J Neurosurg 1:3–22, 1944.
33.   Key A, Retzius G: *Studien in der Anatomie des Nervensystems und des Vindegewebes.* Stockholm, Samson & Wallin, 1875/1876.
34.   Martin P, Cushing H: Primary gliomas of the chiasm and optic nerves in their intracranial portion. Arch Ophthalmol 52:209–241, 1923.
35.   Matson DD: Neoplasms, in Matson DD, German WJ, and a committee of the American Association of Neurological Surgeons (eds): *Harvey Cushing, Selected Papers on Neurosurgery.* New Haven, Yale University Press, 1969, pp 104–105.
36.   McClure R: Hydrocephalus treated by drainage into a vein of the neck. Bull Johns Hopkins Hosp 20:110–113, 1909.
37.   Thomson EH: *Harvey Cushing. Surgeon, Author, Artist.* New York, H Schuman, 1950.
38.   Weed LH: Studies on cerebro-spinal fluid. J Med Res 31:21–117, 1914.
39.   Weed LH: The development of the cerebro-spinal space in pig and man. Contrib Embryol Carnegie Inst 5:1–116, 1917.

Comments

This article serves to remind the neurosurgical community of Dr. Cushing's early attempts at treatment of disorders of the pediatric central nervous system. Although his seminal descriptions of childhood brain tumors are recognized widely, Dr. Cushing's efforts to treat neonatal hemorrhage and hydrocephalus deserve the detail that these authors give. His sponsorship of Weed's experimental work is outlined correctly, along with his personal difficulties with the talented Dandy and Bailey. Dr. Cushing had a unique tendency to be "at the right place at the right time"; this article proves the point. His pervasive expertise influenced a variety of clinical and experimental work involving diseases of the central nervous system in children.

William C. Hanigan
Peoria, Illinois

Drs. Canale and Longo have again reminded us of our indebtedness to Dr. Harvey W. Cushing. Cushing's talents encompass many fields, and he pursued all of them with great vigor. The authors have outlined Dr. Cushing's contributions to pediatric neurosurgery, and there were many.

Neoplasms eventually became his major interest, and through meticulous record keeping with the assistance of many fellow investigators, he was able to develop an orderly classification of many of these lesions. This was particularly noted for tumors of the posterior fossa in childhood and adolescence. Through his endeavors, it became evident that these lesions were not hopeless and now could indeed be addressed with success by the neurosurgeon. It must be appreciated that Cushing approached these tumors without the benefit of special diagnostic equipment such as magnetic resonance imaging or computed tomography. He was also without the help of antibiotics, banked blood, or osmotic diuretics. One could only wonder what he would have done with a surgical microscope. We must admire his courage, skill, and resourcefulness.

All too often we tend to forget those to whom we owe a debt. And sadly, particularly for many just beginning a career in neurosurgery, the names of our forefathers are just that—merely names. It is to be hoped that through papers such as this, we will be reminded of their contributions.

Children must have held a special place in Dr. Cushing's heart, and most assuredly he received great satisfaction and joy from his accomplishments in pediatric neurosurgery. This is perhaps best illustrated in a story told by Dr. James C. White:[1]

> I never worked on Harvey Cushing's service, but I shall never forget his charm and unexpected kindness when my three-year-old daughter fell out of a window and landed on her head on the brick sidewalk six feet below. This happened when I was only a third year Harvard Medical Student. How he heard about it I have never been able to ascertain, but he arrived at our house in Boston within a hour, spent a long time examining her and then reassured my wife and me that all was well. So it proved and we both remained everlastingly grateful.

T. Glenn Pait
Washington, District of Columbia

1. Heyl HL: A selection of Harvey Cushing anecdotes. *J Neurosurg* 30:365–376, 1969.

❧ Miscellaneous Topics

William Osler's Departure From North America

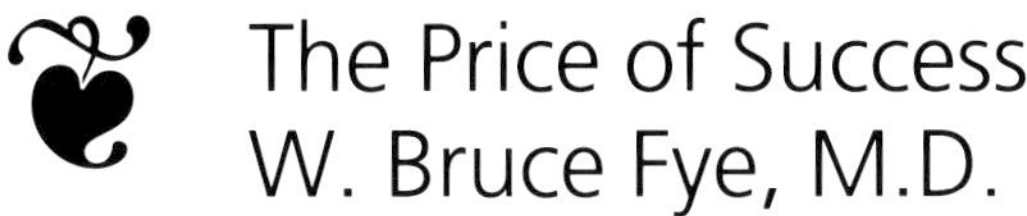 The Price of Success
W. Bruce Fye, M.D.

William Osler was widely acknowledged to be the most influential physician in the English-speaking world at the turn of the century. Born in 1849 in Bond Head, Ontario, he was educated in Canada and Great Britain but emigrated to the United States in 1884 to occupy the chair of clinical medicine at the University of Pennsylvania. Two decades later Osler decided to leave North America to become Regius Professor of Medicine at Oxford. Several considerations influenced his decision to go to Oxford, but the main reason he left America was that his success had made it difficult for him to enjoy life. He sought a simpler and less stressful existence that would provide more time and opportunity for his interests in medical history and book collecting. Osler's autobiographical notes, which are preserved at McGill University, and his letters to friends and colleagues provide valuable insight into his acceptance of the position at Oxford.[1]

In 1889, at the age of 40, Osler arrived in Baltimore after five brief but productive years in Philadelphia. During the 16 years he spent in Baltimore, he married, had a son, made major contributions to the development of the Johns Hopkins Hospital and Medical School, and gained fame through his writings, his active involvement in medical societies, and his popularity as a consultant. Despite enormous energy, a keen sense of organization, and the ability to put odd moments to good use, Osler grew tired of the demands he faced in response to his growing fame. Moreover, he expected a great deal of himself; he always felt pressured to publish and often thought himself delinquent in his literary activities.

Speaking of Osler's years in Baltimore, his successor Lewellys Barker recalled,

> In addition to his heavy executive duties in the hospital and medical school,
> he divided his time so as to participate in teaching, in practice in the hospital

Presidential Address. Read at the annual meeting of the American Osler Society, April 16, 1989.

Reprinted with permission from *The New England Journal of Medicine, 320:*1425, 1989 and in outside consultations, in personal original research and in the stimulation of others to investigate, in literary work, in the making of public addresses, and in the cultivation of friendly and helpful relations with the medical profession in Baltimore and in the country at large.[2]

Success came almost at once to Osler and to the Johns Hopkins Hospital. Ten months after the hospital opened, he informed Daniel Gilman, the university's president, "We have now had nearly 1000 inpatients & over 11,000 out-patients! To-day the ward Population is 130 & the income from private patients over $360."[3,4] The growth of the institution and Osler's personal accomplishments set the stage for his departure. He was soon a very popular man; patients, doctors, and institutions wanted William Osler.

Although he did not leave Baltimore until 1905, Osler had several earlier offers from other medical schools. In 1891, he was offered the chairs of medicine at Jefferson and Harvard. In 1892 McGill attempted to bring him back to fill the chair once held by his mentor, Palmer Howard. A Montreal journalist boasted, "Dr. Osler . . . has become as famous in the United States since his connection with the Johns Hopkins University as he was in Toronto and Montreal."[5]

After several delays due to financial difficulties, the opening of the medical school at Johns Hopkins was made possible by a gift of $500,000 from Mary Garrett and her friends. Two weeks after this endowment was formally accepted, Osler declined the offer from McGill. He told his former resident Henri Lafleur, "I am too comfortable here to think of any change, and I hope to fill out my twenty years and then crawl back to Montreal to worry the boys for a few years."[6]

There would be more offers, however—and some of them were tempting. In 1895, McGill tried once again to recruit Osler, this time as president of the institution. Newspapers inaccurately reported that he had accepted the offer. William Pepper wrote from Philadelphia, "I have known that the presidency of McGill has been offered to you. I assume that the announcement in last evening's paper is authoritative as to your acceptance. It is a magnificent position of commanding dignity and influence. You are truly a 'Wandering Willie,' but as long as your peregrinations carry you only from one peak on to a higher one, your friends and admirers can only rejoice in your continued progress, while they symphathize with the loss that each place you would leave must long feel."[7]

The newspaper reports were false, and Osler remained at Johns Hopkins. Still, other institutions tried to lure him away from Baltimore. He informed the British physiologist Edward Schäfer in 1897, "I have just had a tempting offer from New York—the Department of Medicine in the United Schools—University & Bellevue—at £2000 salary, with of course splendid prospects for consultation work. I have however such exceptional facilities here and we are so comfortable, that I have declined."[8]

The following year Osler's good friend and former colleague in Philadelphia, Weir Mitchell, tried to persuade him to return to Pennsylvania to fill the chair of William Pepper, who had recently died. Osler told his associate at Johns Hopkins, William Sidney Thayer, "Mitchell insists that I shall not say nay until after the Faculty have met but I should only be worried to death by practice in Philadelphia."[9]

Osler had long been concerned that he might be consumed by medical practice, and he sought to limit this aspect of his career. Speaking of Osler's years in Philadelphia, his friend James Wilson remarked in 1905, "We at once sought to make a practitioner of him. But of that he would have none.

Teacher, clinician, consultant, yes, gladly; but practitioner—no! And that with emphasis. This was partly due to his knowledge of affairs, partly to his temperament."[10]

Although these North American opportunities failed to induce Osler to leave Johns Hopkins, he came close to accepting the chair of medicine at Edinburgh in 1900. He informed his sister Charlotte, "So sorry not to have written before but . . . I have never been so busy or so much pressed particularly with arrears of literary work." Mentioning the Edinburgh opening, he told his sister, " 'Tis a great temptation & if it is offered to me I may accept."[11]

Osler's colleagues mounted an intense campaign to keep "the chief" in Baltimore. He told Schäfer, "I was quite unprepared for the outburst which followed the announcement to my colleagues that I was a candidate for the Chair. I had no idea that they would make it such a personal matter. . . . I suppose I should have counted on a strong local opposition but I had no idea that I should have to yield. . . . It is in many ways a great disappointment to me as 1 feel that I could have been very happy in Edinburgh. Mrs. Osler, too, is quite disturbed. She was very willing to go."[12] In another letter to Schäfer, Osler acknowledged that he and his wife hoped to have their son Revere, then 4 years old, educated in England, and that he planned to retire there in 8 to 10 years.

Osler's colleagues were relieved. The pathologist William Welch informed Daniel Gilman that he was delighted Osler would remain at Johns Hopkins. He attributed Osler's decision to the severity of Edinburgh's winters, the "necessity of going back to old fashioned methods of teaching," and less attractive hospital opportunities than he had at Hopkins. Welch wrote, "The position at Edinburgh is, I think, the most distinguished one in medicine in Great Britain. . . . It is most gratifying that the offer came to him, but we should have been brokenhearted if he had gone and never could have filled his place."[13]

Four years later Osler would decide to leave Johns Hopkins and North America for a less demanding life in Oxford. Before giving Osler's explanation of this decision, it will be helpful to review his final years in Baltimore. The many facets of his career included major commitments to teaching, writing, and participation in medical societies. And all of this was complicated by progressive bibliomania. The activity that Osler tried hardest to control was his practice, which grew dramatically in Baltimore. His manuscript day-books are a rich source of information about this aspect of his career.[14,15]

In 1893 Osler usually saw two patients a day in consultation. By the close of the century, his practice had grown remarkably. In 1899 he complained to his former resident Charles Camac, "I have been much driven this winter—so much on hand and so many calls."[16] Recalling Osler's activities, Harvey Cushing, a resident in surgery at the time, claimed, "From January to May of [1899] consultations were incessant—his afternoon hours filled, and many demands from out of town."[17]

By the spring of 1904, Osler was seeing five or six patients in consultation each day, more than twice as many as a decade earlier. Occasionally, he would see as many as eight patients in an afternoon. Although most of his consultations were performed on weekdays, he often saw one or two patients on Saturday and Sunday during his final years in Baltimore. A practice of this volume was not what Osler desired, although the fees it generated were welcome.

According to Lewellys Barker, "private practice was never more than a subsidiary activity in his busy life." Barker continued, "After his text-book attained wide distribution, physicians throughout Canada and the United States referred patients to him, and often requested him to travel long distances for consultations . . . . In Baltimore he restricted his consultations with physicians in the city to the late afternoon hours; but the number of patients thus seen, in addition to those who entered the private rooms in the hospital under his care, soon became a serious load. He got the reputation, too, of being the 'doctor's doctor'; no small proportion of his total private clientele was made up of medical men and members of their families. It was finally the increasing pressure of the burden of practice that made him decide to accept the Oxford call in 1905."[18] At one point Osler informed Barker, "I am living 'a life of the hunted' at present. Infernal nuisance & yet it seems very difficult to limit one's legitimate work."[19]

Osler's autobiographical notes provide insight into his activities in 1901:

> My life has got into a routine of teaching and practice. I get up at 7 a.m., breakfast at 7:30 and at 8:30 a.m. Monday, Wednesday and Friday go to the hospital where I make a ward visit until 11, or 11:30. Then I see the private patients and get back about 12:30, after luncheon at 1:30 I see patients by appointment from 2:30 to 5 p.m., have tea and see a few friends socially, after which there are generally a few consultations outside. On Tuesday, Thursday, and Saturday, I remain at home until 11:45 and these hours I try to devote to my literary work. At 12 I take the 3rd year students at the outpatient clinic.[1]

Osler was very interested in the statistical and financial aspects of his practice. In his autobiographical notes for 1901 he wrote, "My professional work increased very much this year. I have analyzed it as a matter of interest. There were 780 new patients (exclusive of private patients at the hospital) of whom 378 came from outside the city." Osler's list reveals that patients from 31 states traveled to Baltimore to see him in consultation. He was out of the city 33 times for professional reasons, most often in Washington.

He continued, "Two consultations at the White House & several Cabinet Ministers are responsible for a considerable increase in patients from the Capital. I went twice to the South—Fla. and Thomasville. Altogether I traveled in the nine months 19,300 miles, making with my summer traveling about 27,000 miles in the year." He noted that in 1901 his income exceeded $40,000 for the first time. Of this, $7100 represented royalties from his textbook and $3000 the fee charged to see a patient in Thomasville, Georgia. In 1989 dollars this represents an annual income of almost $650,000.[1]

The pace was beginning to take its toll on Osler, however. He wrote to Barker in the spring of 1901, "Greetings! When do I chat at Chicago? All well here. Horribly busy!"[20] That fall, he informed his longtime friend and former Montreal colleague Francis Shepherd, "All goes well here except that I am bothered to death with practice—hard to keep it within decent limits so as to have time for teaching and private work."[21]

Although teaching medical students was one of Osler's favorite activities, he had to forgo it during his first years at Baltimore. The Johns Hopkins Medical School did not open until 1893, and Osler only began to teach medical students there when the first class entered its junior year in 1895. The class was small; there were only 17 junior students. Before 1895, Osler had to satisfy himself with postgraduate teaching at Hopkins. His courses were popular and attracted physicians from around the country and abroad.

Osler enjoyed the intimacy of his small classes at Johns Hopkins. The success and growth of the medical school, however, made it difficult for him to maintain his close relationship with the students and for them to participate in his ward rounds. Osler complained to William Howell, the medical school dean, in April 1902, "No, I cannot possibly take more than twenty-five men [in the postgraduate course]. . . . All through May we have the undergraduates as well, which makes too great a crowd altogether in the wards."[22,23]

Osler was not alone in his frustration about this overcrowding. Walter Baumgarten, a postgraduate student at the medical school, informed his father: "Dr. O[sler]'s rounds are assuming frightful proportions; on Monday I counted 48 people, not including the interns, the staff, and the nurses; of the 48 sixteen were fourth year students for whom the teaching rounds are primarily given. You may imagine how much is seen at the bedside. I slip off & follow Dr. McCrae. I see more."[24]

In 1902 Osler entered in his diary, "I had a very hard winter and never before felt the work to drag particularly as the spring came with the postgraduate work and on some days a congestion of patients." In 1903 he wrote, "It becomes more and more difficult to meet outside demands. Early in May I was unusually hard-pressed—so many calls to Washington and so many people from a distance. During the week of the Triennial Medical Congress in Washington I was much driven. Returning from Cleveland on the 2nd, I had a call to go to Beury, W.Va. from Dr. Davis, on the 7th one from Roanoke, Va.; on the 10th a call to Athens, Ga., on the 14th one from Dr. Prevost to Ottawa to see one of the Ministers; on the 16th a call to New York to see Mr. Stickney & on the 17th one from Dr. Olmstead of Hamilton Ontario to see Mrs. White. I sent Thayer to Athens & Futcher to Roanoke."[1]

Speaking to members of the New Haven Medical Association in 1903, Osler addressed the plight of the busy practitioner: "Greater sympathy must be felt for the man who has started all right . . . but as the rolling years have brought ever-increasing demands on his time, the evening hours find him worn out yet not able to rest, much less to snatch a little diversion or instruction in the company of his fellows whom he loves so well. . . . Many good men are ruined by success in practice."[25] The following year, with a mixture of frustration and pride, Osler informed his friend John Musser, "I have been swamped with work lately—& the wards are surcharged—we reached a high water mark in the private rooms—30 this week."[26]

In this context of increasingly burdensome demands, an opportunity arose that lured Osler away from Johns Hopkins and North America. In 1904, he wrote in his diary,

> Early in the year I had a letter from my old teacher Sir John Burdon-Sanderson asking if I would consider the possibility of accepting the Regius Professorship of Medicine at Oxford, which he had just given up. This seemed to offer the chance of escape from an ever increasing pressure of work. I could not bear to give up teaching and become a mere money-machine and yet the Hospital work, the exacting practice and the many calls of outside affairs were telling on my strength. In spite of the most careful regulation of my time and health I was often utterly 'used up' at the end of the week, and the question was how long could I hold out at the high pressure.

He continued,

> The Oxford position was attractive from the leisure it was sure to give, and the prospect of finishing a lot of literary work. I had reached the stage when I was always in arrears and it seemed impossible to get time for serious work. On the other hand it seemed cruel to leave all my dear friends, and the young fellows with whom I had become so intimate, and the profession of America which

> had done so much for me. I wrote to Sir John saying that it did not seem
> possible to leave my present position, which I regarded as the premiere place
> in clinical medicine in the English speaking world. He replied that there was
> no hurry, and that we could talk matters over when I came to the B.M.A. in
> July. At Oxford, where I was given the honorary D.Sc., I went over the whole
> ground. The position was purely academic, largely executive—the head of the
> medical school, with no hospital work, and only by statute sixteen lectures;
> but in the profession and socially in England the place was one of dignity and
> importance. About July 31st I had a letter from Mr. Balfour, the premier,
> formally offering me the place, after an exchange of cables with Mrs. Osler I
> accepted.

On the page opposite this entry Osler wrote, "Mrs. Osler cabled me 'do
not procrastinate, accept. Better go in a steamer than go in a pine-box.' " He
elaborated,

> All along she was in favor of the change, feeling that the pace of my present
> life could have but one ending—a serious breakdown. I arranged to spend the
> session in Baltimore. There was a perfect chorus of lamentations, lay and
> medical, in America. In England the news of the appointment was very well
> received, tho all my friends wondered not a little that I should give up such a
> splendid clinical position for a comparative sinecure. Financially, of course, it
> meant a tremendous sacrifice.[1]

Grace Osler recalled her feelings when she first learned of the opportunity: "As I read [Sir John's letter] . . . I felt a tremendous weight lifted from my
shoulders as I had become very anxious about the danger of his keeping on at
the pace he had been going for several years in Baltimore."[27] She wrote to her
husband's longtime Canadian friend Henry Ogden, "Oxford is our fate as of
course you know. I have always wondered how Dr. Osler could get away
without a good excuse from the J.H.H. and the enormous amount of work.
Sometimes he has been nearly dead. This was something I have thought of. We
do not have to leave until May. Do pray ask all Dr. Osler's friends to make it
easy. He will find it so hard to say adieu."[28]

Harvey Cushing, who lived next door to the Oslers beginning in 1901,
was a "latch-keyer" who had free access to their home and library. He claimed,

> As the Baltimore years rolled on he had become more and more
> overwhelmed with strictly professional work, and in the spring of 1904 it had
> almost reached the breaking-point. Recognized from Hudson Bay to the Gulf,
> from Nova Scotia to California, as the doctor's doctor, even though he might
> curtail the number of ordinary professional consultations this could not be
> done when some member of a physician's immediate family was concerned.[29]

Overwork and concern about the consequences of his hectic pace led
Osler to accept the Regius Professorship in 1904. But Oxford had long
appealed to him. A decade earlier he informed Lewellys Barker, "We have
been enjoying the British Association [meeting] here so much. I have lost my
heart to Oxford & I feel like the Queen of Sheba after Solomon had displayed
all the treasures of his house."[30] Osler's longtime friend Archibald Malloch
claimed, "There was much to attract him in England and he knew it well from
life in his post-graduate days and from numerous trips in the summer vacation.
England offered him, in many ways, things that he could not find in the New
World, and not least among these was Bodley's Library. And as he once said: 'It
was always my wish to live within an hour's run of the British Museum.' "[31]

Osler's decision was made known to many of his close friends and
colleagues in letters written aboard the S.S. *Cedric* as he was returning to

America in August 1904. The letters contain common themes that provide further insight into Osler's decision to leave Johns Hopkins. It seems likely that he informed his colleagues in this manner to avoid the kind of lobbying that had led him to pass up the opportunity in Edinburgh four years earlier.

To Henry Barton Jacobs, another "latch-keyer," Osler wrote,

> You will be disgusted to hear that I have accepted the chair of medicine at Oxford—not to leave tho, until next May or June. 'Tis a purely academical position in which one can do as much or as little as one wishes. Two things have influenced me. First, the feeling that I could not possibly last long at my present pace. I have had warnings that the pressure has been too high & it does not seem possible to lower it—at least I tried hard last winter & failed. Secondly, Oxford is a quiet restful place for a man of my habits and tastes and there is much in the life there that appeals to me. It will be a hard wrench to part with all my good friends & you dear boys at the Hospital. Mrs. Osler is strongly in favor of it, largely on my account as she has been much worried about the racket of my present life. . . . Please do not scold me—I really feel it is the best thing to do under the circumstances.[32]

Grace Osler played an important part in her husband's decision to go to Oxford. She informed Charles Camac, "You can never know what a struggle it has been and such hard work for me to encourage Dr. Osler to do what I knew was really the best for him—I am sure he can never regret this—but we both anticipate woeful days."[33] Osler told Camac, "I have accepted the Chair of Medicine at Oxford. Virtually it is a retirement as there is no Clinical School but a purely Academic berth. With as little or as much teaching as one likes. I am tired of the strain of the past few years which could have only one end—a breakdown."[34]

In his letter to Judge Henry Harlan, the president of the board of trustees of Johns Hopkins, Osler acknowledged that he was leaving "the best equipped medical clinic in the English speaking world" and giving up a lucrative practice.[35] He confessed to the university's new president, "I have reached the end of the session of late years thoroughly done up. I tried hard this winter to limit my outside work, but without much success—it only grows—and I have less and less time for teaching and for my literary work."[36]

In his letters to his colleagues at Johns Hopkins, Osler revealed his concern about his hectic life. He told William Sidney Thayer, "I am on the downgrade, the pace of the last three winters has been such that I knew I was riding for a fall. Better to get out decently in time, & leave while there is still a little elasticity in the rubber."[37–39]

Osler confessed to his friend Weir Mitchell, who had written extensively on the emotional dangers of overwork, "I am tired of the incessant racket of my present life. I tried hard last winter to cut off some of the work but without any success, and I am often on the edge of a break-down."[40] Mitchell responded,

> I read your letter with very mingled feelings. . . . [but] I think you are wisely counselled to go. Twice in the last year I was on the point of writing to ask you to consider whether you are not being worked beyond your strength. . . .
> When I read your letter to my wife, she said isn't it splendid? and I—isn't it sorrowful?—for of course this does take you out of my life. . . . As to Jn. Hopkins—perhaps you do not know that the med. school at J.H. is or was Wm. Osler.[41]

Osler left family members as well as friends when he went to Oxford. His mother was 97 when she learned from him that he was going to England. He reassured her, "It is a nice comfortable berth without very arduous duties. . . . It will be much better for the boy in every way, and I will have a quieter life. We can come out every year and I daresay see more of you than we have done of late."[42]

Osler's announcement produced an outpouring of ambivalent feelings from his friends and colleagues. Henry Hurd, a psychiatrist and superintendent of the Johns Hopkins Hospital, expressed his disappointment but added, "I have thought for a long time that you were driving the machine much too hard and that you must inevitably break down if you did not find some way to slow up." Hurd addressed the impact of Osler's departure on the institution they had worked hard to develop: "But what are we to do here in the Hospital and Medical School and in the community at large where you have done so much and are likely to leave so much to do that nobody can do so well? . . . I feel that the success of the Hospital and Medical School has been largely your achievement."[43]

William Welch, Osler's longtime colleague, told him, "Your letter drove me into a fit of the blues. . . . Your going will be an irreparable loss to us in a multitude of ways. . . . It is a blessing that you remain through this year and you must help us in choosing your successor; of course your place never can be really filled by any one else."[44,45]

In many of his letters, Osler referred to his concern that he was heading for a breakdown. Although the implication is that he was concerned about the nervous effects of overwork (he was well aware of the concept of neurasthenia and thought physicians were predisposed to it), there is reason to believe that he was also worried about his cardiovascular system. His brother, Britton Bath Osler, 10 years his senior, died in 1901. Osler informed his friend Francis Shepherd that Britton "went off with coronary disease. He has had slow pulse with syncopal attacks for a year. 'Twas a mercy that he died suddenly as he dreaded a long illness."[46,47]

There is evidence that Osler thought he had angina pectoris. In 1902 he entered in his diary, "In May I had a severe coryza for a week with involvement of the frontal sinuses. I had too, when hard pressed, several days of sub-sternal tension, a warning of too-high pressure."[1,48] Osler's autobiographical notes for 1907, two years after his arrival in Oxford, include the comment, "I have been very much better in health since coming here—no cardiac irregularities, or substernal tension."[1]

In his 1897 monograph on angina pectoris, Osler noted the frequency of this symptom in physicians. He claimed,

> In the worry and strain of modern life arterial degeneration is not only very common, but develops often at a relatively early age. For this I believe that the high pressure at which men live, and the habit of working the machine to its maximum capacity, are responsible, rather than excesses in eating and drinking, or than any special prevalence of syphilis. Angeio-sclerosis, creeping on slowly but surely, 'with no pace preceived,' is the Nemesis through which Nature exacts retributive justice for the transgression of her laws—coming to one as an apoplexy, to another as an early Bright's disease, to a third as an aneurysm, and to a fourth as angina pectoris, too often slitting 'the thin spun life' in the fifth decade, at the very time when success seems assured.[49]

In Osler's Lumleian lectures on angina pectoris in 1910, he called angina the "morbus medicorum" to emphasize its frequency among physicians. In recounting the cases of a number of prominent doctors who had died after attacks of angina he mentioned his good friend William Pepper, who "died with coronary arteries like pipe-stems." Speaking of Pepper, Osler could have been describing his own career. He referred to his departed Philadelphia friend as "a universally sought consultant, an enthusiastic teacher, a prolific author, in him was incarnate the restless American spirit, which drove him into a premature grave at the height of his career at the comparatively early age of 55."

Osler emphasized the uncertainty of the prognosis in cases of angina:

> Much depends on the patient himself—on the life he has led—the life he is willing to lead. The ordinary high-pressure business or professional man may find relief, or even cure, in the simple process of slowing the engines, reducing the speed from the 25 knots an hour of a Lusitania to the 10 knots of a 'black Bilbao tramp.' The difficulty is to induce a man of this type to lessen the race. . . . We doctors are notorious sinners in this respect, but it is so hard to lessen work when in full swing, so much harder than to give up altogether, and how few of us at 50 or 55 are able to do this![50]

At 55, Osler was willing to try. He went to Oxford.

A decade after his departure from Baltimore, Osler recalled the strain of his final years there. He told an audience at St. Bartholomew's Hospital, "William Pepper, my predecessor in Philadelphia, died of angina at 55; John Musser, my successor, of the same disease at 53! After listening to my story [about medical teaching at Johns Hopkins] you may wonder how it was possible to leave a place so gratifying to the ambitions of any clinical teacher: I had a good innings and was glad to get away without a serious breakdown."[51]

Another reason Osler preferred Oxford to Baltimore was his bibliomania. He had long loved books and wanted to be close to libraries and booksellers. In 1891 he wrote to Charles Fisher, the librarian of the College of Physicians of Philadelphia, "I miss the Library very much. For it alone it would be worth returning to Philadelphia."[52] Although the libraries of the Medical and Chirurgical Faculty of Maryland and the Johns Hopkins Hospital were growing rapidly in sophistication and quantity, they could not match the great collections in Oxford and London. Moreover, Oxford afforded ready access to the book dealers on the continent. Osler was well aware that the collectors of medical books found most of their treasures in European bookshops. Cards and letters written during his frequent summer trips to Europe from Baltimore mentioned recent acquisitions. Writing from Amsterdam in the summer of 1901, Grace Osler informed one of the "latch-keyers" that her husband was having a great time book hunting. In her words, he "became utterly disgusted at every place where old books were not forthcoming and promptly wanted to leave."[53]

In his valedictory address at Johns Hopkins, delivered in 1905, Osler told his many friends and colleagues that his years in Baltimore had been exceptionally happy. He publicly explained his departure:

> Neither stricken deeply in years, nor damaged seriously by illness, you may well wonder at the motives that have induced me to give up a position of such influence and importance, to part from colleagues so congenial, from associates and students so devoted, and to leave a country in which I have so many warm friends, and in which I have been appreciated at so much more than my real worth.

He continued,

> After years of hard work, at the very time when a man's energies begin to flag, and when he feels the need of more leisure, the conditions and surroundings that have made him what he is and that have moulded his character and

abilities into something useful in the community—these very circumstances ensure an ever increasing demand upon them; and when the call of the East comes, which in one form or another is heard by all of us, and which grows louder as we grow older, the call may come like the summons to Elijah, and not alone the ploughing of the day, but the work of a life, friends, relatives, even father and mother, are left to take up new work in a new field.

Osler considered the effect his departure from Johns Hopkins would have on the institution. "This is not a university that men care to leave," he told his audience. But, he assured them, "I do not see that the departure of any one has proved a serious blow." He claimed that a professor could stay too long in one institution: "We are apt to grow stale and thin mentally if kept too long in the same pasture." Periodic change benefited both the person and the institution.[54]

Osler left Baltimore on May 15, 1905, and traveled to New York, where four days later he and his wife boarded the S.S. *Cedric* for their journey to England and a new, and they hoped less rigorous, life. A few months after his arrival in Oxford, Osler informed his lifelong friend Ned Milburn, "I have settled down into a quiet life here and like it very much. We are finding some difficulty in getting a suitable house, but I think we shall like everything here very much. Of course, the life is very different but very restful after the sort of racket I have had for some years."[55]

In 1906 Osler entered in his diary,

> Today finishes my first year in Oxford. On the whole I have stood the change better than I expected. It was very hard at first. I missed my old associates and young men with whom I had become as intimate. We were both homesick for a week or two, and I confess to one or two restless and sleepless nights, and yet it seemed unreasonable to worry and I set my face steadfastly toward the east, resolved to make the best of the new circumstances. The term was nearly over when we arrived, so I did not lecture. Everyone was most kind, particularly the local physicians.[1]

Osler spent the last 14 years of his life in Oxford. It was not the life of a man who had retired; he remained active in teaching, writing, and consulting. Nevertheless, the pace was slower, and he had more time for his son and for his historical and literary interests. Osler never regretted his decision to leave America. At the height of his career "the chief" became the Regius Professor to preserve his emotional and physical health. Today, we might term Osler's tribulations over his decision to leave Johns Hopkins "midlife crisis" or "burnout." He succeeded, however, in his attempt to find a more suitable lifestyle in a position that brought him continued fame, but at less cost.

I am indebted to the archivists of the Trent Collection at Duke University, the Alan M. Chesney Archives of the Johns Hopkins Medical Institutions, the Osler Library at McGill University, and Washington University for their help and for granting permission to incorporate manuscript materials from their collections in his article.

References

1. Bensley EH, Bates DG. Sir William Osler's autobiographical notes. Bull Hist Med 1976; 50:596–618.
2. Barker LF. Osler at Johns Hopkins. Can J Med Surg 1920; 47;135–46.
3. Osler to Gilman, 6 March 1889. In: Cushing H. The life of Sir William Osler. Vol. 1. London: Oxford University Press, 1925:325.

4. Chesney AM. The Johns Hopkins Hospital and the Johns Hopkins University School of Medicine, a chronicle: early years, 1867–1893. Vol. 1. Baltimore: Johns Hopkins University Press, 1943.

5. Cushing H. The life of Sir William Osler. Vol. 1. London: Oxford University Press, 1925:373.

6. Osler to Lafleur, 12 January 1893. In: Cushing H. The life of Sir William Osler. Vol. 1. London: Oxford University Press, 1925:375.

7. Pepper to Osler, 10 January 1895. In: Grace Revere Osler's scrapbook. Montreal: Osler Library, McGill University.

8. Osler to Schäfer, 14 May 1897. In: Cushing H. The life of Sir William Osler. Vol. 1. London: Oxford University Press, 1925:451–2.

9. Osler to Thayer, [12 August 1898]. In: Cushing H. The life of Sir William Osler. Vol. 1. London: Oxford University Press, 1925:477–8.

10. Wilson JC. Dr. Osler in Philadelphia, teacher and clinician. [1905]. Int Assoc Med Museum Bull. 1926; 9:243–6.

11. Osler to [Charlotte] Lisbeth Osler Gwyn, [c February 1900]. In: Cushing H. The life of Sir William Osler. Vol. I. London: Oxford University Press, 1925:515.

12. Osler to Schäfer, 27 March 1900. In: Cushing H. The life of Sir William Osler. Vol. 1. London: Oxford University Press, 1925:519.

13. Welch to Gilman, 27 March 1900. Ballimore: Alan M. Chesney Archives, Johns Hopkins Medical Institutions.

14. Osler W. Daybooks 1874–1918. Montreal: Osler Library, McGill University.

15. Harrell GT. Osler's practice. Bull Hist Med 1973; 47:545–68.

16. Osler to Camac, 9 February 1899. In: Nation EF, McGovern JP. Student and chief, the Osler-Camac correspondence. Pasadena, Calif.: Castle Press, 1980:11–2.

17. Cushing H. The life of Sir William Osler. Vol. 1. London: Oxford University Press, 1925:490.

18. Barker LF. Osler in America: with especial reference to his Baltimore period. Can Med Assoc J 1935; 33:353–9.

19. Osler to Barker, c 1901. Baltimore: Barker papers, Aian M. Chesney Archives, Johns Hopkins Medical Institutions.

20. Osler to Barker, 4 April 1901. Baltimore: Barker papers, Alan M. Chesney Archives, Johns Hopkins Medical Institutions.

21. Osler to Shepherd, 18 October 1901. Montreal: Shepherd folder, Osler Library, McGill University.

22. Osler to Howell, 22 April 1902. In: Cushing H. The life of Sir William Osler. Vol. 1. London: Oxford University Press, 1925:576–7.

23. Chesney AM. The Johns Hopkins Hospital and the Johns Hopkins University School of Medicine, a chronicle: 1893–1905. Vol. 2. Baltimore: Johns Hopkins University Press, 1958.

24. Walter Baumgarten to Gustav Baumgarten. 23 April 1902. Baumgarten papers. St. Louis: Archives, Washington Universily School of Medicine.

25. On the educational value of the medical society. In: Osler W. Aequanimitas: with other addresses to medical students, nurses and practitioners of medicine. Philadelphia; Blakiston, 1904;345–62.

26. Osler to Musser, 1 May 1904. In: Cushing H. The life of Sir William Osler. Vol. 1. London: Oxford University Press, 1925:637.

27. Grace Revere Osler [to Harvey Cushingl. In: Cushing H. The life of Sir William Osler. Vol 1. London: Oxford University Press, 1925:644.

28. Grace Revere Osler to Ogden, 25 August 1904. In: Weistrop L. The life & letters of Dr. Henry Vining Ogden, 1857–1931. Milwaukee: Milwaukee Academy of Medicine Press, 1986: 111–2.

29. Cushing H. The life of Sir William Osler. Vol. 1. London: Oxford University Press, 1925:636.

30. Osler to Barker, 14 [August 1894]. Baltimore: Barker papers, Alan M. Chesney Archives, Johns Hopkins Medical Institutions.

31. Malloch A. Sir William Osler at Oxford. Int Assoc Med Museum Bull 1926; 9:363–77.

32. Osler to Jacobs, 8 August 1904. Baltimore: Jacobs collection. Alan M. Chesney Archives, Johns Hopkins Medical Institutions.

33. Grace Revere Osler to Camac, [August 1904]. In: Nation EF, McGovern JP. Student and chief, the Osler-Camac correspondence. Pasadena. Calif.: Castle Press, 1980:31.

34. Osler to Camac, 14 [August 1904]. In: Nation EF, McGovern JP. Student and chief, the Osler-Camac correspondence. Pasadena, Calif.: Castle Press, 1980:30.

35. Osler to Harlan, 6 August 1904. Baltimore: Alan M. Chesney Archives, Johns Hopkins Medical Institutions.

36. Osler to Ira Remsen, 6 August 1904. Baltimore: Alan M. Chesney Archives, Johns Hopkins Medical Institutions.

37. Osler to Thayer, 6 August 1904. In: Cushing H. The life of Sir William Osler. Vol. 1. London: Oxford University Press, 1925:651.

38. Osler to George Dock, 10 August 1904. Montreal: Dock folder, Osler Library, McGill University.

39. Osler to Mall, 8 August 1904. Baltimore: Mall papers, Alan M. Chesney Archives, Johns Hopkins Medical Institutions.

40. Osler to Mitchell, 8 August 1904. Durham, N.C.: Trent collection, Duke University Medical Center.

41. Mitchell to Osler, 14 August 1904. In: Cushing H. The life of Sir William Osler. Vol. 1. London: Oxford University Press, 1925:651–2.

42. William Osler to Ellen Osler, 6 August 1904. Montreal: Osler Library, McGill University.

43. Hurd to Osler, 14 August 1904. Montreal: Osler Library, McGill University.

44. Welch to Osler, 30 August 1902. Baltimore: Welch papers, Alan M. Chesney Archives, Johns Hopkins Medical Institutions.

45. Welch WH. A great physician and medical humanist. Sat Rev Lit 1925; 2:309–10.

46. Osler to Shepherd, 11 February 1902. In: Cushing H. The life of Sir William Osler. Vol. 1. London: Oxford University Press, 1925:548.

47. Wilkinson A. Lions in the way: a discursive history of the Oslers. Toronto: Macmillan, 1956.

48. Golden R. Sir William Osler's angina pectoris and other disorders. Am J Cardiol 1987; 60:175–8.

49. Osler W. Lectures on angina pectoris and allied states. New York: D. Appleton, 1897.

50. *Idem*. The Lumleian lectures on angina pectoris. Lancet 1910; 1:697–702, 839–44, 973–7.

51. *Idem*. An address on the medical clinic; a retrospect and a forecast. Br Med J 1914; 1:10–6.

52. Krumbhaar EB. Additional notes on Osler in Philadelphia. Arch Intern Med 1949; 84:26–33.

53. Cushing H. The life of Sir William Osler. Vol. 1. London: Oxford University Press, 1925:558.

54. Osler W. Valedictory address at Johns Hopkins University. JAMA 1905; 44:705–10.

55. Osler to Milburn, 11 November 1905. In: Holley HL. A continual remembrance: letters from Sir William Osler to his friend Ned Milburn, 1865–1919. Springfield, Ill.: Charles C Thomas, 1968:83.

The Oslers' Son—Revere

 George T. Harrell, M.D.

William and Grace Revere Osler married relatively late in life.[1] What sort of person was the only surviving child of these world famous, devoted, and often overly solicitous parents? Grace's first pregnancy while married to Osler had resulted in a son who lived only seven days. The second, and last pregnancy, was marred by an attack of peritonitis in the mother during the first trimester. On December 28, 1895, Edward Revere Osler was delivered by Howard A. Kelly at the Osler's home in Baltimore. The boy weighed seven pounds and was blue-eyed and fair-haired like his mother. She was 42 and his father 46. Osler was very excited, but waited five days before he kissed the child. He then began the role he followed over the years of proud parent who showed off his child at every opportunity and wrote about him in letters to family and professional friends.[2]

Childhood

From the beginning Revere was described as a happy, gentle, shy, sweet child who never gave any trouble. The black mammy who originally cared for him was quickly replaced by a Scotch governess when Osler heard Revere at age four order: "Hist dat window."[3] His father already had registered him for British citizenship and was determined he should be educated in England. The boy was very close to his mother, but he also spent much time with his father when the family went on trips to Canada and abroad. When he was six, he went to England for the first time. He was introduced to cricket at eight on Guernsey where he promptly knocked a ball through a window. During his childhood his father had begun to read Milton's "Ode on the Morning of Christ's Nativity" to his son on Christmas Eve.[4] During his whole life he was

Read at the annual meeting of the American Osler Society meeting, April 29, 1980.

Reprinted with permission from *Bulletin of the History of Medicine, 54*:561, 1980

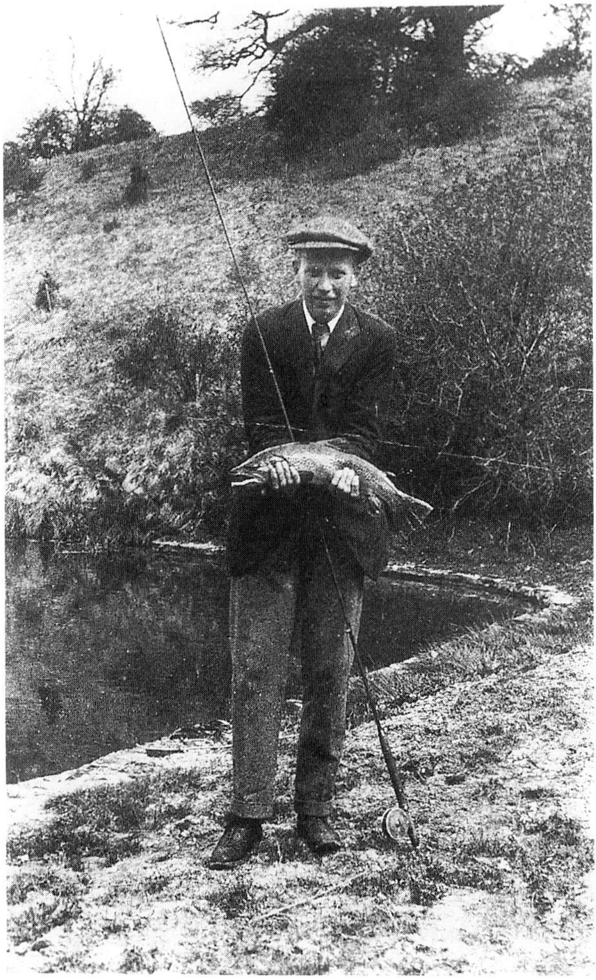

FIGURE 1 Revere with trout at Cornbury Park lake.

exposed to English literature and encouraged to follow his father's interest in the books of the classics.

Schooling

Little is known of Revere's early education in Baltimore. The Oslers moved to Oxford when he was ten, and he entered the Dragon school. He began playing football there. His father repeatedly noted that the boy was not interested in schooling or formal studies and would not become a scholar. For a few years, he had an interest in stamps. His parents took him abroad to Paris, Florence, other cities on the Continent and also back to North America. By age fifteen he had grown taller than his father and was entered at Winchester. For the first time he was on his own away from his family. His academic performance was mediocre, and he required tutoring, especially in Latin and Greek. He played cricket and happily plunged into the life of an English public schoolboy.

By 1913 he was age 18, but had not decided on a future career. He failed on his first attempt to pass the entrance examinations for Oxford, though he had been tutored the winter before. He repeated the exams, this time passing them successfully and in October 1914, entered Christ Church College where he lived in. Revere was proud of his college and included its crest in the bookplate he designed. The war and its pressures already were disrupting the lives of most young men. His parents and family in Canada urged him to continue his education as long as he could, but he was very uneasy about not being in uniform. His formal education ended in January, 1915, after he turned 19, when he withdrew from college to enter the military.

Friends

Little is known of his friends in Baltimore. Occasionally a child would be invited by his parents to lunch. On moving to Oxford, Revere played with the Max Müller boys from whose family the first house at 7 Norham Gardens was rented.

During the first summer vacation after entering Winchester, he had a friend, Raleigh Parker, with his sister as guests for fishing. Mrs. Osler always had girls around the house and a French girl spent a year with them. Two Canadian sisters were special friends over the years. On her death, Lady Osler left a ring to the quieter, younger one whose first long dress she had made for the girl to go to a dance with Revere. That friendship persisted into college, and the young lady gave great comfort to his mother after Revere's death. A friend, Bobby Emmons of Oxford, was a frequent companion during the college and war years. He participated in one of Revere's rare practical jokes played on his father in a fictitious letter about rare books. The very close ties with his parents and their friends, the fact that he was an only child, and by nature shy, apparently did not lead to many strong friendships. Revere's chief interests and hobbies were solitary ones he could pursue alone.

Fishing

Revere's consuming life-long passion was fishing which he pursued at every opportunity. He became entranced with the sport at age nine in Murray Bay, Quebec. The next year in Oxford he caught a variety of fish, including a pike of record size. Thereafter, family vacations and holidays anywhere were planned with opportunities for fishing in mind. His father encouraged him and often went with him. His mother went occasionally. Professional instruction was arranged, and his father's friends sent rods and advice. Some of the boy's most charming letters, which reflected his mother's style and literary skill, were written to thank them and describe his fishing experiences. Osler seized on this interest as a means of stimulating his son to emulate his own deep concern with books and bought him first editions of Izaac Walton's writings. His father used Isaac or Ike as the most frequent nicknames for Revere. When he designed his bookplate, Revere included fishing tackle and described himself on it as "Discip. IZ. WA."

He fished for some years before he caught his first salmon on August 30, 1913, in Elder's pool, Kirksig River, Sutherland. It weighed nine and three-quarter pounds. The family excitement was so great that a formal dinner for nine guests was arranged the next day at the Culag Hotel, Lochinver, North Britain. The handwritten menu to which the actual fly used is attached still exists.[5] Another sheet of paper has the signatures of the guests with a drawing of the fish, signed E. Revere Osler, and a childish sketch showing the landing with a second kneeling figure holding a boathook. These memorabilia are pasted in Revere's copy of a reprint of Walton's *Compleat Angler* presented to him in September, 1913. A photograph is preserved of two trout weighing four and one-quarter and four and one-half pounds caught with a fly June 21, 1914. In May, 1917, while on leave in England, he caught a record trout at Cornbury Park Lake (Figure 1).

Osler apparently also used Revere's interest in fishing to try to develop a wider one in natural history in general such as he had had in Canada while young. In 1908 while in Paris, he borrowed a microscope for a joint field excursion. The following year Osler and Revere investigated a pond in Oxford, but neither occasion kindled the boy's interest. Osler concluded Revere would never be a scientist.

Cabinet work

At an early Christmas in Baltimore, probably 1898 when he was three, Revere was given a set of carpenter's tools. A letter from his mother describes the son and father happily driving nails into the floor and furniture. A reply from the grandmother supposes the early use of tools will later turn his attention to architecture, an interesting prediction in view of his etching subjects as a teenager.[6] No other written record has been found on this long term interest in carpentering, but Revere included some tools on his bookplate. A letter by Osler in August, 1912, mentions Revere as a "good carpenter." He more properly should be considered an amateur cabinetmaker, as judged by several existing pieces of his work. Members of the Revere family in Massachusetts have a dark finished chair-side carved magazine or book rack, and a small light finished chest on tall slender legs with two inlaid doors over three narrow drawers. A larger dark finished chest with hinged lid similar to those used to store toys or blankets at the foot of a bed is in the Tudor and Stuart Club room on The Johns Hopkins University Homewood campus in Baltimore. The sides are carved in a vertical pattern similar to the magazine rack (Figure 2). The work table he used, said to be Jacobean, is in the Osler Library at McGill University in Montreal.

Art

Revere was a direct descendant of the famous American silversmith, Paul Revere. His mother did some simple sketches to illustrate letters, so his artistic interest and talent had a long family background. Early examples of his work are simple line drawings of a head and the wings of insects, probably done in Oxford during the summer of 1910. He had been avidly collecting butterflies and moths from age 12. Several simple drawings of fish have been preserved.

During the spring of 1912, the family visited northern Italy and Osler introduced his son to some features of architecture. Revere made sketches in Florence and took photographs in Venice of friezes, gargoyles and other details, but none of these were found. This interest grew after the family returned to England and Revere expanded his interests to etching. Miss

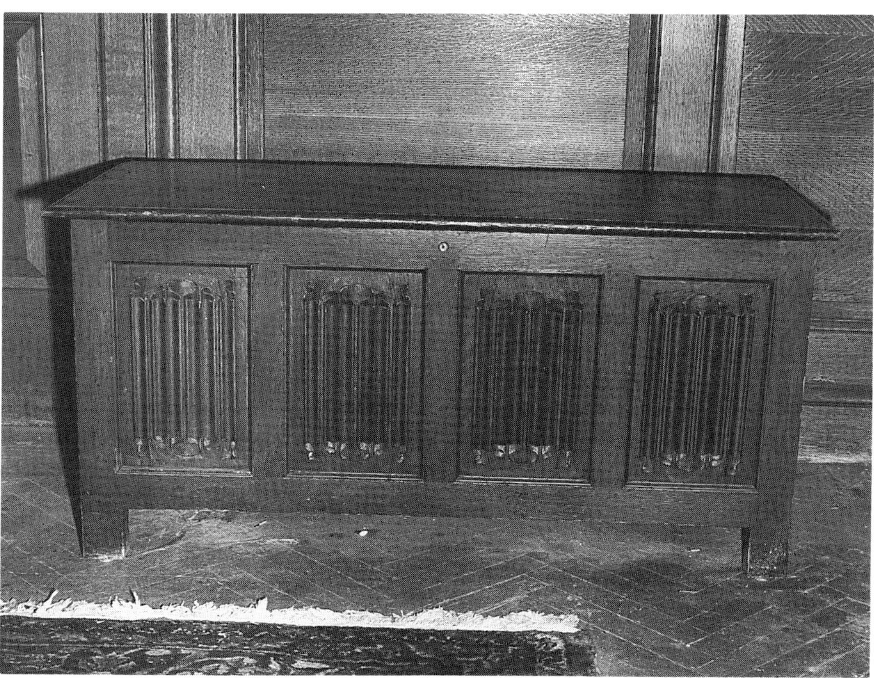

FIGURE 2   Chest in Baltimore.

Marion Wright, a young Canadian student in Oxford, was a close friend of Revere whom she described as artistic. He etched in his room at Christ Church College and often had her critique his work. Miss Margaret Revere, a niece of Lady Osler, inherited a print of one of his etchings, the only known surviving one made by Revere himself (Figure 3). The print is unsigned, the subject is not identified on it, nor did Miss Revere know what it was. A photograph of the etching was made and sent to various people in England, Canada and the States, asking if they recognized the subject. It was assumed to be a doorway in Oxford, possibly at 13 Norham Gardens, but all replies were negative for "The Open Arms" as the location and no one in Oxford could identify a similar place in the colleges.

While reviewing the books in the Tudor and Stuart Club room, it was discovered that a cardboard box which might contain memorabilia was in the files of the English Department. When examined, this box was found to contain six small manila envelopes which held copper plates of etchings not previously recognized. On the front of each in an unidentified handwriting was the statement that the plates were done by Edward Revere Osler. The plates vary in size from $8 \times 4^1/2$ to $3^1/2 \times 2^1/2$ inches. The subject of the largest is identified as Merton College, Oxford, with other envelopes being labeled Oxford Castle, Norfolk, Doorway in Norwich. Two plates are not identified and one of these is labeled "cancelled." That plate is scored with parallel lines across it and contains several spots which might have been caused by acid drops. The envelopes are not dated, but the etchings probably were done between 1913–14 when Revere was 18–19 years old. All are of architectural subjects and the print of Miss Revere's was from the Norwich plate which measures $7 \times 3^1/2$ inches.

This information was transmitted to Dr. A. H. T. Robb-Smith who had tried unsuccessfully to identify the subject of Miss Revere's print in Oxford. He recalled that Revere had been tutored in the Norfolk-Norwich area. He had in his library a book containing water colors by E. W. Hazelhurst, including one of Stranger's Hall, originally a 15th-century home of a merchant and now a folk museum. He identified it as the subject. A photograph of the painting shows that Revere etched the doorway so that the print is a mirror image with a few small deviations in the windows.

Osler had predicted in letters that his son would become an architect or an artist, since he was not a scholar. In one he mentions that Revere was etching from sketches, but does not identify the subjects. Osler wanted prints to send as Christmas gifts, but Revere refused. It is possible that Sir William saw prints of one or more of the plates found. No plates or prints of etchings of known Italian subjects have been located, or are known actually to have been made. If they were, Revere must not have been satisfied with them. It is also possible that the cancelled plate and the other unidentified one might be of Italian rather than English subjects. The six plates were transferred in late 1979 from the Homewood campus to the Alan Mason Chesney Archives of The Johns Hopkins Medical Institutions.

In 1913, at age 18, Revere drew his bookplate.[7] The wood-mounted metal cut of the original is with the etching plates. In January, 1916, after his interest in books had grown, he began a small volume with blank pages to list his new accessions. He noted the date, place of purchase, author, title, price and occasionally other comments. The last entry is May 12 of the same year. The title page is beautifully done by pen in sepia ink. It is interesting that he used his first name Edward here, since on other occasions he signed himself E. R., E. Revere Osler, or simply Revere.

Books

From early childhood, Osler took Revere on his book hunting expeditions. He always had hoped that his son would be infected with his own enthusiasm for collecting classics. The interest was a long time developing. Revere's first purchase at an auction resulted from a bid in December, 1913, of £1 to Sotheby's for Landor's *Pericles and Aspasia*. Poetry, especially that of Spenser and Shelley, appears to have interested him. There is no documentation of earlier gifts or purchases in the 1916 list.

After Revere's death, on October 30, 1918, Sir William and Lady Osler gave to The Johns Hopkins University an endowment of securities realizing between $1500–$2000 per year to encourage students in the study of English literature of the Tudor and Stuart periods. The gift was a memorial to their son in recognition of the family's happy years in Baltimore. Revere's books were to be donated as the nucleus of an English departmental and literary club library. They were sent in March, 1922, and the club was started in early 1923. The books were mainly English literature and history, poems and sonnets and included four volumes of Spenser and a number by and about Shelley. Osler added some of his own books on general literature, including ones by Milton, Shelley, Keats and Fuller. Many books were about fishing, including ones by Walton. Revere's Bible and the 100,000th copy of Osler's *Textbook* which his father had given him were sent. On her death, Lady Osler willed an additional £2000 to the endowment and sent 79 more of Revere's books. The collection now included some volumes on drawing, engraving, architecture, war, the priesthood and Walt Whitman.

The club room was fitted out in Stuart style by Mrs. Robert Brewster with oak paneling and a fireplace. A portrait by Marie Page of Boston of Revere in uniform was hung January 22, 1926 (Figure 4). The club still sponsors an annual lecture. Its archives included, in addition to items mentioned previously, Revere's two army commissions, scrolls and letters about his death, three medals with ribbons, and a program of the memorial service held January 20, 1924, at St. James Church, Dundas, when a tablet was dedicated to

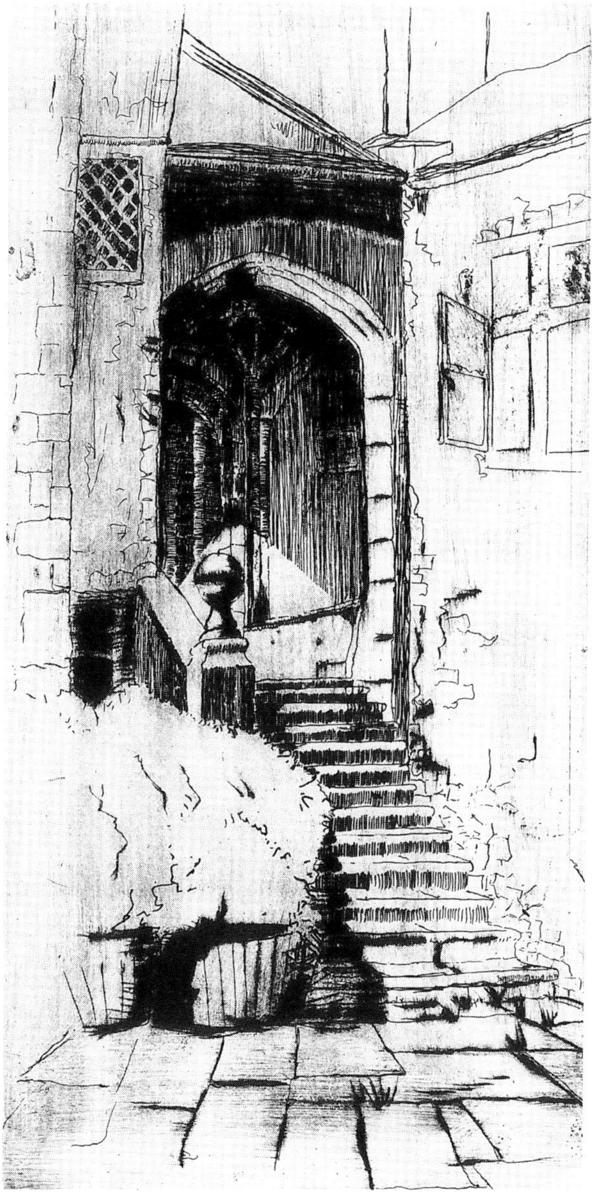

FIGURE 3   Etching now in Baltimore.

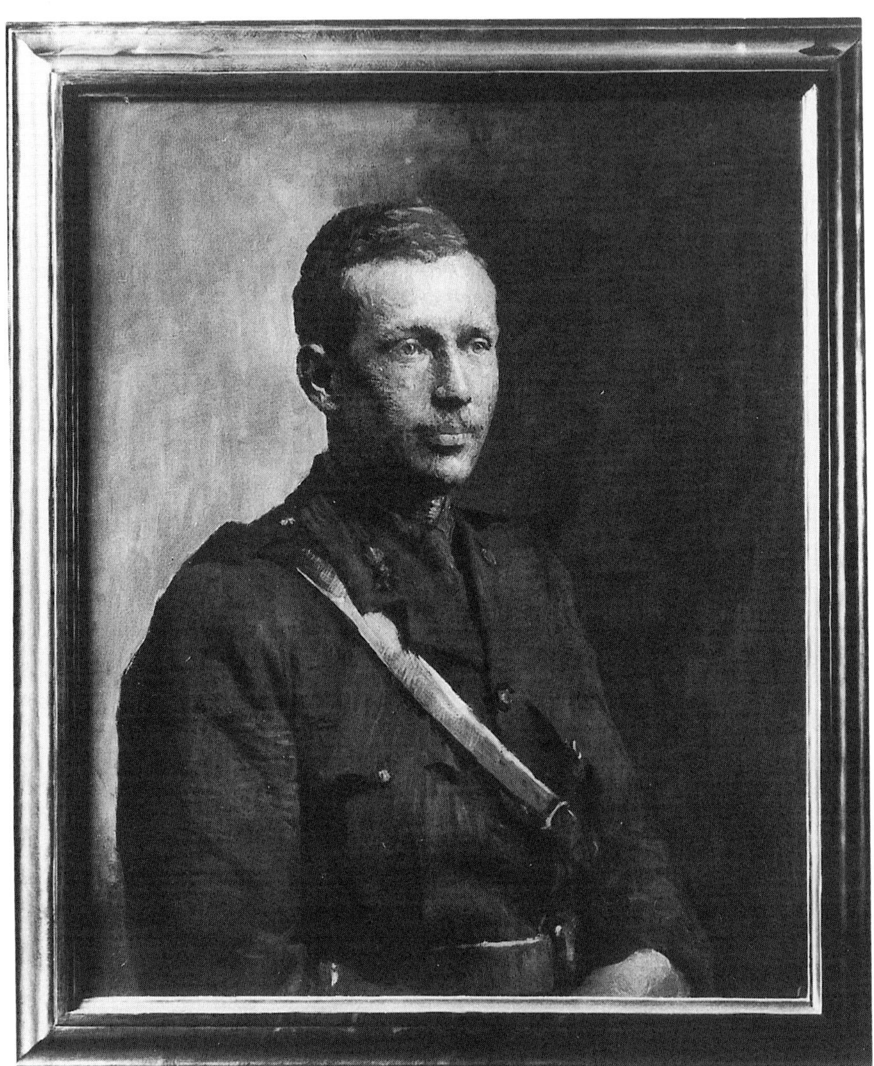

FIGURE 4 Portrait in the Tudor and Stuart Club, Baltimore.

three Oslers. These memorabilia were transferred in 1979 to the medical school archives along with the etching plates.

Military service

From the beginning of the war, both Sir William and Lady Osler had premonitions that it would bring tragedy. Many students at Oxford, sons of Canadian relatives or friends, were being killed or wounded. Revere was urged to enter and remain at Christ Church but the pressures of the times weighed heavily on his conscience. He could not talk to his father about it, but confided in his mother. In September, 1914, he entered the Officer's Training Corps in Oxford and attended the Public Schools camp at Salisbury. His first try for a commission failed, since he was judged "too immature." In January, 1915, he intended to enlist as a private in the Universities Public School Regiment. (Revere in a letter calls it "Public

Schools batallion'' (sic), while Cushing lists it as Inns of Court Corps.) His parents had learned that the McGill Hospital unit was organized and scheduled to come to England in the spring. By cable, Revere was offered an appointment as orderly to the Commanding Officer. On February 15, 1915, a commission was issued to "Revere Osler, Gentleman" as Honorary Lieutenant (Temporary) in the Canadian Militia. He was assigned as a quartermaster for supply duty to the base in Cliveden where the unit came in May. The hospital moved to France in June, but Revere was not happy with the lack of action. He applied for assignment to an ambulance corps in December, but continued to press for transfer to a fighting unit.

On April 28, 1916, a commission was issued to "E. R. Osler," 2nd Lieutenant in the Land Forces. It is stamped TEMPORARY at the top in red. On the folded front, the branch is listed as Royal Horse and Royal Field Artillery. Revere returned to England for training, then went back to France and immediately into action. In spite of living in trenches and his revulsion at the death and destruction around him, he seemed happier. Many letters addressed to "Muz or Dad" about his war experiences are preserved. On August 29, 1917, the day was quiet and Revere was helping bridge a shell hole to move his battery closer to the front lines near Ypres. Without warning about 4:30 in the afternoon, a 4.2 inch shell, which none of the 20 men working had heard coming, made a direct hit. Revere was severely wounded along with his commanding officer and six men. One fragment of the shell traversed the upper abdomen cutting holes in the colon and mesenteric vessels. Another penetrated the chest just above the heart and two others the thigh, but the femur was not fractured. Cushing was notified, which Revere's mother had expressed hope for in a letter several weeks earlier, and came immediately to aid Revere. A transfusion was done and the abdomen opened about midnight to stop the bleeding, but Revere died about seven the next morning. He was buried near Poperinghe in Belgium. The original wooden grave marker has been replaced by a stone one.

Osler was working in his library late in the afternoon when the telegram came telling of the wound. A phone call at nine that evening confirmed Revere's death. Neither parent ever recovered from the tragedy. Though Osler considered having the body exhumed, cremated, and the ashes sent to the Tudor and Stuart club library, Lady Osler did not agree and it still remains buried in a Flanders Field.

Acknowledgements

Miss Marilyn Fransiszyn of the Osler Library, McGill University, Montreal, has furnished invaluable assistance in the collection of material for this paper, including photographs. Miss Margaret Revere, Chestnut Hill, Massachusetts, furnished photographs of cabinet work and presented the author with the print of the Norwich etching. Miss Marion Wright, Montreal, graciously consented to interviews. Dr. A. H. T. Robb-Smith, Woodstock, Oxfordshire, England, identified the subject of the Norwich etching. The English Department, The Johns Hopkins University, permitted review of the books and kindly furnished photocopies of material in the Tudor and Stuart club archives. John E. Sparks, Head of the Department of Prints, Maryland Institute College of Art, Baltimore, cleaned the plates and made new sets of prints.

Notes

1. George T. Harrell, "Lady Osler," *Bull. Hist. Med.*, 1979, *53:* 81–99.
2. Harvey Cushing, *The Life of Sir William Osler* (New York: Oxford University Press, 1940) has many scattered, brief references to Revere.
3. Edith Gittings Reid, *The Great Physician: A Short Life of Sir William Osler* (New York: Oxford University Press, 1931), pp. 145–286.
4. Anne Wilkinson, *Lions in the Way: A Discursive History of the Oslers* (Toronto: Macmillan, 1956). pp. 198–224.
5. The menu was as follows:

Clear Soup
Scotch Broth

———

Boiled Salmon, Hollandaise Sauce
a la Revere (added in pencil)

———

Saute of Kidney
Curried Prawns

———

Roast Chicken
Roast Beef

———

Bachelor's Pudding
<u>Trifle</u>!!!! (exclamation points and underlining
added in pencil)
Compote of Pears

———

Cheese Dessert

6   E. Osler to Grace Revere Osler, letter (copy) 1899. Acc. 417/95, the Osler Library, McGill University, Montreal.
7   Thomas E. Keys, "Edward Revere Osler: 1895–1917," *Arch. Int. Med.*, 1964, *114:* 284–293.

William Osler's Experiences with Smallpox

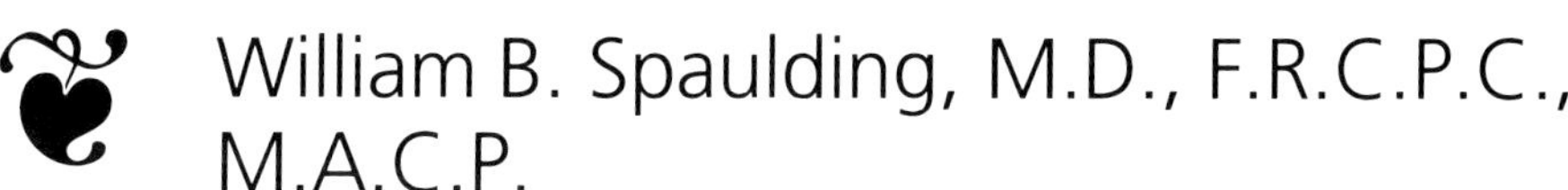William B. Spaulding, M.D., F.R.C.P.C., M.A.C.P.

Summary

William Osler had extensive first-hand experience with smallpox. Soon after his appointment to the Faculty of Medicine at McGill, he became Physician to the Smallpox Department of the Montreal General Hospital. His first major clinical publications dealt with the initial rashes and the uniformly fatal hemorrhagic form of smallpox. In his textbook, he wrote extensively about the disease, drawing on personal experience, and describing the devastating epidemic in Montreal in 1885. Later, he spoke out publicly against the powerful anti-vaccinationist lobby, likening his challenge to that of Elijah confronting the priests of Baal. He placed classic publications on smallpox in the first rank or Prima section of the Bibliotheca Osleriana, which describes his library of medical history. Osler's involvement with smallpox shows his versatility as master clinician, writer of the most successful medical textbook of his time, educator of the public and medical historian.

When Osler graduated at age 22 from McGill University in 1872, he had neither a job nor prospects of future employment. True, his performance as a medical student ensured that Palmer Howard, his professor of medicine, appreciated his remarkable potential. Despite that, no academic doors swung open. In July, he sailed to the British Isles and Europe, accompanying his brother Edmund, who helped finance the venture. During nearly two years away, he did important work on the platelet, in London, and visited the leading institutes and clinics of Great Britain and the continent.

In the spring of 1874, he returned to the family home in Dundas, still

Presidential Address. Read at the annual meeting of the American Osler Society, April 12, 1986.

Reprinted with permission of *The Annals of The Royal College of Physicians & Surgeons of Canada*, 19:445, 1986

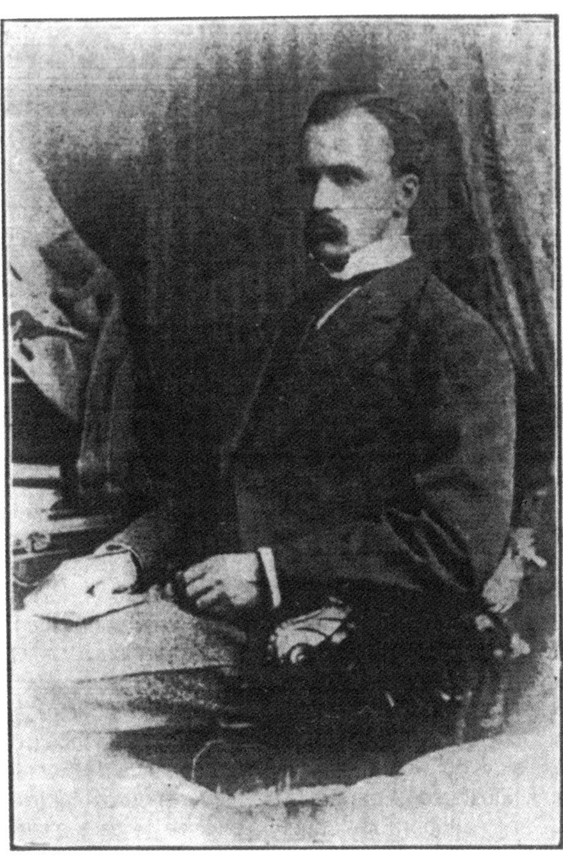

FIGURE 1 Osler as a student at McGill, 1871.

without a job. He spent time in Dundas as a locum tenens, and then a month as Resident Physician at the Hamilton City Hospital. In July, he was offered and accepted a position at McGill as Lecturer in the Institutes of Medicine. The job, which began in the autumn of 1874, called for the delivery of four lectures a week in physiology, and practical demonstrations in histology.[1]

Later in 1874, Osler applied for and was granted the position of attending physician to the smallpox wards of the Montreal General Hospital—his first major clinical responsibility. By looking at his published case reports, some of which are dated, one can be reasonably sure that he assumed duties in early 1875 and carried on until autumn, when the wards were closed, because two special hospitals for smallpox were opened elsewhere in the city.[2,3]

In Figure 1, we see Osler as a medical student. Figure 2 shows the young professor 10 years later.[4]

TABLE 1   SMALLPOX DEATHS IN MONTREAL[5]

Year	Number of deaths
1872	897
1873	228
1874	647
1875	590
1876	703
1877	506
1878	728
1879	472

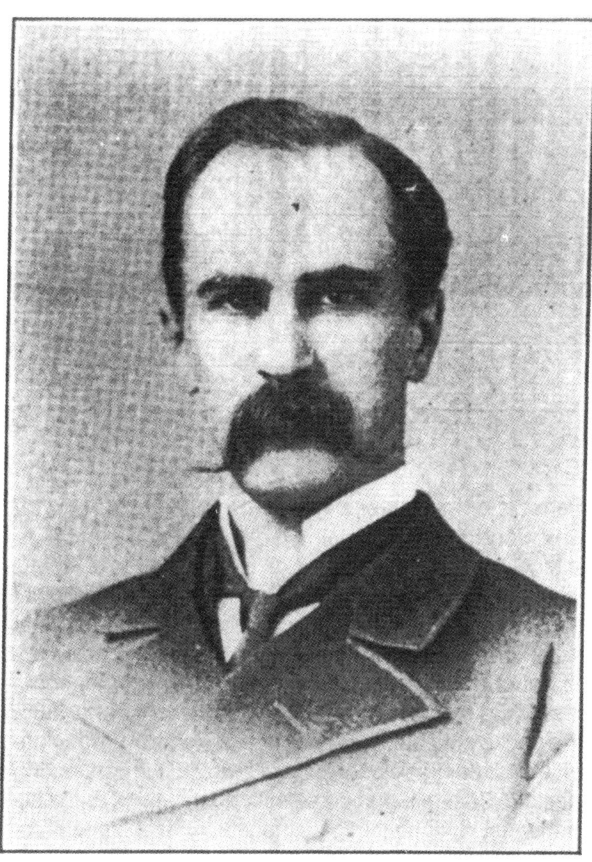

FIGURE 2   Osler in 1881.

At that time, Montreal, a city of 150,000 with a fine port, many factories and industries, and thriving trade, had a dismal record in infectious diseases. The press had branded Montreal as the "most unhealthy city in the world." One editorialist wrote, "We boast a Board of Health, salaried Health officers, and paid Health constables—but of what earthly use are all these when we are plainly told by them that they receive no information concerning the commencement, rise and spread of infectious diseases, and that they have no power to inspect premises, order removals, make improvements, or otherwise interfere to preserve the health of any place or district."[5]

In those days, and for years to come, Montreal was embroiled in a battle over vaccination. The English-speaking Protestants, led by their doctors and leading citizens, favored vaccination, compulsory if needed. The French-Canadian Catholics were less enthusiastic; some, including a few doctors, were vehement in their opposition.

Each year, hundreds died of smallpox in the city (Table 1).[6] For half a century, the Montreal General Hospital had been the leading centre in the city for the institutional treatment of smallpox (Figure 3).[7] At first, beginning in 1822, smallpox patients were treated in the main hospital building. To prevent the cross-contagion that occurred, a separate Fever Hospital was opened in 1868 behind the main building. The Fever Hospital had two public wards, which contained 40 beds, used mostly for smallpox, of which 150 cases were admitted in the first year. In 1871 and 1872, when another smallpox epidemic swept the city, some citizens and the leaders of the Montreal General Hospital campaigned unsuccessfully for a separate civic isolation hospital.

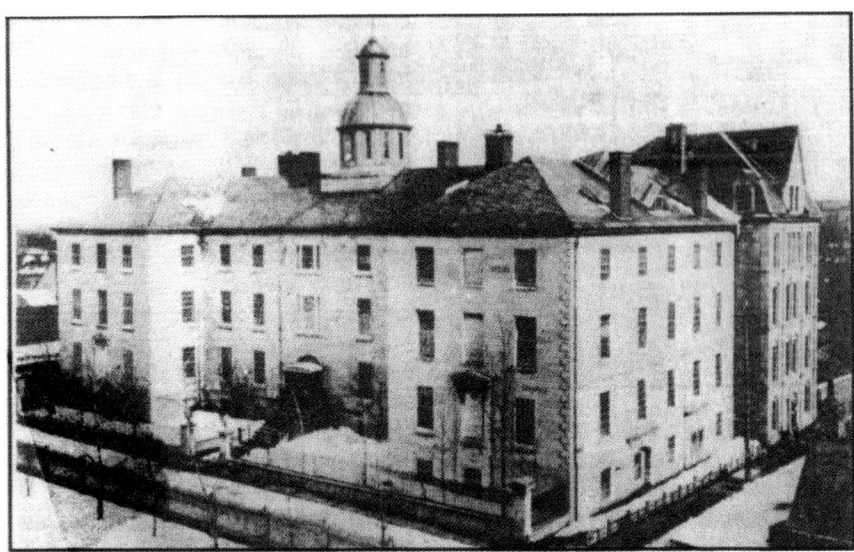

FIGURE 3 Montreal General Hospital as it was at the time of Osler's service, showing the cupola and sloping roof erected in 1822.

At the Montreal General Hospital, the Fever Hospital building was divided by a brick wall into two sections, one exclusively for smallpox and having a separate entrance from the street. Even these measures did not prevent occasional cross-infection from the smallpox section to other parts of the hospital, a fact that kept the Montreal General Hospital leaders pressing for a separate smallpox hospital off the grounds.

In 1873, the care of smallpox patients at the Montreal General Hospital no longer fell to the regular attending physician but became the responsibility of a special physician. The first appointee was Dr. Simpson, to be followed by William Osler, who combined these duties with his teaching and his work carrying out autopsies at the Montreal General Hospital.[3] The governors of the hospital paid the physician in charge of the smallpox service what they called "a fair sum," namely $600. In return, they insisted that the doctor visit twice daily throughout the wards, a duty that was reported to have been thoroughly performed.[8] Osler put the money toward the cost of 15 microscopes, which he had purchased previously out of his pocket, to allow students to learn the microscopic changes in normal and diseased tissues.[9]

As a result of assuming clinical responsibility in the smallpox wards, Osler became an expert on the disease, publishing several new observations. He began a lifelong interest in the clinical, public health and historical aspects of smallpox, and he later caught smallpox himself.

Fortunately, his case proved mild. He was supposedly immune but though repeatedly vaccinated, he had never had a successful take. Before the illness, he had mingled freely with relatives and friends, thinking that there was no danger of giving them the disease. In a letter dated January, 1876, he described the attack as, "a wonderfully light one, the pustules numbering sixteen, all told, and of these only two . . . . on my face; so that 'my beauty has not consumed away.' I have been out of Hospital now a week and am regaining my strength rapidly. The disease has been and is very bad. You need not be afraid of this letter. I will disinfect it before sending."[10]

His first paper reporting a personal experience with smallpox, published in 1875, described the case of a nine-year-old girl convalescing in hospital from

TABLE 2   INITIAL RASHES OF SMALLPOX

Ages 14 to 29

Varieties of rash

•diffuse erythema
•measly or macular
•petechiae, purpura or ecchymoses

1/11 died of hemorrhagic smallpox

smallpox. She developed scarlatina (scarlet fever) with a bright red, diffuse rash, which went on to feature small, miliary vesicles "the size of No. 4 shot" filled with creamy fluid. After detailing day-to-day changes, Osler described the condition as scarlatina pustulosa and discussed the differential diagnosis.[11] The clinical description fits that of streptococcal infection and scarlet fever, yet it was published five years before Louis Pasteur discovered streptococci.[12] In the case report, Osler identifies himself as the likely carrier of the infection, for he had attended another patient with scarlet fever 18 days before.

In 1877, Osler published two extensive studies, one on the initial rashes of smallpox and another on hemorrhagic smallpox.[13,2] In these papers, he identified himself as a Fellow of the Royal Microscopical Society, London, late Physician to the Smallpox Department of the Montreal General Hospital, and Professor of the Institutes of Medicine, McGill University, for he had been promoted to the rank of professor within a year of joining the faculty. These two papers constituted the first extensive clinical observations published by Osler. Before that, he had produced case reports and accounts of autopsies, but it was his smallpox papers that signalled the arrival of the consummate clinician.

Table 2 summarizes the major features of the paper on the initial rashes of smallpox. A variety of prodromal rashes could precede the characteristic pustules. Each point in the paper is documented from the medical literature. In the paper on hemorrhagic smallpox, he refers to the epidemic that had raged for five years and featured a high prevalence of the fatal hemorrhagic variety. Between December 1873 and July 1875, 260 cases were admitted under Dr. Simpson and himself, of which 10 per cent died of hemorrhagic smallpox (Table 3).[2] Osler carried out what he described as seven "carefully performed autopsies." He thanked Sister Rosalie, apothecary at the Roman Catholic Civic Smallpox Hospital, for notifying him about two of the cases.[2]

Meanwhile, the lack of effective public health measures and the antipathy to vaccination, made effective prophylaxis and control impossible. In 1876,

TABLE 3   HEMORRHAGIC SMALLPOX

27 cases, ages 4 to 53, 21 males, 6 females

All died, days 3 to 9

Autopsies: 7

Bleeding sites:

•skin
•nose, stomach, bowel
•bladder
•lungs
•uterus

the Mayor of Montreal and Chairman of the Board of Health was William H. Hingston, MD. He addressed the issue at a meeting of public vaccinators, other physicians and citizens. He described the prevalence of smallpox as disturbing the tables of mortality of the city, affecting its reputation and injuring its trade. Then, he reviewed the evidence from many countries that vaccination was effective. He quoted at greater length from continental than from British authorities because "it has been asserted by a certain orator who inveighed against vaccination at public gatherings in this city, that it was an 'English remedy, and that Englishmen had a pride in engrafting their "beastly" virus on the Christian children of fair Canada' ".[14] The certain orator was probably Dr. Coderre who led the anti-vaccination forces, which included some priests and Roman Catholic doctors who advised their parishioners and patients to boycott public health campaigns advocating vaccination.

Dr. Coderre, a vociferous, single-minded opponent, was convinced that vaccination did much harm. He let his views be known in the public press and also founded a medical journal entitled "L'Antivaccinateur Canadien-Français."[15]

The following is a translation into English of a portion of Dr. Coderre's statement introducing his journal.[15] "This journal is published in the interest of public and private health. . . . Doctors wishing to make known the truth about the protective action of vaccine cannot recommend this practice without committing the most serious error and being unpardonably ignorant about the disastrous results of vaccination."

The journal only survived for three issues with what must have been a limited circulation, for no copies have been found in Canadian medical libraries.[16]

Dr. Hingston found that such anti-vaccination views were advocated by a small, ceaselessly active section of medical and legal thought. To understand why Montreal had such a high prevalence of smallpox, he focused on the success of many cities and countries in Europe and elsewhere in programs of widespread vaccination. After citing the excellent records of nearby Canadian communities such as Quebec City, Trois-Rivières and Toronto, he asked, "And why does the disease visit Montreal so severely? WE NURSE IT." He noted that in Montreal, "the mortality is immensely greater among that nationality whose beautiful language has been made to serve as a vehicle for the dissemination of a most fatal error." He referred to Dr. Osler who had kindly handed him the records of the Smallpox Department of the General Hospital from December 14, 1873 to July 21, 1875, the period during which it was under Drs. Simpson and Osler (Table 4).

By 1876, Montreal had two civic hospitals for smallpox, one run by Protestants, the other by Roman Catholics. When the figures were analysed between November 1874 and November 1876, the results were as shown in Table 5. Dr. Hingston circulated a notice, which he called a Pronunciamento of Physicians in Montreal who were in favor of vaccination; 146 signed,

TABLE 4   SMALLPOX DEPARTMENT, MONTREAL GENERAL HOSPITAL

	Death Rate (Per cent)
Admitted (261) Died (73)	28
Vaccinated	17
Unvaccinated	59

TABLE 5   FIGURES FROM TWO MONTREAL CIVIC HOSPITALS

Hospital Run by Protestants

	Admitted	Died	Per cent
	168	34	20
Unvaccinated	54 (32 per cent)	25	46
Vaccinated	114	9	8

Hospital Run by Catholics

	Admitted	Died	Per cent
	396	127	32
Unvaccinated	165 (42 per cent)	89	54
Vaccinated	231	38	16

including William Osler. Some of the names were French-Canadian, reminding us that many French-Canadian doctors favored vaccination.[14]

In the early 1880s, Montreal had a brief period of freedom from the disease. Vaccination continued to be neglected, with the result that a large group of children, predominantly French-Canadian, grew up unprotected. By this time, Osler had accepted an invitation from Philadelphia to become the Clinical Professor of Medicine at the University of Pennsylvania. He moved in late 1884, only a few months before the horrendous smallpox epidemic, which made 1885 a black year for Montreal. When Osler prepared the first edition of his "Principles and Practice of Medicine," published in 1892, he drew on his experiences and knowledge of events in Montreal to describe the disease.

As he noted, "Perhaps the most remarkable instance in modern times of the rapid extension of the disease occurred in Montreal in 1885." On February 28, a Pullman car conductor arrived from Chicago, where the disease had been slightly prevalent. He was admitted to Hotel-Dieu Hospital in Montreal thought to be suffering from chickenpox. No attempt was made to isolate him and, on April 1, a servant in the hospital died of smallpox.

What happened next appalled Osler, for he wrote, "Following her decease, with a negligence absolutely criminal, the authorities of the hospital dismissed all patients presenting no symptoms of contagion, who could go home. The disease spread like fire in dry grass, and within nine months there died in the city, of smallpox, 3,164 persons." Osler emphasized that although "Small-pox is common at all ages, it is particularly fatal to young children; thus in the Montreal epidemic. . . . . 86 per cent of the deaths were children under 10 years."[17]

As the epidemic spread, the conflict over strict public health measures intensified. One French-Canadian doctor who favored firm measures of control was the Medical Health Officer, Dr. Laberge. Against the opposition of many merchants, manufacturers and priests, he deployed his small staff to placard factories, stores and homes, in attempts to quarantine patients and contacts, and persuade contacts to be vaccinated. As the year wore on, smallpox and its control became a hot political issue, enmeshed in a national conflict between francophone Catholics and anglophone Protestants.

In the Northwest Rebellion, the Metis, a mixed breed of French-Canadians and Indians, joined with prairie Indians in an attempt to secede and establish an autonomous country in western Canada. The federal government reacted by sending an army to quell the rebellion. Louis Riel, a French-Canadian Catholic, led the rebellion and ruled the embryonic nation. Riel became a folk hero for French-Canadians in Quebec. By the summer of

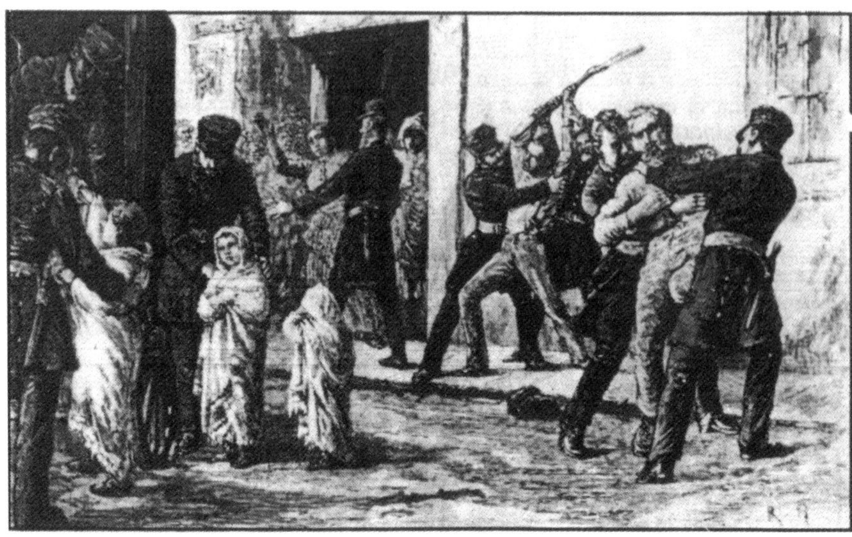

FIGURE 4 "An incident of the Smallpox Epidemic in Montreal." From Harper's Weekly, November 28, 1885. Many families in Montreal violently resisted control measures during the deadly 1885 epidemic. Similar riots erupted in Norfolk, Va., in 1768–1769, and in Milwaukee, Wis., in 1894–1895.

1885, he had been captured, tried and jailed to await sentence. At this time, smallpox raged in Montreal and the lists of dead lengthened. Dr. Laberge's campaign to introduce tighter control measures met with open defiance. Placards were torn down and cases of smallpox deliberately were not reported to the Medical Health Officer.

Matters reached a crisis in September with the introduction of compulsory vaccination in the city, at the same time that Riel was sentenced to death. With these two announcements, mob violence broke out against Dr Laberge and his hated measures of control. Unruly crowds stormed the health office; they stoned Laberge's house and threatened to kill him. With shouts of, "Bravo Riel! Vive la France! Hurrah Canadiens Français!" they rushed through the streets, defying the police. Only when the militia was called was order restored[6] (Figure 4).[18]

Years later, Osler described a medicolegal autopsy that he had performed on a case of traumatic aneurysm resulting from the riots. In a major paper entitled "Arterio-Venous Aneurysm," published in the Lancet in 1915, he described one of his cases of 30 years previously. "A soldier during the vaccination riots in Montreal gave a man a prod with his bayonet, which passed through the top of the left lung and cut the subclavian artery just as it leaves the arch to curve over the pleura."[19]

Efficient methods of producing enough vaccine from calves to immunize large numbers of people were introduced into Montreal and other areas of Canada in the 1880s. Before that, one had to use dried material from pustules of recently vaccinated individuals. When Osler published his textbook in 1892, he wrote a section on the disease vaccinia or cowpox, describing how to prepare vaccination material and use it properly.[17]

Paradoxically, the more effective preventive measures became, the better organized and militant the anti-vaccination movement became. In England, the National Anti-Compulsory Vaccination League constituted a political lobby powerful enough to influence elections and modify vaccination legislation.[20] Led by such prominent figures as Alfred Russell Wallace, co-discoverer with Charles Darwin of the theory of evolution, and George Bernard Shaw, the witty gadfly, the English anti-vaccination movement provided an example for many North Americans who considered compulsory vaccination to be not only harmful but a violation of civil liberties.

Osler, who had learned by bitter experience the power of a hostile press when he delivered the address on the "Fixed Period" in 1905, kept out of the fray over vaccination as long as he could. Finally, he was goaded into making a public statement in an attempt to neutralize the virulent campaigning of the anti-vaccination forces.

At Edinburgh in 1910, in a lay sermon entitled "Man's Redemption of Man" (Figure 5), he confronted the issue with these words, "A great deal of literature has been distributed, casting discredit upon the value of vaccination in the prevention of smallpox. I do not see how any one who has gone through epidemics as I have, or who is familiar with the history of the subject, and who has any capacity left for clear judgment, can doubt its value. Some months ago, I was twitted by the Editor of the Journal of the Anti-Vaccination League for maintaining a curious silence on the subject. I would like to issue a Mount Carmel-like challenge to any ten unvaccinated priests of Baal. (He referred to the dramatic confrontation between the prophet Elijah and the priests of Baal, taunting them to make their god send fire to roast their sacrificial bull, and vanquishing them when hours of their prayers went unheard, whereas Elijah's God sent fire to burn up his sacrifice.) I will take ten selected vaccinated persons, and help in the next severe epidemic, with ten selected unvaccinated persons (if available). I should choose three members of Parliament, three anti-vaccination doctors, if they could be found, and four anti-vaccination propagandists. And I will make this promise—neither to jeer nor jibe when they catch the disease, but to look after them as brothers; and for the three or four who are certain to die, I will try to arrange the funerals with all the pomp and ceremony of an anti-vaccination demonstration."[21]

Pursuing a profound interest in the literature of medical history, Osler

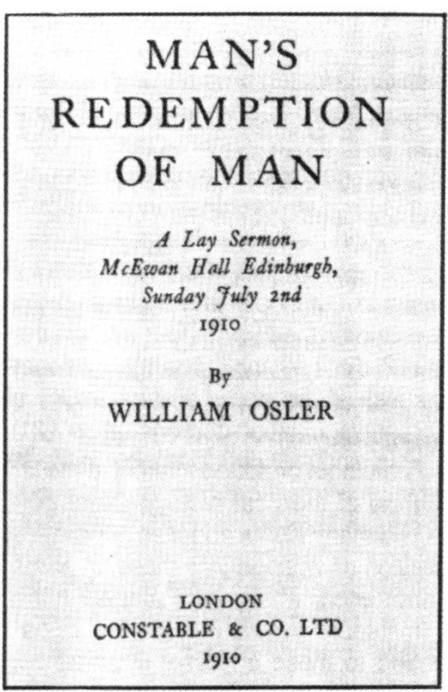

FIGURE 5 Cover page of Osler's lay sermon "Man's Redemption of Man."

TABLE 6   BIBLIOTHECA PRIMA

Rhazes: first authentic description
?850–?923
Sydenham on confluent Variola
1624–1689
Jenner: 44 items
1749–1823

collected many works about smallpox. His division of writings into those of prime importance, which were placed in the Prima section of his Bibliotheca, as opposed to those of lesser importance, appearing in the Secundum section, displays his personal evaluation.[22]

The cardinal writings on smallpox were featured in the Bibliotheca Prima (Table 6). Osler hailed Jenner's discovery of vaccination as a landmark in the history of preventive medicine. In his Silliman Foundation Lectures delivered at Yale University in 1913, later published as "The Evolution of Modern Medicine," he said, "Thanks to Jenner, not a single person in this audience is pockmarked! A hundred and twenty-five years ago, the faces of more than half of you would have been scarred."[23]

In conclusion, we can divide Osler's interest in smallpox into four phases. The earliest arose from his first major clinical responsibility as Physician in the Smallpox Department of the Montreal General Hospital. His familiarity with the disease resulted in several important papers. The second phase featured the author of the most successful medical textbook of his time including in the work a definitive account of smallpox and cowpox derived from his experience in Montreal. The third concerned the public health aspects of control and his decision to break silence by speaking out forcefully, in public, against the antivaccination point of view. The final phase shows us the bibliophile evaluating his collection of the key publications that led to the control of the disease, and placing them in the first rank of historical importance.

References

1. Cushing H. The life of Sir William Osler. London, New York, Toronto: Oxford University Press, 1940.
2. Osler W. Haemorrhagic small-pox. Can Med Surg J 1877;5:289–304.
3. Stewart RC. The Montreal General Hospital and the care of contagious diseases, 1822–1897. Can Med Assoc J 1940;43:282–4.
4. Abbott ME, ed. Bulletin of the International Association of Medical Museums and Journal of Technical Methods (Sir William Osler Memorial Number). Privately issued at 836 University St., Montreal. Printed by Murray Printing Company, 1926;9:174
5. Sanitary authority (Editorial). Can Med Surg J 1874;3:235.
6. Guyot M. A brief history of the small pox epidemic in Montreal from 1871 to 1880 and the late outbreak of 1885. Public Archives of Canada.
7. Abbott. Bulletin, 190.
8. Our civic small-pox hospital. (Editorial). Can Med Surg J 1877;5:237.

9. Cushing. Life, 143.

10. Cushing. Life, 142–3.

11. Osler W. Case of scarlatina miliaris. Can Med Surg J 1875;4:49–54.

12. Garrison FH. An introduction to the history of medicine. 4th ed. Philadelphia and London: W.B. Saunders Company, 1929.

13. Osler W. The initial rashes of small-pox. Can Med Surg J 1877;5:241–55.

14. Hingston WH. Remarks on vaccination. Montreal: Printed by Louis Perrault and Co., 1876.

15. Coderre, JE. L'Antivaccinateur Canadien-Français 1885–1886;1 (1–3).

16. Roland CG, Potter P. An annotated bibliography of Canadian medical periodicals 1826–1975. The Hannah Institute for the History of Medicine, 1979.

17. Osler W. The principles and practice of medicine. New York: D. Appleton and Company, 1892:47–8.

18. Hopkins DR. Princes and peasants. Smallpox in history. Chicago, London: University of Chicago Press, 1983; plate 35.

19. Osler W. Remarks on arterio-venous aneurysm. Lancet 1915;1:949–55.

20. MacLeod RM. Law, medicine and public opinion: The resistance to compulsory health legislation 1870–1907. In: Griffith JAG ed. Public law. London: Stevens and Sons, 1967.

21. Osler W. Man's redemption of man. London: Constable and Co. Ltd., 1910.

22. Osler W. Bibliotheca Osleriana. Montreal and London: McGill-Queens University Press, 1969.

23. Osler W. The evolution of modern medicine. New Haven: Yale University Press, 1922:199.

William Osler and Arthur Conan Doyle Versus the Antivivisectionists: Some Lessons from History for Today

 Jack D. Key, M.A., M.S. and Alvin E. Rodin, M.D.

The word "vivisection" has an obvious meaning: the cutting into of a living body. The dictionary provides a more specific definition: "the practice of subjecting living animals to cutting operations, esp. in order to advance physiological and pathological knowledge."[1] Common usage has now expanded the term to include all experimentation, surgical or nonsurgical, on animals.[2]

Before the nineteenth century, vivisection was not unusual. For example, Erasistratus, a 3rd century B.C. anatomist in Alexandria, is considered the first experimental physiologist because of his study of the functions of the nervous system and heart in living bodies,[3] including those of humans.[4] The greatest physiologist of ancient Greece, Galen, operated on mammals, including primates, to determine the results of such a surgical procedure as severing the spinal cord.[5]

The seminal figure for modern physiology, however, was William Harvey, who in the seventeenth century wrote that "special care must be taken that you know things well, and have investigated them through frequent dissections of animals."[6]

Read at the annual meeting of the American Osler Society, May 3, 1983.

Reprinted with additions with permission from Mayo Clinic Proceedings. *59*:189, 1984

Antivivisection

Reactions against research on living animals became quite evident during the latter part of the eighteenth century and gained momentum during the latter part of the nineteenth century.[7] Some reactions were even somewhat vicious (Figure 1). Such a movement cannot be understood *in vacuo,* so to speak, but requires knowledge of the society in which it was manifested.

The antivivisection movement had its roots in several characteristics of British society during the eighteenth and nineteenth centuries. Cruelty to animals in general was widespread. This was effectively satirized by Hogarth in 1750, in his engraving depicting various types of torture to animals.[8] Illustrated are releasing a cat with artificial wings to make it fly, watching two suspended cats clawing at each other in fright, burning out the eye of a captive bird, plunging an arrow into the anus of a dog, tying a bone to a dog's tail, setting a dog upon a cat, and aiming a stick to throw at a cock (Figure 2). Bullbaiting and cockfighting were popular sports. Such senseless cruelty to animals eventually disturbed sensibilities to such an extent that the reaction was against any manipulation, including vivisection. The eighteenth century

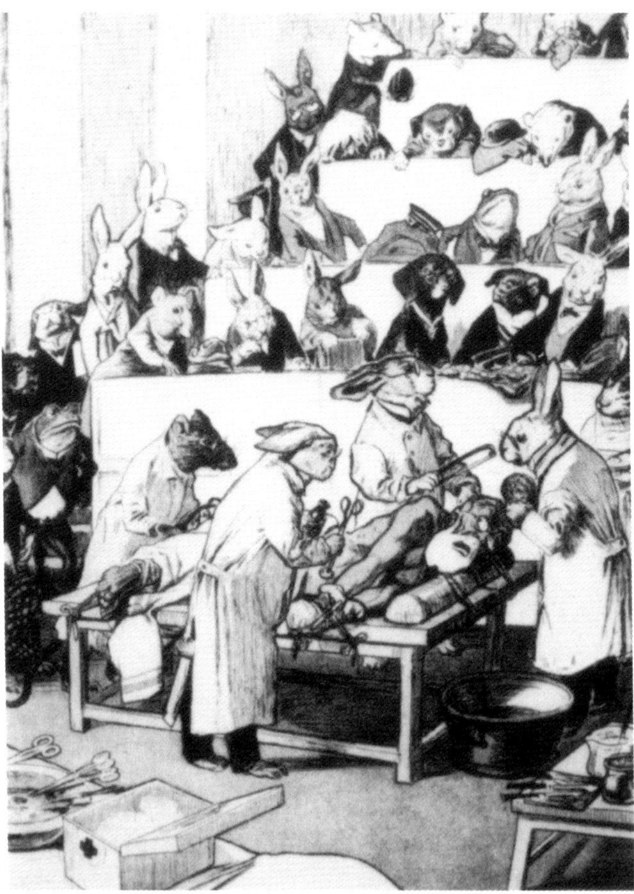

FIGURE 1 Die Vivisektion der Menschen. (*From Halländer E: Die Karikatur und Satire in der Medizin.* Stuttgart, Von Ferdinand Enke Verlag, 1921, p. 397. (Reproduced with permission.)

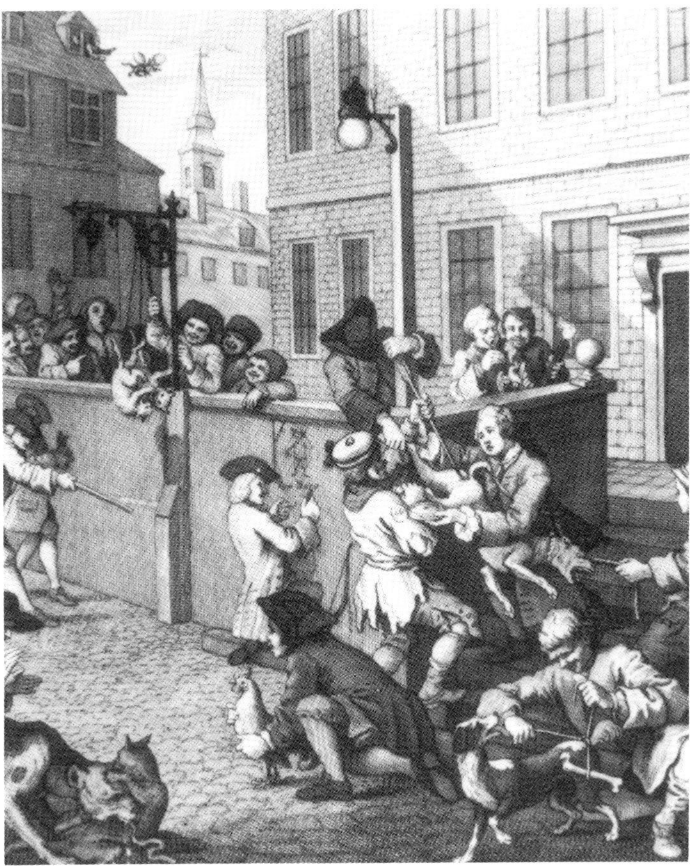

FIGURE 2   First State of Cruelty, by William Hogarth, 1750. (Used with permission of Dover Publications, Inc.)

also saw the development of evangelism, humanitarianism, and romanticism, including the cult of the pet, with its sentimental anthropomorphism.[9] It appeared to some that materialism was leading to the affliction of pain on defenseless creatures that had feelings, consciousness, and even souls.

The Victorian era was characterized by an abhorrence of biologic reality and of man's physical self. Vivisection appeared to emphasize these lower aspects of the human race. It also was part of the rapid rise of science in the nineteenth century, a rise that threatened long-standing institutions, such as the church, conflicted with established ways of thinking, and tampered with the order of things.

Antiscientism focused on several major developments in this period. Best known are the violent tirades against Darwin and Huxley for their advocacy of the evolutionary theory[10] and the use of anesthesia to relieve the pain of childbirth, which appeared to directly confront the biblical dictum[11] resulting from Eve's disobedience.

Not as well known, but more closely related to the antivivisection movement itself, was the extensive opposition to Jenner's development of smallpox vaccination. Some of this opposition was related to the imagined effects of Jenner's cowpox, as caricatured by Gillray in his engraving *Cow Pock,* which included bovine features and excrescences.[12] Reactions against smallpox vaccination, as against vivisection, were due more to fundamental and pervasive elements in Victorian society than to any fear of acquiring brutish features. Indeed, many individuals who opposed vaccination were also anti-vivisectionists.[13]

Vivisection in the nineteenth century was related primarily to the search for physiologic knowledge. In Britain, the development of physiology was considerably behind that in Europe proper, being hampered by several constraints that were more prominent there.[14] Traditional medicine was conservative and clinically oriented.[14] Sir Charles Bell, a leading anatomist and physiologist of the time, explained function on the basis of anatomic studies.[9] His bias against vivisection led him to conclude in 1811 that the anterior spinal roots subserve voluntary behavior and the posterior ones subserve involuntary behavior. Bell considered the motives for animal experimentation to be egotism and self-aggrandizement.

The lack of anesthesia before the mid-nineteenth century was less of a deterrent to the sensibilities of Europeans than to those of the English. Magendie of France, for example, demonstrated correctly in 1822 that the anterior spinal roots are motor and that the posterior ones are sensory. This was done by vivisection on a litter of eight puppies, but only by the infliction of considerable pain.[3]

Relatively early in the nineteenth century, a strong anticruelty to animals movement began to take an organized form in Britain.[15] In 1822, Martin's Act, which outlawed cruelty to larger domestic animals, was passed by Parliament. In 1824, the Royal Society for the Prevention of Cruelty to Animals was formed.

Given these characteristics of Victorian society, it is not surprising that British physiology lagged behind that of the rest of Europe. The second and third quarters of the century saw the development of strong support both against and for vivisection. The former included literary figures, such as Tennyson, Browning, Carlyle, and Ruskin, and especially Queen Victoria. The latter included prominent figures in the scientific world, such as Darwin, Huxley, Burdon Sanderson, and Joseph Lister.[16] One example of the effect of the strong opposition to vivisection in Britain was Lister's need to go to Paris to conduct experiments with sutures in living animals.

In 1874, an event occurred that greatly strengthened the forces against vivisection. At the annual meeting of the British Medical Association, a French experimentalist named Eugene Magnan injected absinthe into two dogs to induce epilepsy.[9] There were objections from the audience at the cruelty of the unnecessary experiment. A protestor cut the restraints of one dog, which staggered about. Two county magistrates were sent for, and the session was disrupted.

This unfortunate incident, widely publicized, further inflamed antivivisection feeling. It was a stimulus for the formation, by Frances Power Cobbe in 1875, of the Victoria Street Society for the Protection of Animals Liable to Vivisection. This group pushed for abolition of all vivisection, whereas the Royal Society for the Prevention of Cruelty to Animals did not oppose vivisection under anesthesia. The intensity of the furor led to the establishment in 1875 of a Royal Commission "on the practice of subjecting live animals to experiments for scientific purposes." The resulting Cruelty to Animals Act of 1876 was actually a compromise. Experimentation on living vertebrates required the following measures by law:

1. Endorsement by a scientific or medical body and by a professor.
2. Application to the Home Secretary.

3. Performance in a place registered and open to inspection.
4. License renewed yearly.
5. Performance only for the advancement of physiologic knowledge and the saving of life.
6. Special permission needed for experiments without anesthesia or for demonstrations.

The fine was £50 for the first offense and £100 for subsequent ones. As might be predicted, the abolitionists were unhappy with the act.

By the turn of the century, the number of vivisections had reached 7,500, and by 1980, more than 6 million. A strong force countering the abolitionists was the formation in 1882 of the Association for the Advancement of Medicine by Research. This association was composed of prominent physicians and citizens.

One way to obtain a better appreciation of the emotions involved in the antivivisection movement is to leave the realm of facts and figures. An example of a particularly effective opponent of vivisection was George Bernard Shaw, who, in fact, railed against many of the activities of the medical establishment. In the lengthy introduction to his play of 1913, *The Doctor's Dilemma*,[17] he suggests that motives for the performance of vivisection by doctors include cruelty for its own sake, the need for a livelihood, and curiosity. "The men whose business it was to discover new clinical methods were coarsening and stupefying themselves with the sensual villaniess and cutthroat's casuistries of vivisection."

A less vitriolic, but as negative, opinion was given by Robert Knox, the Edinburgh anatomist who was so motivated in teaching by dissection of corpses that he accepted without question bodies sold by the infamous murderers Burke and Hare.[18]

> I have, all my life, had a natural horror for experiments made on living animals, nor has more matured reason altered . . . the belief that for the most part they are wholly unnecessary, and therefore highly to be reprobated.[18]

His basic scientific premise was that of many of his era, that is, "Physiologic knowledge can be derived from morphologic appearance." Such a dedication to the antivivisection position was undoubtedly also emotional, being influenced by Knox's express love for animals, as it was for many others.

Sir Arthur Conan Doyle and Vivisection

Another mode in which the emotional aspects of the vivisection controversy surfaced is that of direct confrontation. Here, an example is provided by the report in the *Portsmouth Times* of April 17, 1886, of a public meeting in support of kindness to animals.[19] The speaker, a minister, denounced Pasteur's torturing of thousands of "poor dumb creatures in order to save us from hydrophobia." Two physicians in the audience objected. Dr. Conan Doyle upheld the need to kill rabbits in order to relieve human suffering (Figure 3). He also objected to a clergyman lecturing on medical science. Dr. Claremont gave a biblical source for the use of animals to relieve human suffering and emphasized the medical importance of vivisection. The lecturer did not reply specifically to these arguments.

Letters to the editor columns in the press were one of the battlefields for

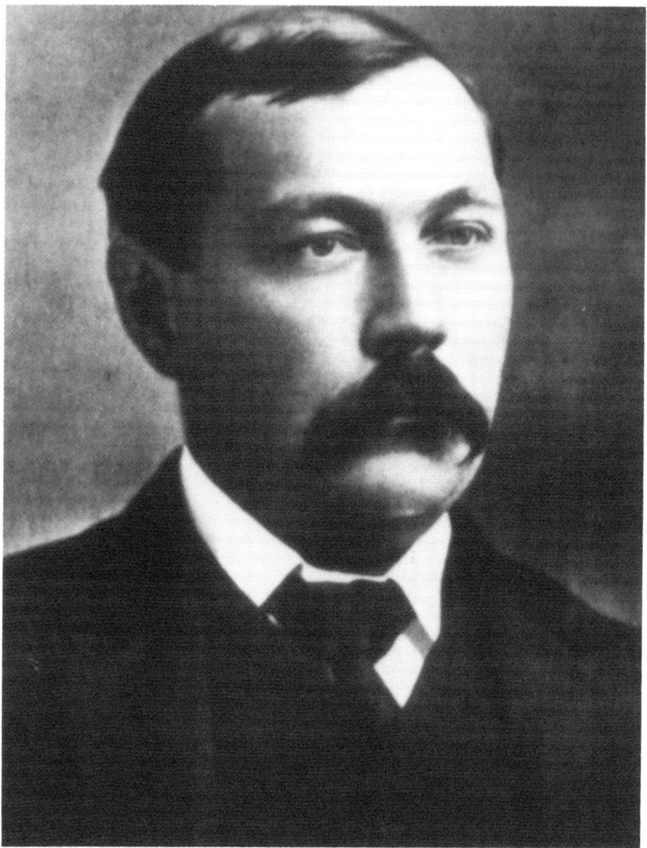

FIGURE 3 Arthur Conan Doyle (circa 1895). (Courtesy of the Wellcome Institute, London.)

the vivisection controversy. The *London Daily Express* of October 29, 1910, contained a letter from A. Wall, honorary treasurer of the London Antivivisection Society.[20] He stated that there was not an atom of evidence that any lives had been "saved by the torture of rabbits or guinea pigs." In quick response, the paper published on November 1 a letter from Arthur Conan Doyle.[21] He referred to the positive statistics in the population of a district of India inoculated against plague, such prevention having been developed in animals. In characteristic rhetoric, he also referred to "the anti-human campaign with which Mr. Wall is associated."

Conan Doyle also made references to vivisection, in the sense of any experimentation on animals, in several of his writings. His master detective, Sherlock Holmes, investigated the death of Drebber in *A Study in Scarlet*, published in 1887, a year after the confrontation with the clergyman.[22] Holmes gave a pill found in the suspect's room to a dog. "It gave a convulsive shiver in every limb, and lay as rigid and lifeless as if it had been struck by lightning." Holmes's conclusion was that Drebber had been poisoned by an alkaloid arrow poison.

In this episode, Conan Doyle felt the need to justify the implicit cruelty of such an act by describing the dog as a poor little terrier in chronic pain. He also referred to a concern for cruelty to animals by Pheneas, the spirit guide for his family's seances.[23] "Animals will be saved from all future suffering and when the spirit first touches the earth that particular suffering will at once be eliminated."

More directly related to experimentation was Conan Doyle's reaction to the research activities of one of his medical school teachers at the University of Edinburgh. His autobiography, published 43 years after his graduation, contains a criticism of William Rutherford, professor of the Institutes of Medicine.

> He was, I fear, a rather ruthless vivisector, and although I have always recognized that a minimum of painless vivisection is necessary, and far more justifiable than the eating of meat as a food, I am glad that the law was made more stringent so as to restrain such men as he.[24]

Such an orientation is characteristic of the more conservative approach to vivisection—a compromise between the desire to help humanity through science and the psychologic revulsion against inflicting pain on living creatures.

Sir William Osler and Vivisection

Another physician, more famous for medical than literary activities, was also involved in the vivisection controversy (Figure 4). The first indication of William Osler's awareness of the controversy was recorded while he was doing graduate studies in London in 1872.

> On the propriety of using the lower animals for the purpose of experimentation Dr. Sanderson said 1st, we are at liberty to use them on the same ground as we do for food: 2nd for scientific investigation are justified in giving pain: 3rd for mere demonstration we are not justified in giving pain.[25]

Burdon Sanderson was one of the more vocal opponents to legislative restrictions on vivisection.

More direct involvement on the part of Osler, but still relatively passive, was the signing in 1896 of a resolution protesting proposed antivivisection legislation.[26] A year later, in a presentation of cretinism and its treatment, he gave credit to animal experimentation.

> That I am able to show you such marvellous transformations, such undreamt-of transfigurations, is a direct triumph of vivisection, and no friend of animals . . . will consider the knowledge dearly bought, though at the sacrifice of hundreds of dogs and rabbits.[27]

Osler provided additional opposition to legislation against vivisection in the United States by testifying at a public hearing of a Senate committee. He considered such regulations "a piece of unnecessary legislation."[28]

Thus, Osler played an important supportive role in defeating antivivisection laws in the United States. He was also involved in the British controversy while Regius Professor of Medicine at Oxford. In testimony to the Royal Commission on Vivisection in 1907, he emphasized that the cure for cretinism by thyroid extract and the prevention of a number of diseases were made possible mainly by animal experimentation.[29]

Osler further extolled the value of vivisection to humanity in a lengthy letter to the *London Times* on March 15, 1909. He concluded an extensive

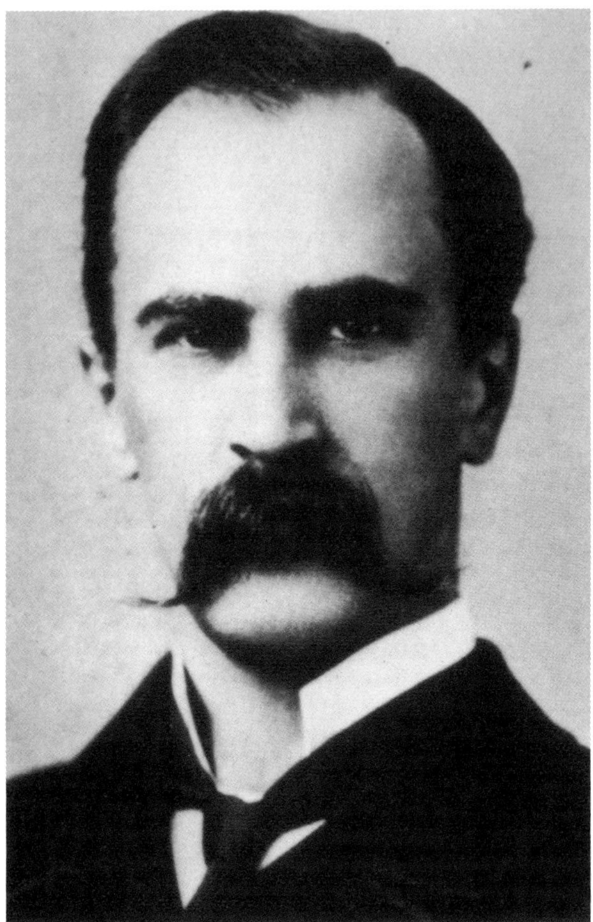

FIGURE 4 William Osler in 1881, when pathologist to the Montreal General Hosptial. (From Rogers EJA: Personal Reminiscences of the Earlier Years of Sir William Osler. [Sir William Osler Memorial Volume] Int Assoc Med Museums 9:163–170, 1929. By permission of Murray Printing Company.)

review of the contribution by Italians to the prevention of malaria with the following:

> And let us not forget that humanity owes this triumph to the men who introduced experimentation into medicine, to the Harveys, the Hunters, the Magendies, and the Claude Bernards—the arch-vivisectors whom it has become fashionable to abuse!—and who have thus enabled us to wring from nature what Harvey called "her closet-secrets."[30]

This is an excellent example of the union of Osler's historical knowledge with his writing skills for a cause.

William Osler was to enter into the breech once more, this time in opposition to the "Dogs' Protection Bill" introduced into Parliament in March of 1919, the last year of his life.[31] The specific restrictions were considered by the medical profession to be a major menace to medical progress,[32] so much so that William Osler made a resolution on the subject at a scientific meeting of the British Medical Association.

> The prohibition of experiments upon dogs would . . . have the deplorable result of hampering the progress of medicine and of rendering Britain alone, among the civilized nations of the world, unable to contribute to progress in a department of medical research in which it has hitherto played a distinguished part.[33]

Osler's involvement helped to rally the British medical profession against such a restriction to research.[34] The results were amendments to soften the bill.[35] The final victory was passage in Parliament of an amendment, proposed by Sir Watson Cheyne, that the House decline to proceed further with the measure.[36]

William Osler's involvement with vivisection differed from that of Conan Doyle in that he also actively engaged in research using animals. He published accounts of three such investigations. The first is found in a review "On the Pathology of Miner's Lung" in the *Canada Medical and Surgical Journal* in 1875,[37] in which he described his experiments conducted on kittens. The objective was "To show the remarkable aptitude of cells to take up granules of various sorts, and, also, to demonstrate the rapidity with which the lymphatic glands are affected."

In one experiment, Osler injected india ink into the axilla of one kitten and the thorax of another. The kittens were killed within 2 to 3 days. Gross and microscopic studies revealed india ink in leukocytes, lymphatic vessels, and lymphatic glands. Osler concluded that extraneous materials, such as india ink and carbon, are quickly rendered harmless by becoming "fixed in cells" and then are carried to lymphatic glands.

Osler did not perform the first animal experiments related to anthracosis.[38] In 1862, Villaret exposed rabbits to inhalation of carbon.[39] In 1867, Knauff exposed dogs to inhalation of both carbon and ultramarine blue.[39] The objectives of these two investigators nevertheless were different from those of Osler. Villaret and Knauff were concerned with proof that carbon in the air could reach the pulmonary parenchyma. Osler's interest, on the other hand, was in the body's cellular defense mechanism against irritating material. His experiments are significant because they were reported in 1875, eight years before Metchnikoff's first report on phagocytosis was delivered at the Odessa Congress in 1883.[40]

William Osler's purpose in carrying out another animal research project was to clarify knowledge of the so-called pig-typhoid.[41] In 1878, there were many opinions about its nature, including anthrax, typhoid fever, and dysentery. He inoculated four sow pigs, each with a different substance from diseased animals. Included were materials from an ecchymotic skin lesion, from an intestinal plaque, from caseous bronchi, and from diseased glands. To a fifth animal he fed minced intestinal plaques.

Daily and detailed clinical observations were made on the sows. All became diseased. High fever developed in the four inoculated ones, and three had diarrhea; all four died within 18 to 25 days. The condition of the one fed the plaques was similar, but it lived for 31 days, when it was bled to death. In each instance, Osler carried out a complete postmortem examination, including both gross and microscopic studies. He also examined the bodies of 19 pigs that had died in an epidemic of the disease.

The major findings were soft plaques and ulcers of the large intestine and bronchopneumonia with a caseous material in bronchi. Osler concluded that pig-typhoid was a distinct entity, related to dysenteric disease in humans but with the additional involvement of skin and lungs. His description and the location of the intestinal lesions certainly suggest an infective disease similar to human dysentery. Pig-typhoid is now known as swine fever or hog cholera, and it is caused by a virus.[42]

The third animal experiment was carried out in collaboration with A.W. Clement, then a student in the Montreal Veterinarian College and later president of the American Veterinarian Medical Association.[43] Osler held an appointment as instructor in this college. The object of their experiment was to determine why cattle infested with the common tapeworm (*Taenia saginata*) seldom appeared to have larvae in the muscles.[44] They fed 50 segments of the worm to a calf and studied the animal both clinically and pathologically. After 51 days of fever, the calf was killed.

Postmortem examination revealed numerous minute encysted larvae 3 to 6 mm in length in lung, heart, kidney, tongue, and muscle. They concluded that larvae are frequent but are often overlooked by meat inspectors because of their small size and only mild opaqueness. Directly related to this study of parasitic disease in animals is the massive study by Osler and Clement of 1,000 hogs for *Trachinella spiralis, Cysticercus cellulosae,* and *Echinococcus* (Figure 5).[45] Osler has been called the "Father of Comparative Pathology in Canada" on the basis of such fundamental and extensive research.[46]

These three instances of Oslerian vivisection are of interest because each made a significant contribution: one to our knowledge of pulmonary phagocytosis, one to our understanding of a swine disease, and one to the prevention of human infestation with tapeworms. These studies were carried out in Montreal, where antivivisection reaction was not strong. But even in Britain, there would have been little comment on experimenting on pigs and cattle. There would have been some objection, however, to the use of kittens, such sentiments being reserved for animals used as pets and for recreation but not as food.

Present-Day Antivivisection Movements

This overview of the history of vivisection and its opposition in the nineteenth century provides some useful insights for our day. It is obvious that emotion often overshadowed reason in the debate between those for and those against vivisection in Britain. It was no different in the United States, where a bill preventing cruelty to animals in general was passed in Congress in 1871.[2] Here, antivivisection support was not as great as it was in Britain. It resulted in legislation relating to the care of laboratory animals but not to vivisection. Perhaps this outcome was the result of the different societal characteristics between a country steeped in centuries of history, tradition, and formality and one not yet emerged from the frontier way of life.

There is direct relevance for the present, because antivivisection activity has again increased, more strongly, as before, in Britain than in the United States.[47] For example, a bill for the protection of animals (scientific purposes) was introduced in the British House of Commons several years ago.[7] Sponsored by the Royal Society for the Prevention of Cruelty to Animals, it precluded use of animals in experiments except to relieve suffering or to prolong life in man and animals.[48] In the United States, the antivivisection sentiment is now even stronger than it was in the last century.[49] In December 1982, a hearing was held by the House Subcommittee on Health and the Environment on a bill entitled "The Humane Treatment and Development of

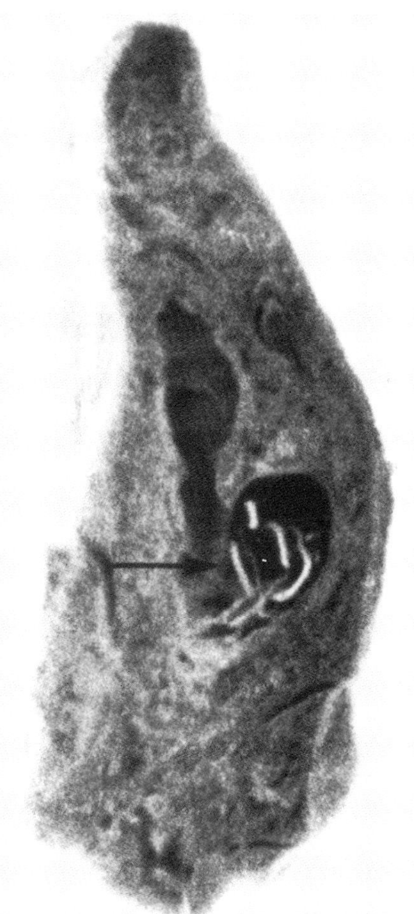

FIGURE 5   Osler's 1877 museum specimen of pig's lung. Parasitic worms (*Strongylus*) block a bronchus (*arrow*) and produce bronchopneumonia. (From Rodin AE: *Oslerian Pathology: An Assessment and Annotated Atlas of Museum Specimens.* Lawrence, Kansas, Coronado Press, 1981, p. 197. By permission.)

Substitutes for Animals in Research.'' Because of opposition by the chairman of the Labor and Human Resources Committee, it did not reach the Senate floor. As recently as late March 1983, amendments to the proposed legislation were approved that would require the National Institutes of Health to develop a plan to reduce the number of animals and the stress to animals used in research.[50]

As in the past, antivivisection is associated with a general antiscience trend, including opposition to vaccination, fluoridation, and scientifically established treatments. The arguments against vivisection today are basically the same as those of a century ago, but with a few additional ones based on new technology and modern consumer products.[51]

1. The LD_{50} (median lethal dose) determined by exposing animals to various substances is not valid, because it does not give a direct indication of acute, short-term toxicity.
2. There are species differences in reactions to substances.
3. Dissections of animals are carried out by school children who are untrained and who may become indifferent to suffering.

4. Many animals are used for nonmedical purposes, for example, testing toxicity of consumer products, such as cosmetics.
5. The price paid for dogs to be used for experimentation is high enough that pets are often stolen for such purposes; there are "children and old age pensioners whose pets disappear in the night."
6. Alternatives now exist to use of animals in biologic research. Examples are computer research, experiments on bacteria, and exposure of tissue cultures to substances. A bill before Congress in 1981 was based on this argument. It would have banned surgical experiments on living animals.[52]

The modern antivivisectionists argue that the use of living animals is no longer necessary in research but is continued because of tradition, secrecy, bureaucratic lethargy, and profit making. Countering these arguments are those who see vivisection as essential.[53] They point out that alternatives have serious limitations; for example, tissue cultures cannot detect the poisonous actions of curare and strychnine. They point out, furthermore, that antivivisectionists do not object to animals being slaughtered for food or furs. Antivivisectionists are selective in their concern for animals, worrying most about dogs and cats, although at present only about 0.6 per cent of all experiments use these two species.[54] Thus, antivivisectionists are inconsistent. They would not refuse a life-saving drug that was developed and tested with the use of dogs—for example insulin, which was discovered by Banting and Best. The provivisectionists further claim that public demand for improved medical care and the testing for safety of new substances has led to a greater use of animals in research.[55] Testing for the safety of commercial products (for example, cosmetics, food additives, and detergents) accounts for about 60 percent of animals used today.[56]

Discussion

Arguments about vivisection voiced 150 years ago continue today, albeit cloaked in new verbiage. Common societal elements in these two eras are protraditionalism and antiscientism. It appears that antivivisection sentiment is caused not only by cruelty to animals but also by tensions related to the place of science and medicine in society.

The very core of the vivisection controversy was expressed by Gallistel in a recent publication.[52] "One should urge the abandonment of animal research in part or in toto only if one believes that the moral value attached to the avoidance of animal suffering is greater than the moral value attached to the enrichment of human understanding and the alleviation of human suffering."

On a more pragmatic basis, to quote from a letter by Conan Doyle on vaccination, "The interests at stake are so vital that an enormous responsibility rests with the men whose notion of progress is to revert to the condition of things which existed in the dark ages before the dawn of medical science."[57] The basic question, then, is whether the ends (knowledge gained by vivisection) justify the means (inflicting suffering on animals). According to Visscher, "The truism that the ends do not justify the means involves very complex moral questions and is not a self-evident principle with universal applicability."[58]

Finally, before anyone embarks on research involving animals, five fundamental questions should be asked.[59]

1. Is the animal the best experimental system for the problem?
2. Must the animal be conscious at any time during the experiment?
3. Can pain or discomfort associated with the experiment be lessened or eliminated?
4. Can the number of animals used be reduced?
5. Is the problem worth solving anyhow?

Vivisectionists need to justify their experiments, and antivivisectionists need to justify their opposition.[60] The issue in part is moral. "The use of animals in research ultimately comes down to whether the benefits and knowledge gained by experimentation justify the taking of animal life or the infliction of pain."[61] Conan Doyle and William Osler were both staunch defenders of vivisection, the latter also a vivisectionist, and both were moral, sensitive, and humane physicians.

Acknowledgments

Leon Z. Saunders, D.V.M., Ph.D., Vice President of Safety Evaluation for Smith, Kline and French Laboratories, was instrumental in obtaining references to Osler's two pig experiments. The staff of the Health Sciences Library of Wright State University tracked down related nineteenth-century publications.

References

1. Stein J (ed): The Random House Dictionary of the English Language. New York, Random House, 1966.
2. Goodrich JE: The first 100 years of antivivisection—1824 to 1924. Mayo Clin Proc 52:257–259, 1977.
3. Garrison FH: An Introduction to the History of Medicine: With Medical Chronology, Suggestions for Study and Bibliographic Data, 4th edition. Pbiladelphia, W.B. Saunders, 1929, p. 103.
4. Scarborough J: Celsus on human vivisection at Ptolemaic Alexandria. Clio Med 11:25–38, 1976.
5. Sarton G: Galen of Pergamon, series 3. Lawrence, University of Kansas Press, 1954, p. 48.
6. Franklin KJ: William Harvey, Englishman. London, MacGibbon, 1961, p. 51.
7. Beaven DW: Morals and ethics in medical research. NZ Med J 81:519–524, 1975.
8. Hogarth W. First stage of cruelty. In Shesgreen S (ed): Engravings by Hogarth. New York, Dover, 1973, plate 77.
9. French RD: Antivivisection and Medical Science in Victorian Society. Princeton, Princeton University Press, 1975, p. 23.
10. Irvine W: Apes, Angels, and Victorians: The Story of Darwin, Huxley, and Evolution. New York, McGraw-Hill, 1955.
11. MacEachen DB: Wilkie Collins' heart and science and the viuisection controversy. Victorian Newsletter 29:22–25, 1966.
12. Gillray J: The Cow Pock (colored etching). Art Institute of Chicago, 1809.

13. Willcox PHA: The trial of Dr. W.R. Hadwen. J R Coll Physicians Lond 4:227–233, 1970.

14. Schiller J: Claude Bernard and vivisection. J Hist Med 22:246–260, 1967.

15. Bryant I: Vivisection: a chapter in the sociology of Victorian science. Ethics Sci Med 4: 75–86, 1977.

16. Fisher RB: Joseph Lister 1827–1912. New York, Stein & Day, 1977, p. 218.

17. Shaw GB: The Doctor's Dilemma: A Tragedy by Bernard Shaw. Baltimore, Penguin Books, 1965, pp. 35–58.

18. Rae I: Knox the Anatomist. Edinburgh, Oliver & Boyd, 1964, p. 17.

19. Discussion on Hydrophobia. Portsmouth Times, April 17, 1886, p. 5.

20. Wall A: Guinea-Pig or Man? Daily Express (London) October 29, 1910, p. 4.

21. Doyle AC: Guinea Pig or Man? Daily Express (London) November 1, 1910, p. 4.

22. Doyle AC: A Study in Scarlet. Beeton's Christmas Annual, 1887.

23. Doyle AC: Pheneas Speaks. (Direct Spirit Communication in the Family Circle reported by Arthur Conan Doyle, M.D., L.L.D.). London, Psychic Press, 1927, p. 108.

24. Doyle AC: Memories and Adventures. London, Hodder & Stoughton, 1924, p. 25.

25. Cushing H: The Life of Sir William Osler. Oxford, Clarendon, 1925, vol. 1, p. 99.

26. Cushing H: The Life of Sir William Osler. Oxford, Clarendon, 1925, vol. 1, p. 434.

27. Cushing H: The Life of Sir William Osler. Oxford, Clarendon, 1925, vol. 1, p. 449.

28. Cushing H: The Life of Sir William Osler. Oxford, Clarendon, 1925, vol. 1, p. 522.

29. Paget S: For and Against Experiments on Animals: Evidence Before the Royal Commission on Vivisection. London, HK Lewis, 1912.

30. Osler W: Malaria in Italy: A lesson in practical hygiene. Times (London) March 15, 1909, p. 5.

31. Dogs Bill. Br Med J 1:390, 1919.

32. The obstruction of medical research: The "Dogs' Protection" Bill. Br Med J 1:455–456, 1919.

33. Protest by the special clinical and scientific meeting of the British Medical Association. Br Med J 1:456, 1919.

34. The Dogs' Protection Bill: Deputation to the home office. Br Med J 1:613–614, 1919.

35. Medical notes in Parliament: Dogs' Protection Bill. Br Med J 1: 684–687, 1919.

36. Medical notes in Parliament: The "Dogs' Protection" Bill: The measure rejected. Br Med J 2:23–24, 1919.

37. Osler W: On the pathology of miner's lung. Can Med Surg J 4: 145–168, 1875.

38. Rosen G: Osler on miners' phthisis. J Hist Med 4:259–266, 1949.

39. Rosen G: The History of Miners' Diseases: A Medical and Social Interpretation. New York, Schuman's, 1943.

40. Metchnikoff O: Life of Elie Metchnikoff 1845–1916. Boston, Houghton Mifflin, 1921, p. 120.

41. Osler W: On the pathology of the so-called pig-typhoid. Vet J Ann Comp Pathol 6 385–402, 1878.

42. Saunders LZ: Some pioneers in comparative medicine. Can Vet J 14:27–35, 1973.

43. Clement AW: Necrology. J Comp Med Vet Arch 22 178–180, 1901.

44. Osler W, Clement AW: Cestode tuberculosis: A successful experiment in producing it in the calf. Am Vet Rev 6:6–10, 1882.

45. Osler W, Clement AW: An investigation into the parasites in the pork supply of Montreal. Can Med Surg J 11:325–336, 1883.

46. Mitchell CA: A note on the early history of veterinary science in Canada: Sir William Osler. Can J Comp Med 3:276–281, 1939.

47. Dennis C: America's Littlewood crisis: The sentimental threat to animal research. Surgery 60:827–838, 1966.

48. Cross BA: Currents and portents in biomedical research. Vet Rec 108:202–206, 1981.

49. Sechzer JA: Historical issues concerning animal experimentation in the United States. Soc Sci Med 15:13–17, 1981.

50. Cooper JAD: Association of American Medical Colleges: President's Weekly Activities Report. No. 83–10, March 10, and No. 83–12, March 24, 1983.

51. Whittaker A: Vivisection: The case against. Nursing Times 75:395–396, 1979.

52. Gallistel CR: Bell, Magendie, and the proposals to restrict the use of animals in neurobehavioral research. Am Psychol 36:357–360, 1981.

53. McMillan B: Vivisection, do we have double standards. Nursing Times 75:397–398, 1979.

54. Editorial: Experiments on living animals. Lancet 2:702, 1970.

55. Payne JP. Animal experimentation. Br J Anaesth 50:871–872, 1978.

56. Editorial: Vivisection. Lancet 2:667–668, 1976.

57. Doyle AC: Compulsory vaccination (letter). Evening Mail (Portsmouth) July 15, 1887.

58. Visscher MB: Animal rights and alternative methods—Two new twists in the antivivisection movement. Pharos 42:11–19, 1979.

59. Lane-Petter W: The place and importance of the experimental animal in research. Proc R Soc Med 65:343–344, 1972.

60. Visscher MB: Medical research and ethics. JAMA 199:631–636, 1967.

61. Nyman J: Moral issues in the use of animals in experimental research from the renaissance to the twentieth century. Anim Regul Stud 2:31–35, 1979.

Sir William Osler, Ageism, and "The Fixed Period" A Secret Revealed

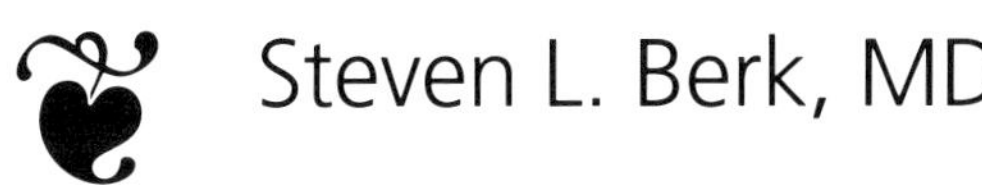 Steven L. Berk, MD

On the occasion of his 70th birthday, a 1919 editorial in the *Lancet* honored Sir William Osler with Oliver Wendell Holmes' comment that "To be 70 years young is sometimes far more hopeful and cheerful than to be 40 years old."[1] Osler continued to be an active teacher, researcher, and statesman until his death.

He lay in state in Wrens Towers at Oxford, his bier covered with a plain velvet pall on which lay a single sheaf of lillies and a copy of *Religio Medici*. He was described as "a man who advanced the science of medicine and enriched literature and the humanities, yet individually he had a greater power. He became the friend of all he met, he knew the workings of the human heart both metaphorically as well as physically. He joyed with the joys and wept with the sorrows of the humblest of those who were proud to be his pupils."[2]

Clinicians and teachers from all specialties can learn from Osler's writings, but to the geriatrician Osler must be considered an enigma. In 1905, while giving a farewell speech to the Johns Hopkins faculty, Osler put forward his views on aging. Osler was only 56 years of age at the time but lived in an era when the median life expectancy was between 45 and 47. To many, his comments seemed out of character. To modern geriatricians this address (later published in an essay entitled "The Fixed Period" after the novel by Trollope) would be diametrically opposed to current principles of gerontology. I will review Osler's essay and propose an explanation for his position.

In the middle of his farewell address, Osler expressed the concern that in the new universities, all professors were growing older at the same time, and only an age limit on professors would prevent an unfortunate situation.

> I have two fixed ideas well known to my friends, harmless obsessions with which I sometimes bore them, but which have a direct bearing on this

Read at the annual meeting of the American Osler Society, April 27, 1989.

Reprinted with permission from *The Journal of The American Geriatrics Society*, 37:263, 1989 important problem. The first is the comparative uselessness of men above 40 years of age. This may seem shocking, and yet, read aright, the world's history bears out the statement. Take the sum of human achievement in action, in science, in art, in literature—subtract the work of the men above 40, and while we should miss great treasures, even priceless treasures, we would practically be where we are today. It is difficult to name a great and far-reaching conquest of the mind which has not been given to the world by a man on whose back the sun was still shining. The effective, moving, vitalizing work of the world is done between the ages of 25 and 40—these 15 golden years of plenty, the anabolic or constructive period, in which there is always a balance in the mental bank and the credit is still good. In the science and art of medicine young or comparatively young men have made every advance of the first rank.

My second fixed idea is the uselessness of men above 60 years of age, and the incalculable benefit it would be in commercial, political, and professional life if, as a matter of course, men stopped work at this age. In his Biathanatos, Donne tells us that by the laws of certain wise states sexagenarii were precipitated from a bridge, and in Rome men of that age were not admitted to the suffrage and they were called Depontani because the way to the senate was per pontem, and they from age were not permitted to come thither. In that charming novel *The Fixed Period,* Anthony Trollope discusses the practical advantage in modern life of a return to this ancient usage, and the plot hinges upon the admirable scheme of a college into which at 60 men retired for a year of contemplation before a peaceful departure by chloroform. That incalculable benefits might follow such a scheme is apparent to any one who, like myself, is nearing the limit, and who has made a careful study of the calamities which may befall men during the seventh and eighth decades. Still more when he contemplates the many evils which they perpetuate unconsciously, and with impunity. As it can be maintained that all the great advances have come from men under 40, so the history of the world shows that a very large proportion of the evils may be traced to the sexagenarians—nearly all the great mistakes politically and socially, all of the worst poems, most of the bad pictures, a majority of the bad novels, not a few of the bad sermons and speeches.[3]

Harvey Cushing, in his biography of Osler, describes the reaction to Osler's speech,

. . . and for days and weeks there followed pages of discussion, with cartoons and comments, caustic, abusive, and worse, with only an occasional word in his behalf lost in the uproar. Day by day there were columns of letters contributed by newspaper readers, none of whom in all probability had read the innocent paragraphs said half in jest that have been quoted above; until to "Oslerize" became a byword for mirth and opprobrium. Knowing nothing of the whimsical reference to Trollope's novel, interposed to mask his own pain at parting, nor of the rather pathetic allusion to his own advancing years, the public at large felt that it was the heartless view of a cold scientist who would condemn man as a productive machine.[4]

Cushing explains Osler's comments in several ways, "Though he loved young people more, and felt the future lay in their hands, his love for the aged was scarcely less. Few men during their lives have gone out of their way farther and more often to pay them tribute."[4] In essence, Cushing accepted that Osler was attempting humor. "It required no great degree of intelligence to distinguish between the serious and the jocular in what Osler had said, and if rightly read, certainly no one's feelings should have been ruffled in the slightest." Those, such as Cushing, who knew Osler well, were aware that his humor could be misperceived. Osler had a childlike mischievous nature. Egerton Y. Davis, a pen name assigned to his fanciful half, had been used to sign tongue-in-cheek case reports written to satirize the pomposity of certain investigators. It is for this reason perhaps that some may see the essay as Oslerian humor. Certainly the reference to chloroform and euthanasia are exaggerations of the theme intended to be humorous.

Cushing emphasizes the respect Osler had for individual elderly patients. Without doubt, Osler's respect and concern for elderly patients pervades his medical writings. His observations on certain disease states in the elderly continue to be valid and useful today.[5]

Cushing's explanation for "The Fixed Period" speech and essay is the most direct available. Joseph Pratt, a student of Osler in his book *A Year with Osler* also addresses the circumstances surrounding the valedictory speech.

> What he said in jest was taken in earnest! The press of the entire country so heartlessly misrepresented him that he became the target for general abuse. Even then he did not lose his equanimity, and those of his household did not know at the time how keenly he felt the sting of such unjust criticism. About two weeks after the delivery of the address he wrote me. "I hope you are hurrying as the years are flying and you will soon be 40." He also remarked that "the way of the joker is hard."[6]

Osler, while his sorrow and regrets about the speech are well documented, appears to have clarified himself on only one occasion. In the second edition of his Aequanimitas, Osler includes "The Fixed Period" essay in the collection, but makes the following comments in the preface:

> To this edition I have added the three valedictory addresses delivered before leaving America. One of these—"The Fixed Period"—demands a word of explanation. "To interpose a little ease," to relieve a situation of singular sadness in parting from my dear colleagues of the Johns Hopkins University, I jokingly suggested for the relief of a senile professoriate an extension of Anthony Trollope's plan mentioned in his novel *The Fixed Period*. To one who had all his life been devoted to old men, it was not a little distressing to be placarded in a worldwide way as their sworn enemy, and to every man over 60 whose spirit I may have thus unwittingly bruised, I tender my heartfelt regrets. Let me add, however, that the discussion which followed my remarks has not changed, but has rather strengthened my belief that the real work of life is done before the 40th year and that after the 60th year it would be best for the world and best for ourselves if men rested from their labours.[7]

Hence, despite Cushing's closeness in time to the event and deep understanding of Osler's life, his explanation of the issue is unsatisfactory in that Osler clearly maintained his position that productivity in life occurs before the age of 40. As a great admirer of Osler's work, I have searched for a better explanation of Osler's views on aging and hoped to find one before my upcoming 40th birthday. The explanation was buried with Osler but it is still available to us.

One cannot overemphasize the influence of Sir Thomas Browne's *Religio Medici* on the life of Osler. Osler had intended to join the ministry as a young man, and Father W.A. Johnson was one of the three most influential individuals in his life. Cushing states,

> It was Johnson's custom to read aloud to the boys in the parsonage, and for this purpose, as Osler recalled in later years, he often selected extracts from such works as the *Religio Medici* "in illustration of the beauty of the English language." But it must have been more than this. That a high-churchman should have cared particularly for Sir Thomas Browne is remarkable enough,

but that he should have been able to transmit this appreciation to a boy of 17 is truly amazing. It moreover is an important thread which from this point weaves its way through Osler's story to the end; and the 1862 edition of the *Religio Medici*, his second book purchase, to which he referred more than once in his published addresses, was the very volume which lay on his coffin 52 years later.[8]

Osler asks all physicians and students to read the *Religio Medici*. When I attempted to do so, I was unable to find any of the timeless humanism that pervades Osler's own work. In fact, I found it a dark and difficult book that seemed to encourage religious intolerance. However, Osler stated about the book,

> As I am on the confessional today, I may tell you that no book has had so enduring an influence on my life. I was introduced to it by my first teacher, the Reverend W.A. Johnson, Warden and founder of the Trinity College School, and I recall the delight with which I first read its quaint and charming pages. It was one of the strong influences which turned my thoughts to medicine and my most treasured copy has been a constant companion for 31 years.[9]

Osler does tell us what he admires about Sir Thomas Browne. He is a man who was denationalized and knew all countries. He was a man who mingled the waters of science with the oils of faith. Osler states, "I know of no one in history who believed so implicitly and so simply in the Christian religion and yet it is evident from his writings that he had moments of ardent scepticism. He also led a perfect life in a simple way."[10]

Osler is attracted to Browne's view of immortality, his appreciation of literature, and his skill in the use of language. Though it is still difficult to understand the essence of this attraction clearly, the *Religio Medici* was of biblical significance to Sir William Osler.

Establishing the importance of this work in Osler's life, I quote from the *Religio Medici:*

> It is not, I confess, an unlawful prayer to desire to surpass the days of our Saviour, or wish to outlive that age wherein he thought fittest to die; yet if (as divinity affirms) there shall be no grey hairs in heaven, but all shall rise in the perfect state of men, we do but outlive those perfections in this world, to be recalled unto them by a greater miracle in the next, and run on here but to be retrograde hereafter. Were there any hopes to outlive vice, or a point to be supernatuated from sin, it were worthy our knees to implore the days of Methuselah. But age does not rectify, but incurvate our natures, turning bad dispositions into worser habits, and (like diseases) brings on incurable vices; for every day as we grow weaker in age, we grow stronger in sin; and the number of our days doth but make our sins innumerable. The same vice committed at 16, is not the same, though it agrees in all other circumstances, as at 40, but swells and doubles from the circumstance of our ages; . . . . . Let them not therefore complain of immaturity that die about 30; they fall but like the whole world, whose solid and well-composed substance must not expect the duration and period of its constitution: when all things are completed in it, its age is accomplished. . . . And truly there goes a great deal of providence to produce a man's life unto threescore: there is more required than an able temper for those years; though the radical humour contain in it sufficient oil for 70, yet I perceive in some it gives not light past 30.[11]

The *Religio Medici* is the foundation for Osler's farewell speech to the Johns Hopkins faculty; the source of his original sin. Osler's ageism as expressed in "The Fixed Period" was not an attempt at humor but a strong feeling based on early religious teachings from the *Religio Medici*. Osler remains a foremost physician and teacher of our time. He was an exemplary geriatrician and his admirers need not apologize for him. The theory I propose can never be validated or refuted, but for Oslerians it might provide a solution to "The Fixed Period" enigma. For me the matter has been laid to rest.

References

1. Cushing H: The Life of Sir William Osler. Oxford, Clarendon Press, 1925. Reprinted for Classics of Medicine Library, Gryphon Eds. Birmingham, Alabama, 1982, Vol. II, p 659
2. Ibid, p 685
3. Osler W: Aequanimitas. The Fixed Period. 3rd ed. Philadelphia, Blakiston, 1932, pp 375–393
4. Cushing, op cit, Vol. II, p 669
5. Berk SL: Bacterial pneumonia in the elderly: the observations of Sir William Osler in retrospect. J Am Geriatr Soc 32:683–685, 1984
6. Pratt JH: A Year with Osler. Baltimore, Johns Hopkins Press, 1949, p IX
7. Osler W: Aequanimitas. Preface to the 2nd edition. Philadelphia, Blakiston, 1932, p VII
8. Cushing, op cit, Vol. 1, p 50
9. Ibid, p 504
10. Ibid, p 589
11. Browne T: Religio Medici. Classics of Medicine Library, Gryphon Eds. Birmingham, Alabama, 1981, pp 100–110

Osler's Brain and Related Mental Matters

 Alvin E. Rodin, M.D. and Jack D. Key, M.A., M.S.

ABSTRACT: Interest in the relationship between the morphology of the brain and mental and behavioral characteristics was evident in the 18th century; it flourished in the 19th century and waned during this century. This concern has been expressed in several activities. The weight and cortical area and gyral patterns of brains have been measured in detail in prominent and highly intelligent individuals, such as William Osler, Thomas Browne, and Albert Einstein, as well as in "average" individuals and in criminals. Phrenology is based on the assumption that various modalities of behavior are localized to specific morphologic areas of the brain. Little credence is now given to the mental, behavioral, and psychosocial significance of brain weight and gyral patterns. Practices based on such concepts are now considered by most to be a manifestation of quackery, though phrenology is still believed in by some.

The brain of Sir William Osler (Fig 1) is still with us, in at least two forms. First, and best known, are the varied products of his brain, namely his extensive medical works and his literary essays.[1] The second form is his actual brain, which is preserved in Philadelphia at the Wistar Institute of Anatomy and Biology in the form of cross-sections, cushioned by cotton and immortalized by preservative fluid (Fig 2).[2] This location is not by chance. When the institute was established in 1892, Osler, with others such as William Pepper, formed The Anthropologic Society.[3] The members of this society agreed to bequeath their brains to the institute for study.

When Osler was dying he made several requests, including that of having his autopsy performed by Dr. A.G. Gibson, having his brain sent to the Wistar Institute, and having his body cremated. Osler died in Oxford on Dec 29, 1919, at 4:30 PM. The autopsy was done at 2:30 PM the following day at his

Read at the annual meeting of the American Osler Society, May 4, 1988.

Reprinted with permission from *The Southern Medical Journal, 83:*207, 1990

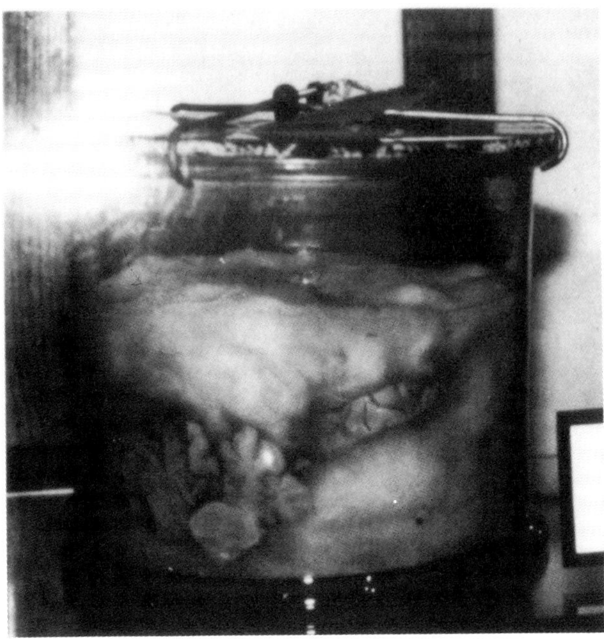

FIGURE 1   Osler's brain in jar at College of Physicians of Philadelphia, on loan from Wistar Institute, April 30, 1987. (Photograph by A.E. Rodin)

home in Norham Gardens (Fig 3).[4] A notation in the Wistar Museum catalog reads as follows: "Brain of Sir William Osler. Presented at his request to The Wistar Institute. Brought from England by Dr. Thomas McCrae, 1627 Spruce Street, Philadelphia, May 17, 1920" (B. T. Clause, written communication, December 1987). Thus it was about $4^{1}/_{2}$ months after the autopsy that McCrae carried the brain overseas.

Examination of Osler's Brain

Two gross examinations of Osler's brain were made, the first by Gibson at the time of autopsy.[4]

> The pia-arachnoid is slightly adherent to the dura over the vertex and the dura again to the calvarium. The falx cerebri and tentorium cerebelli thickened. Frontal lobes large, squarish in transverse outline. Atheroma of the basilar arteries and circle of Willis. No external abnormality. Preserved for further examination.

The second gross examination was done at the Wistar Institute (Fig 4). The brain had a normal weight of 1,396 gm. The features described at Norham Gardens are noted, and further detail is provided as follows:

> The superior surface shows the left hemisphere to be appreciably larger than the right with some suggestion of atrophy over the postfrontal and precentral areas on the left with a more diffuse but less distinct atrophy over the right hemisphere . . . . The parietal area of the left side is much more prominent than the right. . . .

Osler's brain was not examined microscopically until 1959 when Wilder Penfield was permitted to borrow it in exchange for agreeing to speak at the

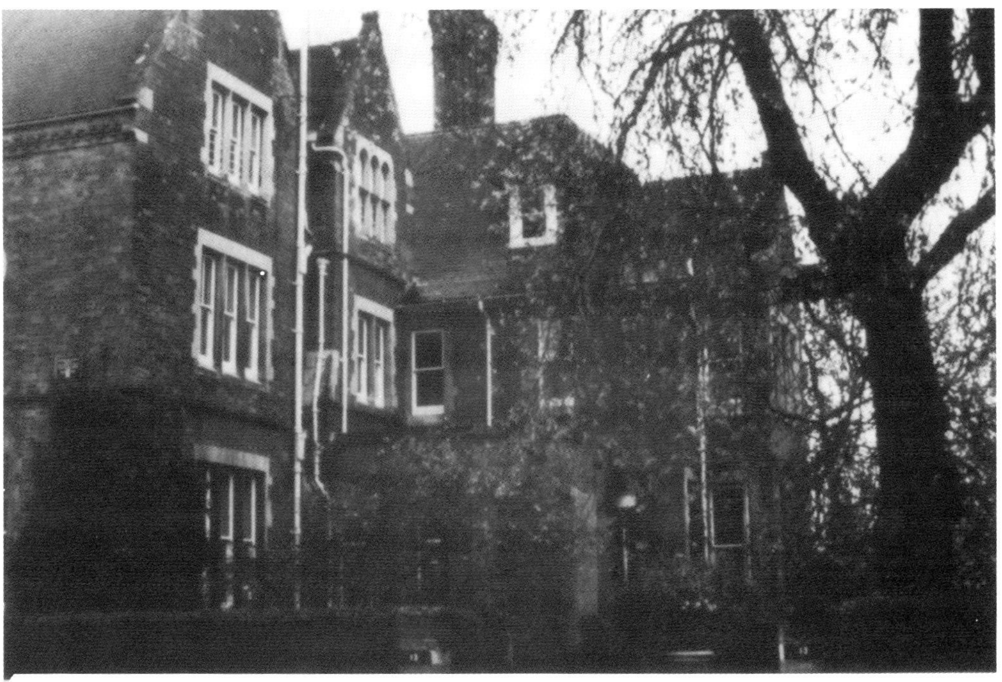

FIGURE 2   Osler's house, Open Arms, at No. 13 Norham Gardens, Oxford, in 1981. (Photograph by A.E. Rodin)

Wistar Institute (A.H.T. Robb-Smith, MD, written communication, June 1988). He then took it to the Montreal Neurologic Institute where samples were taken from the frontal lobes, pons, medulla, and cerebellum. The consequent microscopic slides were examined by Dr. G. Mathieson,[5] neuropathologist, who reported that "A survey of different regions has failed to show any significant histopathologic changes."

It is not surprising that there were no microscopic abnormalities found in Osler's brain. Today one would not make too much of its gross appearance. Atheroma would be considered "normal" for the brain of a 70-year-old man, and the presence of some atrophy, of little consequence. But much more has been made of the external morphologic features of brains in both ancient and recent history.

Historical Interpretations

The size, shape, weight, and convolutions of the brain have long been considered as having some relationship to mentality—either intelligence or character or both. Measurement of cranial capacity of skulls is a frequent method used in studies of the origins of man. Anthropoid apes have a much smaller capacity than does modern man—400 to 500 ml as compared with 1,550 ml.[6] This considerable difference is due to evolutionary development of the frontal lobe of the brain, with a resultant marked increase in intelligence of *Homo sapiens*.

Between 1900 and 1930 several studies were conducted on brain size as determined by external measurements of the head.[7] A direct correlation with

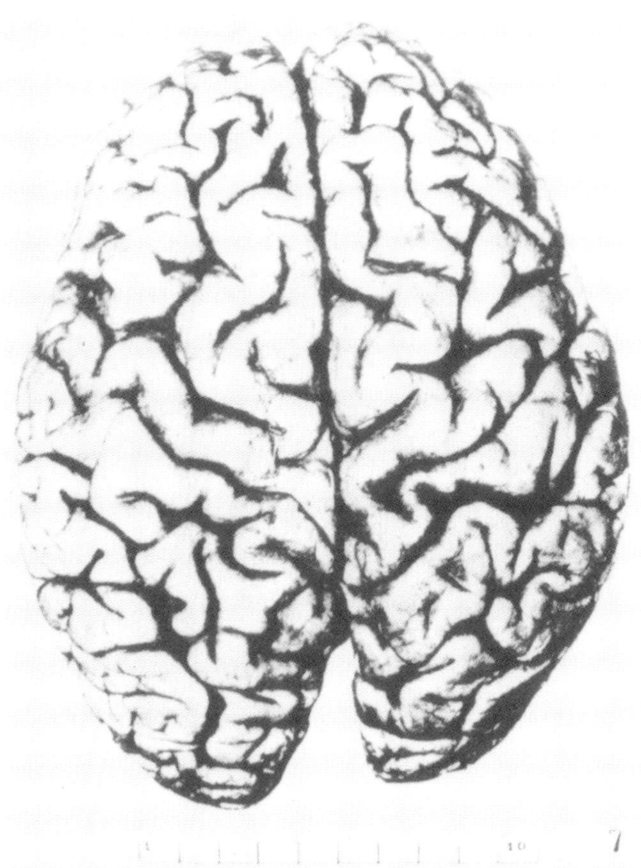

FIGURE 3   Superior surface of William Osler's brain. (From Donaldson and Canavan.[2])

intelligence was suggested in some instances. More recently, in 1979, Passingham[8] found only a slight correlation between brain size and intelligence.

Literature, being a reflection of society, has not been exempted from the brain size/intelligence controversy. An example is Conan Doyle's creation, Professor Challenger, the egocentric and brilliant scientist who led an expedition to *The Lost World*.[9] Professor Summerlee, Challenger's protagonist, estimated that his head contained a large brain that functioned as "a big engine running smooth, and turning out clean work."

In addition to brain size, brain weight has also been considered to have a direct correlation with intelligence. Tilney[10] reported in 1928 that "Statistics indicate that the brain weight of distinguished and talented individual members of the race is somewhat in excess of the average adult brain." Valen,[7] in a 1974 review of many studies, found as high a correlation as 0.3 between brain weight and intelligence. Some authors, however, have objected on the basis that there are other correlates of brain weight, such as age, height, and sex.[11] The definitive word may well have been given by Simms[12] 83 years earlier (1887) when he reviewed the brain weight, body weight, and height of many individuals. His conclusion was that "A great mind may belong to a person who carries a very small, a medium sized, or a very large brain, the size and weight neither adding to the mental power nor detracting from it, provided only that the encephalon is sufficient to give due support to bodily life."

There have been other extrapolations from brain weight. A considerable furor was caused in 1887 by William Hammond (1828–1900), a neurologist and former Surgeon General of the United States.[13] He wrote, "It is the height of absurdity to attempt . . . the education of girls according to the same method as pursued by boys."[14] His rationale was that the female brain is on the average about 5 ounces less in weight than the male brain (49 vs 44 oz) and with less frontal development. He therefore considered it an absurdity to teach them certain subjects, such as mathematics.

The various areas of the brain surface have also been extensively studied. Franz Joseph Gall (1758–1828) established phrenology as a science early in the 19th century.[15] Its basic premise is that there are 27 personality traits, each one being situated in its own distinct area of the brain (or *organ*, as labeled by phrenologists) (Fig 5). The size of the area determines the prominence of the mental trait and the shape of the overlying skull. Heads of many individuals were carefully measured by calipers, and various deductions were made. Two examples will suffice from an 1877 handbook, *How to Read Character: A New Illustrated Hand-Book of Phrenology and Physiognomy.*[16]

> **Amativeness** (amorous): Aaron Burr (third vice president of the United States) was noted for his debauchery. His skull from below the occipital process to the mastoid process was protuberant. This is compared to the smallness of this area in George Bancroft, the American Historian who had never married.

The cerebellum was considered by phrenologists to be the organ of sexuality,[17] thus accounting for the increased size of the overlying part of the skull in the licentious Aaron Burr.

> **Parental Love:** Queen Victoria was considered to be overfond of her children. The back of her head had a fullness due to enlargement above the occipital protuberance, indicative of parental love. This area was not developed in Andrew Johnson, 17th president of the United States, who was a bachelor and stated to have no love for children or women.

Many prominent individuals supported the science of phrenology. Horace Mann (1796–1859), known as the father of American public education, looked "upon phrenology as the handmaiden of Christianity. Whoever disseminated true phrenology is a public benefactor."[16] Alfred Russel Wallace, the great biologist, predicted in 1899 that "in the coming century phrenology will assuredly attain general acceptance. It will prove itself to be the true science of the mind."[15] Many famous people had their heads calibrated. For example, a phrenologist examined the head of Arthur Conan Doyle in 1897.[18] Prominent in his brain were the "organs" that are necessary for a successful writer of medical, mystery, and historical works: "Human Nature, Comparison, Individuality, Form and Size, together with large Constructiveness and Imitation to give power to adapt and assimilate ways and means." Anyone could come to the same conclusion today by merely reading the works of Conan Doyle.

There are no writings on phrenology by William Osler to be found in Abbott's bibliography of his works.[19] However, Osler's *Bibliotheca Osleriana*[20] includes nine books on the subject, the earliest one published in 1817. Phrenology was rejected by the scientific establishment during the latter part of the 19th century. It is now considered to be a form of quackery which preys upon the gullible.[21]

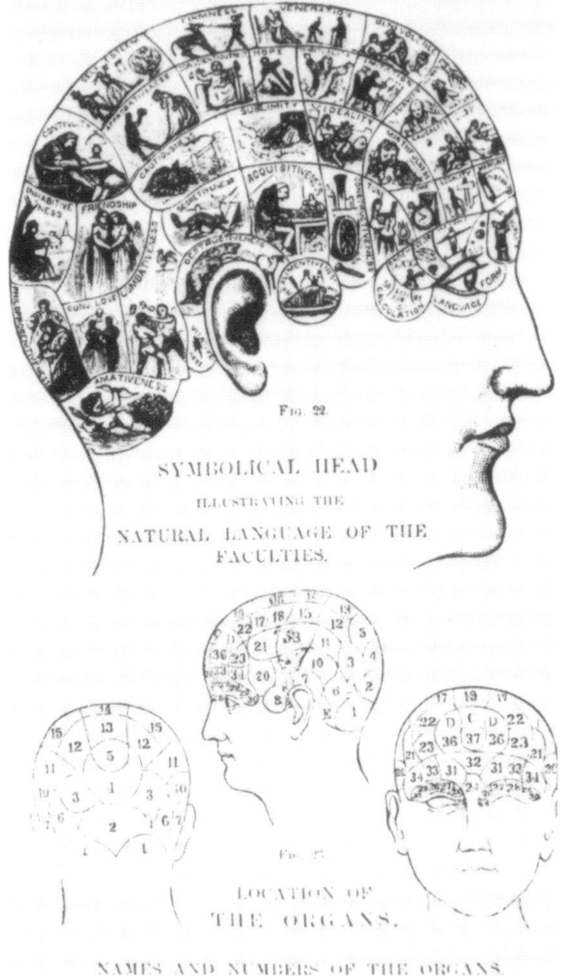

FIGURE 4 Phrenology's 27 "organs" of the brain, as depicted in 1877.[16]

Brains of Criminals

The brain has also been studied to determine differences between criminals and noncriminals. In 1879 Moriz Benedikt[22] (1835–1920) published a major book on this subject, *Anatomic Studies Upon the Brains of Criminals,* which was translated into English in 1881. Benedikt was a Viennese medical scientist who is better known for his work on electrotherapy and for the Benedikt syndrome.[23] He made a detailed study of the brain surface of 22 criminals. They had a generalized "deficient gyrus development—and a consequent excess of fissures, which are obviously fundamental defects." He stressed that these abnormal fissures of criminals were more confluent with each other than normally.

In 1882, Osler published a detailed study "On the Brains of Criminals,"[24] to ascertain the validity of Benedikt's conclusions. Complete details are given of the history and brain morphology of a murderer and of a half-witted Frenchman. Osler obtained permission from the Canadian government to attend their executions and to perform autopsies,[25] but he sent a medical student instead. For comparison, Osler also studied the cerebral hemispheres of 34 patients who had died at the Montreal General Hospital. In a further paper, Osler detailed the brains of two other notorious murderers that were sent to him, one by a physician and the other by a medical student.[26]

The results of Osler's studies differed from those of Benedikt in that he found as large a number of confluent fissures in noncriminals as in criminals. Osler ended his morphologic report on an ethical and psychosocial note. He questioned "What degree of responsibility can be attached to the actions of a man with a defective cerebral organization?" Osler answered his own question by contrasting the deterministic view of Spinoza (that there is no such thing as absolute or free will) with the intuitionistic one as expressed by Shakespeare's Iago: "Tis in ourselves that we are thus and thus." Osler upheld the latter because "to let this anthropological variety (as Benedikt calls criminals) know positively that punishment will follow the commission of certain acts, should prove an effectual deterrent in many cases. . . ." This is similar to Benedikt's statement that the abnormality he described "does not signify actual disease, but a predisposition to it only."

Osler's interest in brain morphology was not limited to that of criminals. He published articles on diseases of the brain,[27] though he preserved fewer specimens of this organ than of others in his pathology museum at McGill University.[28] His interest in veterinary medicine was reflected in the study of animal brains. According to the *Canadian Record of Science* of 1884,[29] Osler made a presentation at a meeting of the Natural History Society of Montreal on the brain of the seal, which was "illustrated by many prepared specimens." Unfortunately, the text was evidently never published.

Brains of Prominent Individuals

Brains of individuals who have made outstanding contributions to humanity have also been studied in detail. An early such report was published in 1860 by Rudolph Wagner, who found no differences in weight or in complexity of the fissural patterns from that of "ordinary" people.[30] Similar studies in the 20th century have been reviewed by Riese,[30] who found more positive than negative results. For example, several investigators have found that the acoustic, superior temporal, and precentral gyri and the occipital lobe were particularly well developed in outstanding musicians. The philosophers Haeckel and von Monakow had enlarged frontal lobes and parietal lobules, with a more complicated fissural pattern.

Attracting more interest has been the brain of Albert Einstein, who died in 1955 of a ruptured aortic aneurysm.[31] His will stated that his body be cremated except for the brain which could be studied but only in the strictest privacy.[32] Much later, samples from the prefrontal and inferior parietal association areas were studied microscopically. These were compared with brains from 11 patients who had died in a VA hospital.[33] The cortex of Einstein's parietal area had a much higher concentration of glial cells, suggesting "a greater neuronal metabolic need [which] might reflect the enhanced use of this tissue in the expression of his unusual conceptual powers."

The brain of Sir William Osler, like that of Einstein, has had detailed study, though not at the microscopic level.[2] In 1928 Donaldson and Canavan[2] of the Wistar Institute published the findings from studies of the brain of three scholars, including that of Osler. The other two were Granville Stanley Hall (1846–1928), who gave impetus to the development of psychology in the United States, and Edward Sylvester Morse (1838–1925), an American zoologist best known for his studies of the Shell Mounds in Japan. These were compared with the brains of three members of the Southard family—the mother and father, who had had limited opportunities for mental development, and their son, who had been a neurologist. Brief biographies are provided for all. Osler's was quite positive.

> His life reveals a man in whom alertness, mental and physical, is seen at every turn. The art of making and holding Friends came to him naturally, and this trait was conspicuous. In him a great carrying power for information, technical and general, was combined with a capacity for selective condensation, as shown in his writings. His influence on the development of clinical medicine during the last forty years was outstanding.

The extensive examination of the six brains began with their weight. Those of the three scholars and the neurologist of the Southard family were heavier. The assumption was that the weight and the quality of the brain relates to the size of the neurons, and the size of the neurons is dependent upon the adequacy of the vascular supply to the brain.

The percentage extent of the cortical surface of the frontal lobes ranged from 39.1% to 44.7% for the three scholars and the neurologist, Southard. Those of Southard's parents were lower. The lower percentage of the cortical surface of the parietal lobe of Morse's brain was attributed to age atrophy. Presumably the greater extent of the cortical surface of the frontal lobes in the scholars and the neurologist indicates superior mental abilities.

Although the number of individuals studied by Donaldson and Canavan is insufficient for any statistically based conclusion, a conclusion is offered:

> From the data on hand we conclude, therefore, that the scholars had brains that were somewhat better grown and therefore better nourished than those with which they were compared and that this favorable nutritional adjustment constitutes a fundamental condition favoring superior performance. For further inferences adequate data are lacking.

They suggested that "It is quite possible that an individual may have an excellent nervous machine and at the same time not be able to use it effectively." This is similar to the caveats of Osler and Benedikt. It implicates the importance of psychologic and educational influences on the postnatal development and functioning of the cerebral cortex. Thus, it is quite possible that William Osler's parents, other relatives, teachers, and cultural milieu had as much influence on his achievements and interests as did the morphology of his brain.

Conclusion

The relationship of brain morphology to mental matters is epitomized by a gift to the museum of the Norfolk and Norwich Hospital from William Osler in 1901. It is an oblong receptacle made of crystal glass to serve as the casket for the skull of Sir Thomas Browne who died in 1682.[34] An endocranial brain cast of the skull, showing convolutionary markings, received a detailed phrenologic study in 1924.[35] The frontal lobes of Thomas Browne were small and the others above average size. On the pedestal of the receptacle for his skull are several plaques with quotations selected by Osler from Browne's own *Religio Medici* of 1643.[36]

> I believe that our estranged and divided ashes shall unite again; that our separated dust, after so many pilgrimages and transformations into the parts of minerals, plants, animals, elements, shall at the voice of God return to their primitive shapes and join again to make up their primary and predestinate forms.
>
> At my death I mean to take a total adieu of the world, not caring for a monument, history, or epitaph, not so much as the bare memory of my name to be found anywhere but in the Universal Register of God.

Not all will agree that Sir William Osler and Sir Thomas Browne achieved a physical form in the other world as implied in the first quotation; but all can agree that neither had the lack of prominence in this world alluded to in the second quotation. And it appears doubtful that the size, weight, and configurations of their respective brains were related to such prominence.

References

1. Osler W: *Aequanimitas With Other Addresses to Medical Students, Nurses and Practitioners of Medicine.* Philadelphia, Blakiston, 1904
2. Donaldson HH, Canavan MM: A study of the brains of three scholars. Granville Stanley Hall, Sir William Osler, Edward Sylvester Morse. *J Comp Neurol* 46:1–95, 1928
3. Cushing H: *The Life of Sir William Osler.* Oxford, Clarendon Press, Vol 1, 1925, p 196
4. Barondess JA: A case of empyema: notes on the last illness of Sir William Osler. *Trans Am Clin Climatol Assoc* 86:59–71, 1974
5. Mathieson G: Neuropathological Report M187. Sir William Osler, age 70. Brain received from Wistar Institute. Montreal, *Montreal Neurological Institute Pathology Records,* 1950
6. Bishop CW: *Man From the Farthest Past.* Washington, DC, Smithsonian, 1930, p 165
7. Van Valen L: Brain size and intelligence in man. *Am J Phys Anthropol* 40:417–424, 1974
8. Passingham RE: Brain size and intelligence in man. *Brain Behav Evol* 16:253–270, 1979
9. Doyle AC: *The Lost World.* London, Hodder & Stoughton, 1912
10. Tilney F: *The Brain From Ape to Man. A Contribution to the Study of the Evolution and Development of the Human Brain.* New York, Paul B. Hoeber, Chap 25, 1928
11. *Brain. Micropedia Encyclopaedia Britannica.* Chicago, Helen Hemingway Benton, Vol 2, 1974, p 228
12. Simms J: Human brain-weights. *Popular Sci Monthly* 31:355–359, 1887
13. Key JD, Bluestein BE: *William Alexander Hammond, M.D. (1828–1900). The Publications of an American Neurologist.* Rochester, Minn, Davies, 1983
14. Hammond WA: Brain-forcing in childhood. *Popular Sci Monthly* 30:721–732, 1887
15. Davies JD: *Phrenology. Fad and Science.* New York, Archon Books, 1971
16. *How to Read Character: A New Illustrated Hand-Book of Phrenology and Physiognomy.* New York, SR Wells, 1877

17. Shortland M: Courting the cerebellum, early organological and phrenological views of sexuality. *Br J Hist Sci* 20:173–199, 1987

18. Stern MB: *The Game's a Head. A Phrenological Study of Sherlock Holmes and Arthur Conan Doyle.* Rockville Center, NY, Paulette Green, 1983

19. Abbott ME: *Classified and Annotated Bibliography of Sir William Osler's Publications.* Montreal, Medical Museum McGill University, 2nd Ed, 1939

20. Osler W: *Bibliotheca Osleriana.* Oxford, Clarendon Press, 1929

21. *"Know Thyself": A Phrenological Character Reading.* Philadelphia, College Physicians Fugitive Leaves, Vol 2, Fall 1987

22. Benedikt M: *Anatomic Studies Upon the Brains of Criminals. A Contribution to Anthropology, Medicine, Jurisprudence, and Psychology.* New York, Wm Wood & Co, 1881

23. Lesky E: *The Vienna Medical School of the 19th Century* (Translated from German). Baltimore, Johns Hopkins University, 1976

24. Osler W: On the brains of criminals. *Can Med Surg J* 10:385–398, 1882

25. Cushing H: *The Life of Sir William Osler.* Oxford, Clarendon Press, Vol 1, 1925, p 195

26. Osler W: Report on the brains of Richards and O'Rouke. *Can Med Surg J* 11:461–466, 1882

27. Osler W: Three cases of brain disease. *Can Med Surg J* 8:295–304, 346–349, 1879

28. Rodin AE: *Oslerian Pathology. An Assessment and Annotated Atlas of Museum Specimens.* Lawrence, Kan, Coronado Press, 1981

29. IX. Proceedings of the Natural History Society. *Can Record Sci* 1:63–64, 1884

30. Riese W: Brains of prominent people: history, facts and significance. *Med Coll Va* 2:106–110, 1966

31. Quasha A: *Albert Einstein. An Intimate Portrait.* Larchmont, NY, Forest Publishing Co, 1980

32. Maranto G: Einstein's brain. *Discover,* May 1985, pp 29–35

33. Diamond MC, Scheibel AB, Murphy GM, et al: On the brain of a scientist: Albert Einstein. *Exp Neurol* 88:198–294, 1985

34. The skull of Sir Thomas Browne. *Br Med J* 1:413, 1922

35. Keith A: *Phrenologic Studies of the Skull and Brain Cast of Sir Thomas Browne of Norwich.* Edinburgh, Oliver & Boyd, 1924

36. Browne T: *Rellgio Medici.* London, Andrew Crooke, 1643

37. Sir William Osler Memorial Number. *Bull Int Assoc Med Museums,* No. 9, 1926, p 204

From Osler to Olafson
The Evolution of Veterinary
Pathology in North America

Leon Z. Saunders, D.V.M.

Summary

Most branches of biological science in North America developed first in the United States, and later were taught and practiced in Canada. An exception was veterinary pathology, which as a discipline taught in veterinary colleges and as a field of research, developed first in Canada, and from there crossed the border to the United States.

Pathology was first taught at the Montreal Veterinary College, founded in 1866 by Duncan McEachran, a graduate of the Edinburgh Veterinary College. From the outset, he formed a close association with the medical faculty of McGill University, permitting his students to attend the same classes in the basic subjects with the medical students. Eventually, the Montreal Veterinary College became formally affiliated with McGill University, as the Faculty of Comparative Medicine and Veterinary Science.

The McGill veterinary faculty was forced to close for economic reasons in 1903, but it left an enduring legacy, particularly in the field of veterinary pathology. The legacy, a novel concept in the 1870's, was that pathology was the cornerstone of a veterinary education; the place where anatomy, physiology, chemistry and botany met with the clinical subjects, and gave the latter meaning. This tradition was formed at the Montreal Veterinary College by the world renowned physician William Osler, North America's leading medical

Read at the annual meeting of the American Osler Society, May 9, 1990.

Reprinted with permission from *Canadian Journal of Veterinary Research*, 51:1, 1987 teacher, whom McEachran had invited to teach at the College in 1876 in addition to his duties in the faculty of medicine. Osler had studied with Virchow in Berlin and applied his methods of autopsy technique and of scientific inquiry to his teaching of both human and veterinary pathology at McGill.

Osler also undertook investigations into various diseases of domestic animals, at the request of McEachran, who doubled as Chief Veterinary Inspector for the Dominion Department of Agriculture.

Osler left McGill University in 1884. Only after that year did other North American veterinary schools adopt pathology as a discipline of instruction. However, by 1884, Osler had already left his indelible imprint on the students (both medical and veterinary) he had taught in Montreal, one of whom took over the teaching of pathology in the veterinary college. Another, who followed Osler's example and also studied in Berlin with Virchow, wrote the first book in the English language on veterinary post mortem technique in 1889.

By the time the United States Bureau of Animal Industry was founded in May 1884, and Theobald Smith hired as its first pathologist, Osler had already done research work on hog cholera (1878), verminous bronchitis of dogs (1877) and Pictou cattle disease (1883) among others. Thus, veterinary pathology was established as an investigative discipline in Canada before the B.A.I. was launched.

The contributions of William Osler in the field of veterinary pathology, both as a teacher and as an investigator of disease in pigs, cattle, horses and dogs are reported. The contributions to veterinary pathology of four veterinarians, who graduated from the Montreal Veterinary College, are identified. Through one of these four, W.L. Williams, Osler's influence can be traced in an unbroken sequence from Canada in the 1870's to the U.S.A. in the 1980's. These historical data are presented as evidence of Canadian priority in establishing the discipline of veterinary pathology in North America.

Key Words: History of Veterinary Medicine; Pathology, veterinary, history; Osler, William; McEachran, Duncan; North America, veterinary pathology.

Ladies and gentlemen!

A.R. Gurney, a contemporary playwright, has said that an important part of living is being aware of what anthropologists call our tribal identity, our identity as a group, as distinct from our individual identity. His allusion to ethnic tribes is equally apposite to professional tribes. Thus, I'm in favor of trying to discover our professional heritage by looking back and exploring it.

This is a historically interesting year for veterinary pathology on this continent, and our meeting place here in Toronto makes it doubly so. Nineteen eighty-four marks 100 years since the death of Joseph Woodward, who published the first scientific paper in the realm of veterinary pathology in North America.[1]

The report by Woodward, a medical officer at the Army Medical Museum in Washington, described the histopathology of pleuropneumonia in cattle, and appeared in 1870. However, it was a lone event and did not

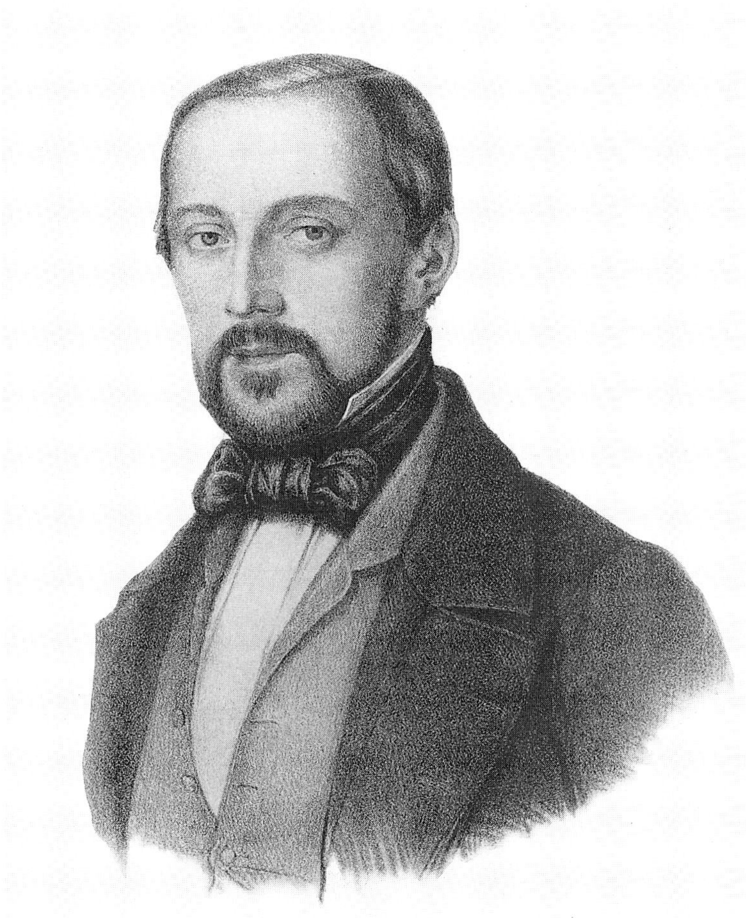

FIGURE 1. R. Virchow.

establish a foothold for veterinary pathology on this continent. Woodward did no further work in the field of veterinary pathology. He left no successors who were interested in veterinary pathology; none of the physicians who worked with him pursued work outside of human pathology. Serious work at the Army Medical Museum (now the Armed Forces Institute of Pathology) was not taken up again until the 1940's, i.e. 75 years later.[2]

This year is also an important milestone for us because of another event that took place a hundred years ago. We are meeting today near the birthplace of a great pioneer who tilled in our vineyard, Sir William Osler, who left the faculties of medicine and of comparative medicine in McGill University in Montreal in 1884, to go to the medical school at the University of Pennsylvania.[3] He departed after eight fruitful years of teaching at the Montreal Veterinary College, (later the faculty of comparative medicine at McGill), in the course of which he established pathology firmly as a discipline of academic instruction in a North American veterinary school. Although the years he spent in our field were few, his influence was profound. It readily crossed the

American border—then as now a peaceful one—and endured long enough to ensure the perpetuation of the discipline in the United States.

I shall discuss how veterinary pathology evolved on this continent, with respect to both the teaching of the subject in veterinary schools, and the development of knowledge within the discipline as the result of scientific investigation. Veterinary pathology evolved as a subject of instruction in Canada, in a veterinary school whose principal thought it should be taught. It also evolved in Canada in the Dominion Department of Agriculture, where the same man, Duncan McEachran, thought that animal diseases should be investigated by pathologists.

McEachran had been a partner with Andrew Smith in the founding of the Ontario Veterinary College in Toronto in 1862. However, it soon became apparent to him that he and Smith held widely divergent philosophies regarding veterinary education.[4] Smith's low standards resulted in third-rate education but attracted numerous students. McEachran (Figure 2) harbored lofty aspirations for the improvement of the veterinary profession. These could only be realized by attracting bright students and providing them with a first-class education. He parted from Smith in 1864, moved to Montreal and in 1866 opened the Montreal Veterinary College as a private venture. We shall touch on McEachran several times in this paper, relative to pathology, but will not repeat the biographical information on him already published.[5-7]

Dominion Department of Agriculture

In addition to his duties as principal and professor at the Montreal Veterinary College, McEachran was appointed Chief Inspector of Livestock by the Dominion government in 1876 and served until 1902. The Ministry of Agriculture opened a quarantine station—the first in the western hemisphere—at Point Levis, Quebec. By inspecting imported animals there, McEachran "... was successful in keeping Canada almost disease-free, despite epidemics plaguing cattle in the United States, England and Europe during those years".[7] It need occasion no surprise that McEachran set just as high a store on the services of pathologists in the investigation of disease as he did on their teaching in his college. As a result, he induced each of the McGill pathologists who taught his students to also investigate diseases: Osler on hog cholera and Pictou cattle disease, Johnston and Adami on the latter, and Adami also on tuberculosis. The tradition which McEachran began resulted in a veterinarian who had been trained by Adami, being appointed the first Dominion animal pathologist when Adami could no longer handle all of the work on a part-time basis. In the same tradition, carried on after McEachran's retirement, the Ministry of Agriculture employed S.B. Wolbach, a famous Harvard pathologist, to work on equine swamp fever during a year that he spent on the staff of the Montreal General Hospital.[8]

I cannot go into detail here about the various diseases which McEachran set the pathologists to investigate. The publications resulting from this work are cited under the individual biographies. Of historical importance is that in Canada, such work began in 1876, and, by the time William Osler left the country in 1884, the discipline of pathology had been applied by a competent pathologist to several diseases.

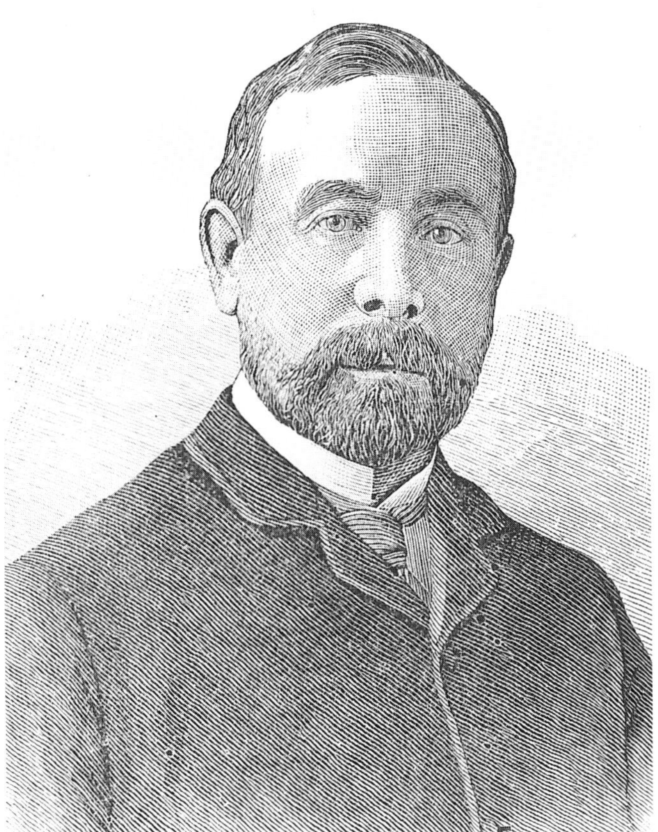

FIGURE 2. Duncan McEachran, from an engraving published in 1888.[5]

By contrast, in the United States, the Bureau of Animal Industry was not founded *until* 1884, and its Division of Pathology not until 1891.[9] Moreover, when this division was organized, there was not a single trained pathologist within its ranks, and no tradition to employ the best pathologists in the country ever developed.

Teaching of Pathology in the Earliest North American Veterinary Schools

In the 1860's, institutions for the education of veterinarians had begun to appear in North America.[10,11] The most important of them were founded by British veterinarians: Andrew Smith (Toronto), Duncan McEachran (Montreal), James Law (Cornell), C.P. Lyman (Harvard) were graduates of Edinburgh and Joseph Hughes (Chicago) a graduate of Glasgow. The dates of founding of the veterinary schools in the nineteenth century are shown in the table:

The following table gives an indication as to which of the veterinary schools of North America taught pathology to the students in the nineteenth century and immediately after the turn of the century. I have not listed the

Teaching of Pathology in the Earliest North American Veterinary Schools

School and Date Founded		Years Pathology Taught and Names of Teachers
Ontario	1862	J. Caven, 1890–1899; D. Smith, 1900–1920
Montreal (McGill)	1866	W. Osler, 1876–1884; W. Johnston, 1885–1891; J. Adami, 1892–1902 [† 1903]
N.Y. Coll. Vet. Surg.	1842	J. Huddleston, 1895 [† 1899]
Amer. Vet. Coll.	1875	Not taught [† 1899]
Columbia	1877	T. Satterthwaite, 1881–1882 [† 1884]
Iowa State	1879	W. Harriman, 1895–1899
Harvard	1882	R. Fitz, 1882–1891; W. Whitney, 1892–1894; L. Frothingham, 1895–1902 [† 1902]
Chicago	1883	A. Edwards, 1894–1900; M. Herzog, 1906–1913 [† 1920]
U. of Pa.	1884	H. Formad, 1884–1891; R. Formad, 1892–1899
Ohio State	1885	Not taught in 19th century
Kansas City	1891	L. Rosenwold, 1894–1900; A. Kinsley, 1906–1918 [† 1918]
National	1892	V. Moore, 1894–1895 [† 1896]
McKillip	1894	O. Schwarzkopf, 1894–1901 [† 1920]
Cornell	1895	V. Moore, 1896–1902; S. Burnett, 1902–1914

†indicates when the institution closed.

smallest of the schools which perished after graduating only a dozen students, such as the University of California. Instead the table shows the schools which were important, either because they graduated thousands of veterinarians (McKillip, Ontario), or because they had high-class teachers even though the schools did not survive (Columbia, Chicago, Harvard). Almost without exception, the first teacher shown at each institution was a physician and in some cases the second one as well. The only veterinarians in the table are Frothingham, R. Formad, Kinsley, Burnett and Schwarzkopf.

Some of the physicians who taught pathology to veterinary students were well trained either in Germany, America or both. Others are so obscure that I have not been able to determine their qualifications. With the exception of the teachers at McGill University, however, none made any lasting contributions to veterinary pathology during the period 1865–1895. In several institutions, it appears that they taught the same course to the veterinary students and the medical students; the instruction in most cases consisted solely of lectures. A few autopsies were done, and reports were even published[12–14] so that the lectures were sometimes based on observations from domestic animals. But, the condition of specialist teaching of veterinary pathology in the nineteenth century in North America was far behind the activity in Berlin, in Berne, in Munich, in Vienna and even in Kazan, Kharkov and Warsaw. In the latter, teachers trained in Germany taught autopsy technique and gross and microscopic pathology to an extent that would not be seen in most North American veterinary schools until about 1910 or even later.[15]

Of the colleges which were founded in the 1860's, the New York College of Veterinary Surgeons did not include pathology in its curriculum. Neither did the American Veterinary College founded in 1875, with which the former institution later merged. During 1895, John H. Huddleston, a physician, served as professor of general and comparative pathology of the N.Y.C.V.S.[11,16], although there is no mention of this in his obituary.[17] That year he reported on a case of neoplasia in the horse to the New York Pathological Society; the only evidence I have found of his veterinary activity.[14] Since he had graduated from medical school only three years earlier and had no training as a pathologist, the impact of his brief fling on veterinary pathology, if any, was miniscule. Thus, this school, along with the contemporary Ontario Veterinary College, cannot compete with the Montreal Veterinary College as a center of activity in veterinary pathology during the 1870's, the critical decade when the discipline came to life in North America.

At the Ontario Veterinary College, founded in 1862, pathology was not part of the curriculum during the 1860's, 70's and 80's.[4] Indeed it could hardly have been taught to the half literate students which Andrew Smith's low admission requirements attracted from both sides of the border. In the 1890's and later, there were lectures by J. Caven and D. King Smith, both physicians and the latter also Andrew Smith's son. The former was a bacteriologist. Smith wrote a couple of pedestrian papers on the submission of specimens for histologic study and on tumors,[18,19] but pathology in his day was a course, rather than a department carrying on diagnostic or research activity. In the last three decades of the 19th century, serious teaching of veterinary pathology by qualified persons in Canada was being done only in Montreal.

In the United States just before and just after the turn of the century, pathology was taught well by Frothingham until 1902 when Harvard closed its doors, by Robert Formad, until he resigned his position, and possibly by V.A. Moore after he had learned the subject himself. Of these, only Frothingham, who had worked in Dresden with Albert Johne, was really well trained, and he left no scientific descendants.

Cornell initially (in 1868) did not have a school, but a one-man veterinary department, under James Law, which offered a four-year course. It graduated only five people, before it became a veterinary college in 1895. Pathology was not taught at Cornell until 1896.[20]

In the decade between 1877 and 1887, while Osler and Johnston were teaching pathology at the Montreal Veterinary College, Iowa State College commenced veterinary instruction in 1879. Like the course at Cornell, the one in Iowa was also a small one-man operation, but in Iowa Milton Stalker offered a two-year rather than a four-year course. While Christiansen identifies this as the first "state supported veterinary college" in the United States,[10] one wonders whether this novel definition of the word college is justified. In the 1890's, pathology was still not taken seriously at Iowa State; thus, the man hired as college physician was also responsible for teaching histology and pathology in the veterinary department.[21] How a person untrained even in human pathology could teach these subjects without a microscope must be left to one's imagination. The history of the school records that as late as 1895, $100 was appropriated for the "Pathology Department." In 1895 when Dr. Harriman (the College physician) asked for $125 to buy a microscope, the trustees of the College demurred—they appropriated $15 to rent one for a year! In 1896, they finally relented, and appropriated the other $110 to consummate the purchase. Four years later, the annual budget for pathology was only $50.[21]

In the period which ended in 1884, pathology was taught by competent, well-trained pathologists only at the Montreal Veterinary College and at Columbia and Harvard Universities. However, Thomas Satterthwaite[22–24] and Robert Fitz,[25] who taught at Columbia and Harvard respectively, did not make any original contributions to veterinary pathology. Even more to the point, they began to teach their veterinary students in 1881 and 1882, respectively, five and six years after Osler had begun to do so in Montreal.

I want to emphasize how few people were engaged in veterinary pathology in North America in the last quarter of the nineteenth century. Both as a discipline taught in the veterinary schools and as one practiced in state or federal government research laboratories, the continuity of veterinary pathology during this time was precarious.

The Montreal Veterinary College

In his Schofield Lecture in 1982, Nielsen said, "The Faculty of Comparative Medicine & Veterinary Science perished in 1903 after 13 years. . ."[26] But it did not perish without leaving a legacy, and it is this legacy that I wish to examine today. It had ramifications so far into the future that it can be traced to the 1980's.

In 1888, Mills, one of the teachers at the Montreal Veterinary College (later a faculty of McGill University), related the history of its first quarter century (Figure 3). The veterinary students had to matriculate, i.e. have completed at least a high school education. They took their pre-clinical subjects, including pathology, with the medical students at McGill University. He added: "The College has a large museum well furnished with models, casts, skeletons, pathological specimens, etc."

> Further, "The lectures and demonstrations in Pathology in McGill University are supplemented at the Veterinary School by special courses on entozoa and cattle pathology. The students of the College have also the opportunity of attending the autopsies on the human subject at the Montreal General Hospital and learning Virchow's methods of making post-mortem examination."

> With respect to pathology, he wrote, ". . . the veterinary students are required to attend the same number of lectures and undergo the same examination as the students of human medicine of McGill University. At these examinations, some of the highest positions have been attained by veterinary students."[5]

The above would seem to be remarkable enough, and to give more than adequate indication as to why the dozen or so students who graduated from McGill each year were so outstanding. But there is more. One of the required courses was six months of histology; this in the 1880's! Mills mentions also two courses of six months each in chemistry and physiology, *with practical laboratory work* (italics mine). More than half a century later, in 1940, our course in physiology at the Ontario Veterinary College consisted solely of lectures, unaccompanied by any laboratory work.

Thus, the claim that the birth of veterinary pathology in North America took place in Montreal, is founded on both the teaching accomplishments of the three well trained pathologists, Osler, Johnston and Adami, who taught it at McGill University and at the Montreal Veterinary College, and on the research contributions of the same three men and of their pupils. The fact that it began in Montreal was, of course, due to the foresight of Duncan McEachran, principal of the Montreal Veterinary College, who recruited Osler to his teaching staff.[5,27,28] But let us think for a moment of veterinary pathology in the broader sense. In veterinary medicine, to a greater extent by far than in human medicine, pathology cannot he considered the exclusive preserve of specialist pathologists. It has always been important for practicing veterinarians to be able to conduct informative postmortem examinations. It was particularly so in the nineteenth century when most veterinarians were

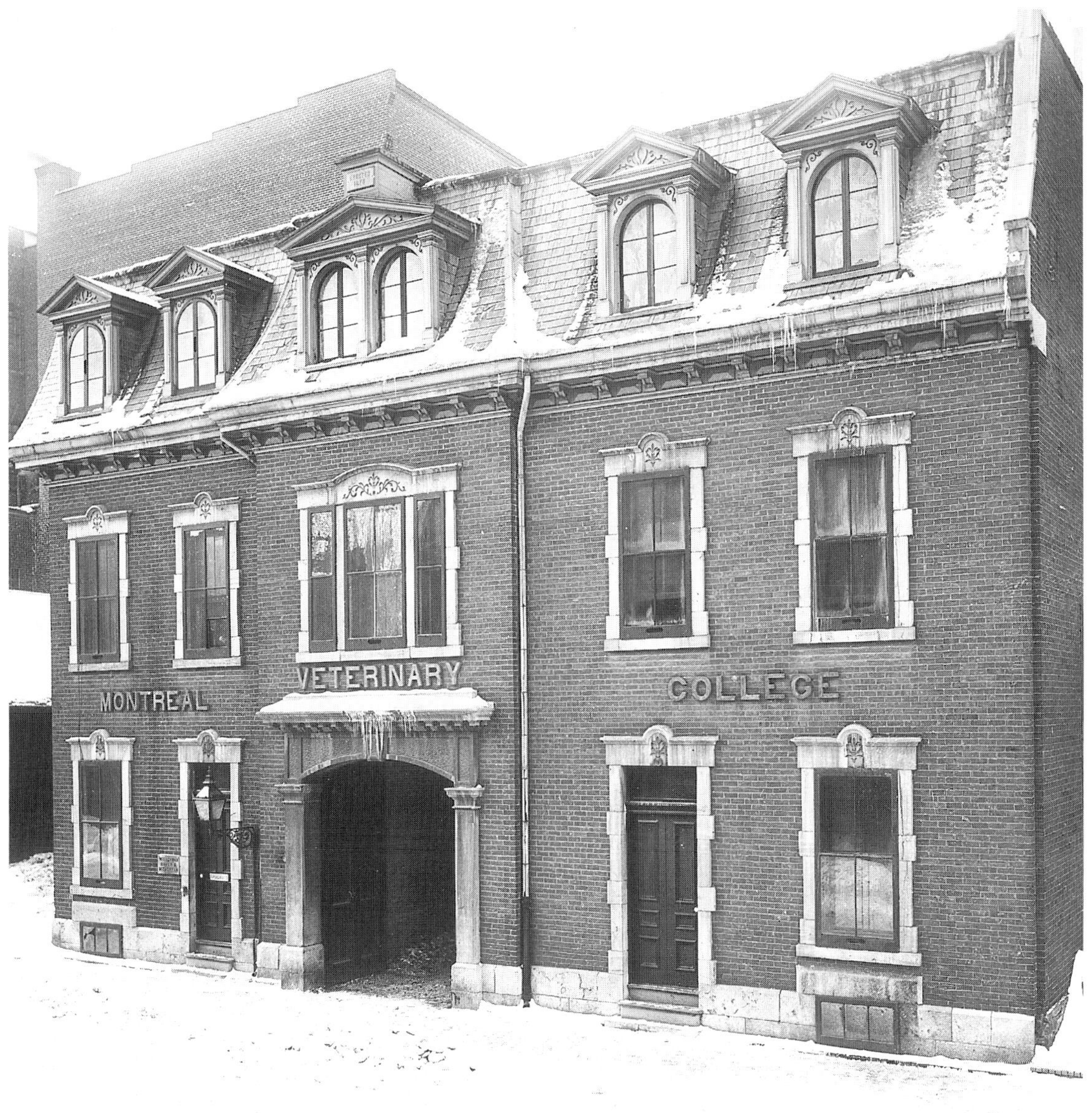

FIGURE 3. The Montreal Veterinary College at 6 Union Avenue in 1895. (By permission of the Notman Photographic Archives, McGill University).

concerned with farm animals. Viewed in this broader context, the supportive attitude of McEachran for pathology is just one more indication of how far ahead he was of his contemporary educators. Here is a most revealing passage, from his commencement address to the graduates of the Faculty of Comparative Medicine at McGill University in 1890:

> "... in your practice acquire a habit of noting cases, record every case of more than passing interest, and study the subject carefully, read every available standard author on it, and in the light of knowledge so obtained, applied to the case under observation, you will soon become masters of your profession.
>
> Never miss an opportunity of making a postmortem examination; nothing aids a man so much in making a correct diagnosis as the repeated corrections and errors disclosed by a post-mortem examination. Never waste a

pathological specimen; think how much good others may gain who succeed you as students of comparative medicine, from even one specimen, accompanied by a carefully recorded history. Museum specimens, accompanied by histories, are of great service in illustrating didactic lectures."[29]

In 1890, there were but few veterinary schools in North America, but I doubt whether there was another whose dean was likely to admonish his students "Never miss an opportunity of making a post-mortem examination." Thus, the fact that veterinary pathology on this continent sprang into life in Montreal stands revealed as no accident. It is what one would expect from a teacher who practiced what he preached, and who himself conducted autopsies, for example, of cattle afflicted with contagious pleuropneumonia.[30] McEachran had advised his students in a previous lecture of the importance of the microscope in supplementing pathologic anatomic examination.[31]

That was in Montreal, however. For the better part of two decades, from 1876 to 1895 the epoch-making scientific advances which were going on in pathology in Germany, and being taught in the veterinary schools of Europe, were ignored in Toronto and in most of the veterinary schools in the United States.

As already mentioned, William Osler, who first taught pathology to veterinary students on this continent, left Montreal in 1884 to continue his career as a teacher of medicine in Philadelphia. Veterinary medicine had been a concomitant interest of his, in which he pursued investigative work in parasitology and pathology and taught students. The beginnings of veterinary pathology as a discipline taught in universities and as a practical pursuit for the investigation of disease can be traced directly to him and to his students. In the 1930's, he had been dubbed the father of comparative pathology in Canada, by Charles Mitchell.[32] However, my examination of the veterinary educational world in the 1870's, 1880's and beyond, has convinced me that Mitchell's claim was unduly modest. Osler is really the father of veterinary pathology in North America.

My purpose is to provide evidence in support of Osler's augmented title, and to show how veterinary pathology began in Canada and later spread to the United States. In tracing Osler's influence, I found that part of it was immediate, concerned with his pupils and with his investigative work. Some of it extended chronologically far beyond the 1870's and 1880's, and can be followed in an unbroken line, through his students to the present. Let us now pick up Osler's trail.

William Osler

Osler's life has been the subject of a two-volume biography, and of innumerable short sketches, articles and bibliographies.[3,33,34] His memory is so revered, and his essays and addresses have so preserved his charisma, that an Osler Society flourishes in North America, whose members are banded together to continue research on the influence of this unique physician. There is another one in England and one in Japan.

Osler was professor successively at McGill University, the University of Pennsylvania, Johns Hopkins University and Oxford University. I deal here only with his veterinary activities, most of which were carried out during his

McGill period. Besides being a pathologist and an incomparable clinician, Osler was also a masterly historian and bibliographer of medicine. We can mention, but cannot enlarge on these aspects of his life; to do justice to them one must read Cushing's fascinating biography.[3]

William Osler was born on July 12, 1849, at Bond Head, Ontario. This was "... at the edge of the great Canadian forest which in those days extended to within a few miles of Toronto."[35] One biographer wrote "During his long and active life he ... played the major part in initiating the greatest revolution in the teaching and practice of medicine—both human and veterinary; he had joined the laboratory to the clinic to help end empiricism."[35] Another wrote that Osler was "... judged by many to be the greatest clinician of our times."[36]

Osler attended the Weston School, near Toronto, and was a pupil of the Rev. W.A. Johnson, who was an ardent naturalist and microscopist. Cameron relates that his enthusiasm soon infected Osler. Through Johnson, Osler met Dr. James Bovell, professor of medicine at the Toronto Medical School, and also an enthusiastic naturalist. Osler spent part of 1867 in Trinity College, preparing to follow his father's career by studying theology. Under Bovell's influence, however, he changed to medicine and commenced his studies at the Toronto Medical School. By this time Osler had already become a proficient microscopist, and developed an interest in the entozoa. Murphy feels that the pattern for Osler's interest in comparative physiology, was set at this time, under the influence of Bovell, who also taught physiology at the Ontario Veterinary College. He writes that Bovell "... no doubt played a large part in forming Osler's ideas with regard to the ubiquity of disease in both man and animal."[28] Osler's first contact with veterinarians came when Bovell encouraged him to study internal parasites in the dissecting room of the Ontario Veterinary College; a room recently described by Barker.[37]

Also influential in shaping the teen-aged Osler was Griffith Evans, who was stationed in Toronto as veterinary officer to the 4th Battery of the Royal Artillery. Evans had recently acquired a medical degree from McGill, while this unit had been stationed in Montreal. He was also an enthusiastic microscopist, who later became famous as the discoverer of *Trypanosoma evansi*, the cause of surra. Evans' biographers write that he took Osler "under his wing and gave him all possible encouragement."[38] They remained life-long friends.

In 1870, Bovell left Canada. Osler went to Montreal to continue his medical studies at McGill University, and graduated in 1872.

That year, Osler undertook advanced studies in Britain and on the Continent. In England, where he studied the blood of people and of various animals, he discovered the platelets in 1873; the first to see them in the circulating blood. When he moved on to Berlin, he encountered its stinking open sewers, which Virchow had just egged the city council into replacing. He waxed eloquent about Virchow, whom he called the master mind that attracts foreign students to Berlin. Obviously impressed with Virchow's intellect and indefatigable industry, Osler described in detail the various lectures, demonstrations and histologic courses in the Pathological Institute. He wrote:

> "Virchow himself performs a post-mortem on Monday morning making it
> with such care and minuteness that three or four hours may elapse before it is
> finished."[39]

His three-month sojourn in Berlin profoundly shaped his life, part of which then followed the footsteps of the master.

Osler moved on to Vienna, chiefly for clinical training, and wrote:

> "After having seen Virchow, it is absolutely painful to attend post-mortems
> here, they are performed in so slovenly a manner, and so little use is made of
> the material."[40]

The impression Virchow made was both profound and lasting. Almost two
decades later, Osler said at the Virchow celebration at Johns Hopkins
University:

> "Surely, the contemplation of a life so noble in its aims, so notable in its
> achievements, so varied in its pursuits, may well fill us with admiration for the
> man and with pride that he is a member of our profession."[41]

Upon his return to Montreal, in 1874, Osler was offered the post of
lecturer in physiology, histology and pathology. The following year he was
made professor, and appointed chief of the pathology laboratory at the
Montreal General Hospital. He introduced the microscope and clinical
chemistry into the hospital and into his teaching. Opie relates that he had but
one microscope; however, he used a small salary from an appointment as
physician to the smallpox ward of the hospital "to order from abroad a dozen
Hartnack microscopes."[42] Bean also emphasizes that "His devotion to pathology and his real concern as a teacher are indicated by the fact that . . . he
purchased first-class microscopes for the use of undergraduate students at
McGill."[43]

In 1876, Osler began teaching parasitology and physiology at the
Montreal Veterinary College. Murphy writes "Osler was able to bring his
famous 'bedside teaching' methods to the stables."[28] Sometime later he also
undertook to teach pathology to the veterinary students, who were already
studying human pathology with the medical students. Osler used human post
mortem material to teach the veterinary students, supplemented by animal
material. He also exhibited lesions from cattle, horses and swine to the
physicians at the Medico-Chirurgical Society in Montreal.[44–46] His mind
already opened to the idea by Bovell,[28] Osler had come to hold the view of
comparative pathology which was put forth by Virchow. Nowhere in the world
were physicians being taught Virchow's maxim, that there is only one medicine, more consistently or more effectively.

At meetings of physicians or veterinarians in Montreal, he exhibited
pathological tissue specimens of disease from cattle, horses and swine as well as
dogs—a wide spectrum of species for a day when cats were still ignored by
veterinarians and sheep did not graze on the streets of this city.

In addition to his teaching duties, Osler delivered the inaugural address
at the Montreal Veterinary College on two occasions. In 1876 his subject was
"The relations of animals to man." He mentioned:

> "You will not be long students before you find out that similarity in animal
> structure is accompanied by a community of disease, and that the 'ills which
> flesh is heir to' are not wholly monopolized by the 'lords of creation'."[47]

Osler gave another inaugural address at the Montreal Veterinary College
on October 1, 1878, on the topic "Comparative Pathology."[48] His hearers
included the newly enrolled student Walter L. Williams of Argenta, Illinois, of
whom we shall say more on a succeeding page. Osler defined pathology as
"the physiology and microscopic anatomy of disease"; a broad and enlightened view in an era where many thought pathology was morbid anatomy.
Williams apparently took careful notes or else had a phenomenal memory—
he cited this definition correctly 65 years later!

In 1878, Osler was a quarter of a century away from his inaugural lecture at the University of Toronto entitled "The Master Word in Medicine," in which he defined this word as work![49] But he was already shaping the idea in 1878, for he urged the veterinary students: ". . . to entertain a

> high appreciation of scientific study, to be regular in their attendance, to adopt a systematic apportionment of their time, and to take advantage of the opportunities afforded them while students here."

Although I have not found Osler's inaugural address at the Montreal Veterinary College in 1882, an advertisement of it appeared in the Journal of Comparative Medicine and Surgery in October of that year (Figure 4). This is on advertising page iv, facing text page 340, in volume III, no. 4, October 1882 with advertisements for two other veterinary colleges of which only one, the oldest, survives today, a century later. The principal of the Montreal Veterinary College, Duncan McEachran, has advertised the opening lecture of the session by Professor William Osler, M.D., M.R.C.V.S.

At the time Osler visited England, many North American physicians who took postgraduate work in England also crammed for the MRCP diploma. Cushing cites Osler as being against this at first but then later (in 1878) deciding to get his own MRCP after all.[3] Osler did not, however, become a member of the Royal College of Veterinary Surgeons. I have this from the Secretary of the College, who wrote in June 1983, "I am at a loss to explain how

ONTARIO VETERINARY COLLEGE,
40, 42 & 44 Tempérance St., Toronto, Canada.

—:MOST:—

Successful Veterinary Institution in America.

PATRONS :—Gov. General of Canada, and Lieut. Governor of Ontario. All experienced teachers. Lessons begin in October. Fees Fifty Dollars per annum. Apply to principal.

PROF. SMITH, V. S., Edin.,
TORONTO, CANADA.

MONTREAL VETERINARY COLLEGE.

ESTABLISHED 1866.

In Connection with the MEDICAL FACULTY OF McGILL UNIVERSITY.
SEASON 1882-83.

INTRODUCTORY LECTURE
—)BY(—

Prof. WILLIAM OSLER, M.D., M.R.C.V.S.
On Tuesday, 3d October, at 8 p. m.

Prospectuses giving full particulars of the course, requirements, fees, etc., sent ree on application to the Principal.

D. McEACHRAN, F.R.C.V.S.,
6 Union Avenue, Montreal.

Columbia Veterinary College
—)AND(—

School of Comparative Medicine,
221 East 34th Street, New York City.

REGULAR TERM OPENS OCTOBER 3d.

FIGURE 4.   Reproduction of advertising page iv from the J Comp Med Surg, Oct. 1882.

the abbreviation M.R.C.V.S. came to be attached to Professor Osler's qualifications. I cannot find his name on any of our Registers either as a member or as an honorary associate or in any other category."

Why is he so listed in this advertisement? It is unlikely that he styled himself MRCVS on his own. Did McEachran do it, or was it a printer's error? Osler was not a surgeon and not a member of the Royal College of Surgeons. But if a printer were going to set a superfluous letter into the abbreviation MRCS by mistake, why would he pick a V, and why would he set it in the only place where it would result in a meaningful abbreviation? If the printer set only what he was told, why would McEachran, a man of unimpeachable probity, advertise a non-existent diploma, especially in a journal in which Osler himself was publishing case reports, and could therefore be counted upon to read the advertisement? I have been unable to come up with answers to these questions.

Osler's publications in the realm of veterinary pathology, while not numerous by today's standards, showed a considerable breadth of interest. His first paper, on parasitic bronchitis in dogs, was excellent, and dates from 1877.[50] Having established the cause of a chronic respiratory condition in foxhounds at the Montreal Kennel Club by careful postmortem work, he named the disease properly, on the basis of its etiology and pathology. He did not succumb to the temptations of certain 20th century veterinarians, who adopted nondescript terms such as "kennel cough" for newly reported respiratory conditions.

His second research paper in 1878, on the pathology of hog cholera, was likewise an outstanding piece of work.[51] Unfortunately, it was ignored by subsequent research workers in the Bureau of Animal Industry and elsewhere. A quarter century before the virus of hog cholera was discovered, Osler stated on the basis of histologic examination, that the disease was not attributable to bacteria. Had Theobald Smith, W.H. Welch and others heeded his report, they could have spared themselves years of futile arguments and bacteriological work.[52]

Always interested in parasitology, Osler's investigation led him from human cases of infestation to the realm of meat hygiene. His mentor, Virchow, had caused microscopic inspection of pork to be instituted in Germany in 1866, some eight years before Osler had come to study in Berlin. In 1882, Osler reported on three cases of human echinococcosis in the Montreal General Hospital. Wanting to know the prevalence of this disease in North America, he undertook a survey of museums, journals and unpublished cases of his correspondents. He wrote:[53]

> "I was led to make this in connection with an annual course of lectures on the parasites of man and the domestic animals which I give to medical and veterinary students. I could not ascertain, from any writings at my command, whether the disease was common on this continent or not. In this section of the country it is rarely met with, and in the inspection of over 800 bodies only three instances have been found."

He also wrote of making "casual visits to butcher stalls and to the shambles" to look for echinococci in meat. He sent a veterinary student to look for them: "One of my students, Mr. A.W. Clement, of Lawrence, Mass., examined 270 hogs at the Montreal abattoir and found 10 animals affected."[53]

Osler's most important veterinary student from our standpoint, Albert W. Clement, was quickly recognized by him as a bright person. He put Clement to work assisting him on several projects, which they later published jointly. They worked together on a study of parasites in the pork supply of Montreal, examining 1,037 hogs.[54] Clement reported later that they had found cysticercus infection in 76 of them.

In 1883, Osler and Clement published case reports on bronchiectasis in a calf, on chronic bronchitis in a dog and pyometra in a bitch.[55–57] It is apparent that Clement was assisting Osler in conducting autopsies on both large and small animals at the Montreal Veterinary College. That same year Osler and Clement also published on the experimental production of tapeworm cysts in a calf. They had conducted the experiment in order to have an actual model demonstrating the life cycle to show the medical and veterinary students.[58]

This contact with the physician of genius, who had himself studied under Virchow, left a deep imprint on Clement's life and professional career. We will recount this shortly.

During his years of activity at the Montreal Veterinary College, Osler was also active in the Montreal Veterinary Association, serving as President during 1879 and 1880.[60] During one meeting he demonstrated a "verminous tumour" on the stomach of a horse, also showing the worms under the microscope.[61] At another meeting, a practicing veterinarian reported on the symptoms of a horse which had been treated by its owner with a large dose of turpentine. He also described the lesions, found at "The post mortem examination, which was conducted by Prof. Osler . . ." who presided at the meeting. The stomach was passed around among the audience. This is perhaps the first instance of a clinicopathologic conference in a meeting of a veterinary society in North America.[62]

Osler still maintained an interest in veterinary medicine after he left Montreal in 1884, but his active participation in veterinary education ceased. During his years in Philadelphia, 1884–1889, he joined the editorial board of the Journal of Comparative Medicine and Veterinary Archives, and contributed occasional editorials[63] or translations from German journals to it (Figure 5). The year before his death in 1919, Osler still identified with the veterinary profession in a review of a book on horses for an Edinburgh veterinary journal.

After Osler's departure, McEachran was able to effect formal incorporation of the Montreal Veterinary College into McGill University, under the designation which Osler had proposed: the Faculty of Comparative Medicine and Veterinary Science.

Osler is thus established as the pioneer in North American veterinary pathology through: (a) his teaching begun in 1876; (b) his investigative work on verminous bronchitis in dogs in 1877, on hog cholera in 1878 and on Pictou cattle disease[59] in 1882; (c) a series of individual case reports between the years 1877 and 1884[44–46,55–57,61–62]; and (d) the work of his students, particularly Johnston, Clement and Williams.

Through having trained Johnston, Osler provided the continuity of teaching and the momentum to help McEachran keep the Montreal school open after 1884. In its last few years, it graduated Higgins and Blair. These men get us well into the present century, where their activities recounted elsewhere in this lecture leave Canada with a national laboratory of veterinary pathology, established in 1902, and the United States' largest zoo with a full time veterinary pathologist also appointed in 1902.

With these three men, however, the thread from Osler, either through his own students or through later McGill veterinary graduates would seem to be broken. Clement left no professional descendant, nor did Higgins or Blair. Each made his own contribution, and while these were enduring, they ended

with the individuals just named. But there is one more man, a student of
McEachran and Osler who graduated from the Montreal Veterinary College in
1879, and who conveyed Osler's influence, like the baton in a relay race, right
up to the mid 1980's. That man is Walter L. Williams, of whom we shall hear at
the end of this lecture.

Osler's Successors

Osler's successors as teachers at the Montreal Veterinary College were Clement, Johnston and Adami; the first two had also been his students. These men
and Charles Higgins, a student of Adami's, were also Osler's successors as
research pathologists for the Dominion Department of Agriculture. Another
student of Adami's, W.R. Blair, was the first pathologist at the New York
Zoological Society. Thus, an unbroken line of graduates of the Montreal
Veterinary College and its successor institution had continued the teaching
and practicing of veterinary pathology to the end of the nineteenth century.
They require individual attention in order to bring Osler's lasting influence
into focus.

Albert W. Clement

Albert W. Clement, Osler's most important veterinary student, was born in
Lawrence, Massachusetts in 1857. He attended the schools of that city, and
then pursued a pre-medical course at Harvard College for two years. He was
obliged to discontinue his studies because of ill-health, and his physician
advised him to seek an outdoor occupation.[64,65] Busying himself with horses,
Clement decided to study veterinary medicine. He entered the Montreal
Veterinary College in 1879, and graduated in 1882. We have already mentioned his selection by Osler as a student assistant and cited some of their joint
work. He remained at the College as a teacher for three years.

In his book "Oslerian Pathology",[66] Rodin illustrates a specimen of
pleurisy from a fatal case of equine pneumonia which Osler and Clement had
presented at the Montreal Medico-Chirurgical Society in 1882.[67] Rodin also
shows specimens of verminous bronchitis in a pig and actinomycosis in a cow's
jaw from the years 1877 and 1884. These were still in the McGill Pathology
Museum in 1980. Although many of Osler's museum specimens had been lost
in the century following his departure, the few which remained in 1980
included these three from his veterinary cases.

I have not discovered which subjects Clement taught during the years
1883–1885 that he remained at the Montreal Veterinary College after graduation. Parasitology was apparently one of them,[68] but there must have been
more. Osler had left McGill for the University of Pennsylvania in 1884. His
successor in the Faculty of Medicine at McGill was Wyatt Johnston, who also
taught pathology to the veterinary students after Osler's departure. Clement
may have taught a clinical subject, assisted Johnston in teaching pathology, or
very likely both.

Two obituaries state that during his years as a teacher at McGill, Clement
was also employed by the Canadian government in investigating contagious
diseases in animals.[64,65] While I have been unable to confirm this, it is in

consonance with the manner in which McEachran, in his capacity as chief inspector of livestock, employed Osler, Johnston and Adami.

In 1885, Clement published his first paper as sole author, and I believe also the first one on pathology by a veterinarian in North America. It dealt with the renal lesions in equine azoturia, and he refers with deference to an aspect of microscopic examination of the urine of the horse which Osler had called to his attention some time previously.[69] Osler had demonstrated the gross lesions at a meeting of the Montreal Medico-Chirurgical Society.[45] Clement's paper is a well-illustrated account of the histologic findings, of a scientific and literary standard which in 1885 had no counterpart from any teacher in any North American veterinary school. The lack of anyone with a comparable knowledge of pathology was particularly true of three veterinary schools then extant which have survived to the present: Cornell, Iowa and Ontario. It is interesting to read in Jones and Hunt's textbook a century later about the renal tubular necrosis; and to learn that the pathogenesis of azoturia is still not really known, although it has a better name: equine rhabdomyolysis.[70]

In the spring of 1885, Clement went abroad for post graduate study in Europe and remained about a year. He studied and worked at the Royal Veterinary College in London, the National Veterinary School in Alfort, France, the pathological institute under Rudolf Virchow at the University of Berlin, the pathological institute under Wilhelm Schütz at the Berlin Veterinary College, and the central slaughter house in Berlin.[71] Pathology is not mentioned in connection with Alfort, and Clement makes clear that no one is concerned with it in London. Most of the article describing his study leave deals with pathology in both the medical faculty of the University and in the Berlin Veterinary College. He writes admiringly of the correlation of the clinical findings with the lesions at the latter:

> "The clinical professor takes his class to the post mortem room and views the organs, pointing out as nearly as possible the relation between the lesions found and the ante-mortem symptoms. On three mornings in the week the pathologist demonstrates the morbid anatomy specimens, and once or twice a week gives instruction in the method of making post-mortems, but in addition to this the students in groups make post-mortems under the direction of the assistants."

In Virchow's Institute, Clement saw essentially what Osler had seen eleven years earlier. At the central slaughter house, which employed 25 veterinarians, one of them a pathologist, he saw a great variety of lesions in food animals. When he returned to Montreal in 1886, he was undoubtedly inspired to apply his newly acquired knowledge, but he did not stay there long. For reasons I have not been able to ascertain, he left Montreal and moved to Baltimore to enter practice.

Clement's greatest contributions to veterinary medicine were his leadership in sanitary science, and in the American Veterinary Medical Association. I have dealt with these in another paper.[72] His most important contribution to veterinary pathology is his monograph "Veterinary Post-mortem Examinations," the first publication on this topic in the English language (Figure 5). In fact, in a broader context, it was the first serious book in the realm of veterinary pathology in the English language.[73,74] It appeared in 1889, as a chapter in a multi-volume reference book on the medical sciences; this was published as a separate book two years later (Figure 5). In the list of authors of the first publication, Clement is identified as being from the Bureau of Animal Industry, United States Government. I have been unable to determine the

VETERINARY

POST-MORTEM

EXAMINATIONS

BY

A. W. CLEMENT, V. S.

NEW YORK:
SABISTON & MURRAY.
VETERINARY PUBLISHERS AND BOOKSELLERS,
916 SIXTH AVENUE,
1891.

FIGURE 5. Title page of Clement's book.

nature of this employment in the several historical publications of the B.A.I. In fact, his name does not even appear therein. However, at a meeting of the U.S.V.M.A., Clement once stated that he was a government inspector in the B.A.I.[75]

In the preface to his book, Clement writes:

"Records of autopsies, to be of any value, should accurately represent the appearance of the tissues and organs so that a diagnosis might be made by the reader were not the examiner's conclusions stated. To make the pathological conditions clear to the reader, *some definite system of dissection is necessary..*" (italics mine).

He explains that he wrote the monograph because of the "The absence in the English language of any guide in making autopsies upon the lower animals . . ." In these prefatory remarks, Clement shows clearly the influence of his exposure to Wilhelm Schütz in Berlin during his sojourn there. A disciple of Virchow's, Schütz had been teaching systematic autopsy procedure since assuming the chair of pathology at the Berlin Veterinary College in 1870. Though advocating such a procedure may seem trite today, it was new when Clement introduced it to American veterinary medicine in 1889.

Clement described the technique for autopsy of the horse and modifications thereof for other domestic animals. He gave detailed instructions for examination of the central nervous system. He was obviously preaching what he practiced, since he had reported lesions of the C.N.S. in a paper antedating his book.[76] He ended the book with a chapter on recording of autopsies, which began:

> "The description of the post mortem appearances should be objective. It is
> not sufficient simply to say that such or such disease is found, but the changes
> in consistence, color, size and shape which the diseased part presents should
> be objectively described."

Again, this sounds trite today, but to advocate this degree of rigor, in a day when most veterinary schools in the English-speaking world did not teach autopsy technique at all, and several lacked a teacher who could conduct an autopsy, was a decided step forward, perhaps even a revolutionary one. Three decades were to elapse before another and more detailed book on the subject appeared in English, and almost two more before systematic autopsies, including the C.N.S., were taught in many veterinary schools in North America.

Clement worked in pathology after he returned to the United States, doing research on hog cholera with William Welch at Johns Hopkins.[75,77,78] All of his subsequent work, in practice, in disease control and in organized veterinary medicine, was based on the application of pathology to clinical and other problems. He served, as did Osler, on the editorial board of the Journal of Comparative Medicine and Surgery (later renamed Journal of Comparative Medicine and Veterinary Archives) (Figure 5). He published both original articles and reviews in its columns.[69,79–85] Like Osler, he translated important articles, such as Kitt's new method of blackleg immunization, from German for this journal.[86]

By any of several criteria, Clement was an outstanding veterinarian, and after Osler, the second of the pioneer veterinary pathologists on this continent. The latter is true despite the fact that he never held a post as a pathologist, and earned his living in private, large animal practice, combined with a part-time position as State Veterinarian of Maryland. By a happy chance for this North American audience, he was an American educated in Canada, so that we can cheerfully lay claim to him no matter which side of the border we hail from. Educated by Osler as a student and as an assistant, later exposed to the best in German veterinary pathology in Wilhelm Schütz's laboratory in Berlin, further trained by collaboration (on hog cholera research) with the famous Welch at Johns Hopkins, Clement was indubitably better versed in pathology than any veterinarian in North America in the last decade of the last century. His book, pointing the way to the future in veterinary pathology, and helping to shape this discipline, is the hallmark of the well-trained man.

Clement practiced pathology as an adjunct to his clinical work, which encompassed horses, cattle and sheep.[79,80,84,85] That this helped to make him a better clinician goes almost without saying, especially to this audience. He reported much of his work in the periodical literature, else we would have no record of the amazing number of autopsies he performed, many of them worked up histologically. Having mixed with the leaders in medicine, he was at ease, and accepted, in medical circles, as his report on a case of human glanders, including the findings in both the human and the horse attests.[81] It is also evidence of his comparative orientation, the imprints of Osler and Virchow, which he enunciated in his presidential address to the American Veterinary Medical Association.[87]

Clement's life was regrettably short, in view of what he might have achieved in a few more years. He began his veterinary career by publishing on pathologic material with Osler while still a student. His interest in pathology never deserted him; near the end of his career, he published with another pathologist, W.G. MacCallum, Welch's successor at Johns Hopkins, the autopsy findings on a tuberculous lion.[88]

During his lifetime, he studied under or worked with outstanding pathologists—Osler and Johnston in Montreal, Virchow and Schütz in Berlin, and five years with Welch and MacCallum in Baltimore.[89] Welch and another Johns Hopkins pathologist, W.T. Councilman, also attended meetings of the Maryland Veterinary Medical Association when Clement was a speaker and supported him during the subsequent discussions.[90] Clement was instrumental in having Welch appointed to Honorary Membership in the AVMA in 1892. It is a pity that Clement was not offered a chair in pathology in a good veterinary school in the 1890's. He returned to McGill for Alumni reunions and for graduations,[91] but he must have seen that there was not a future for his alma mater.

On March 3, 1901, Clement died of cardiac disease in the Johns Hopkins Hospital, of which his old friend and mentor William Osler was physician-in-chief.[65] A career beginning with pathology and informed by it in everything clinical which he did later had been Osler's hallmark. The identical attribute characterized the life of his pupil, Albert Clement. The fact that this professional descendent of Osler's did not teach veterinary students after 1885, meant that he left no such descendants of his own in veterinary pathology. With his last report, on the tuberculous lion in 1900, Clement brought the Osler legacy of veterinary pathology into the twentieth century. It remained for others to bring it further.

Wyatt Johnston

After Osler's departure from McGill University in 1884, his appointment as head of pathology at the Montreal General Hospital, and as teacher of the subject at the University, was taken over by a young physician who had been a student of his.[92] Johnston was born in Sherbrooke, Quebec, in 1863, and educated at Bishop's College in Lennoxville, Quebec. He entered McGill University in 1880 and graduated as a physician in 1884. He became interested in pathology while an undergraduate medical student, and assisted Osler at autopsies and in preparing gross specimens for demonstrations.[93] To further this interest, Johnston went to Berlin in 1885, where he spent the summer working in Virchow's laboratory. The following year he returned to Germany, to work with Paul Grawitz in Greifswald, the pathologist who had first described the embryonal nephroma.

In 1885, Johnston was appointed demonstrator in pathology in the faculty of medicine at McGill, which also entailed teaching the veterinary students at the Montreal Veterinary College. To prepare himself further, he returned to Europe a third time to work on comparative pathology in Munich and also at the London Zoo. Although the year of his third trip is not given,[93] it would have been while John Bland-Sutton, a noted comparative pathologist was the prosector at the Zoo. Johnston may have worked with Otto Bollinger in Munich. My inquiry at the Munich veterinary faculty whether Johnston had worked with Theodor Kitt, drew the reply that there is no record of his having done so.

In a lecture on methods of teaching pathology given in 1900, Adami, Johnston's successor, described how to improve the teaching of postmortem pathology: "... if,

> after the method pursued by my colleague, Wyatt Johnston, such students be given each an organ, be made to describe its appearance, to make or study

sections from the same, to study the descriptions given by standard authorities kept for this particular purpose in the adjoining laboratory, and noting the descriptions to write a diagnosis stating how far the appearances correspond to or depart from the described state, then the postmortem-room becomes the first of all laboratories, the instruction there received the most valuable, whether from the point of view of pure pathology, or of the development of the good physician."[94]

It is apparent from this quotation that Johnston's teaching, like Osler's, was strongly tinged with the systematic approach that each had acquired from his European mentors. Once again, the veterinary students in Montreal were being taught pathology by a master, incomparably better trained than the teachers of most veterinary students elsewhere in North America. Only Fitz and Formad, at Harvard and Pennsylvania had comparable training in pathology during the period 1885–1891 that Johnston taught veterinary students in Montreal.

Like Osler before him, Johnston was recruited by McEachran to do investigative work on Pictou Cattle Disease in 1891, and he published a report of his work the following year.[95] In 1893 he presented a summary of this work, based on autopsies of 35 cattle, at the 30th annual meeting of the U.S.V.M.A. in Chicago.[96] Johnston showed gross lesions at this meeting and made it clear that it was chiefly a disease of the liver, the counterpart of the lesion known in man as cirrhosis. Johnston was the first to describe the histologic lesions in the liver, and he confirmed Osler's previous finding of submucosal edema in the abomasum.[59] Johnston reported that in cattle which had been ill more than a month, ulceration of the abomasal mucosa was present in addition to the edema.

Johnston was more active in veterinary medicine than merely having the veterinary students attend his course for the medical students would have required. He attended the meetings of the Montreal Veterinary Medical Association and participated in presenting cases and showing specimens of diseased tissue.[97] He offered a cash prize to the veterinary student showing the greatest proficiency in post mortem and microscopic pathology.[98] Proposed by Clement for membership, Johnston joined the U.S.V.M.A., gave a paper in Boston in 1892 on tuberculosis in a bull,[99] and another one, on Pictou disease mentioned above.[96] Immediately after joining the U.S.V.M.A., Johnston was appointed the corresponding secretary for Canada.

When J.G. Adami was brought to McGill from England to fill the newly created chair of pathology in 1892, Johnston gave up teaching this subject. I have not discovered why he had not been selected for the new chair. While teaching pathology, he had augmented and organized the museum specimens in the collection begun by Osler, which included material from domestic animals.[100] At least three of these specimens were still in the McGill museum in 1980. Sometime after 1893, Johnston withdrew from veterinary activities. He had a distinguished career in bacteriology and forensic pathology thereafter and eventually was promoted to professor of hygiene at McGill.[101] Unfortunately, he did not live very long to enjoy this recognition.

The obituary written by Osler related that Johnston died of pulmonary embolism from thrombosis of a femoral vein resulting from an infection.[102] He described Johnston as a "genial, warm-hearted man, full of enthusiasm for his work. . .". He deserves remembrance in this lecture, because he continued to 1891 the tradition of high quality teaching of veterinary pathology in Montreal commenced by Osler in 1876.

J. George Adami

The third teacher of pathology at the Montreal Veterinary College, Adami was born in England in 1862 and graduated as a physician from Cambridge University in 1890.[103] He was invited to occupy the first chair of pathology at McGill University in 1892, when that discipline was elevated to independent status. Esmond Long, the historian of American pathology, writes that during his tenure at McGill Adami was the outstanding pathologist in Canada and one of the leading pathologists on the continent.[25] He became particularly well known for his monumental book "Principles of Pathology," published in two volumes in 1908 and 1909.[104] This and a revised edition became the standard textbook in North America for many years and was widely used elsewhere in the English-speaking world. He was a productive research worker in many fields of pathology and influential in training Canadian pathologists of the generation that followed him.

After Adami's arrival in Montreal, McEachran also recruited him to investigate Pictou Cattle Disease,[105] and to work on tuberculosis for the Dominion Department of Agriculture.[106–108] Adami taught the veterinary students, published papers on veterinary aspects of pathology,[109–111] and above all, participated actively in the affairs of the Faculty of Comparative Medicine. He donated a prize of $50 each year, a large sum in those days, for original research in pathology. The winner was selected from students in both human and comparative medicine. In 1896 the prize was split between C.H. Higgins and R.H. Martin, one from each of these faculties.[112]

In the university session which opened in October 1894, Adami gave the inaugural address to the new students in the Faculty of Comparative Medicine.[113] He exhorted the veterinary students to mingle with their fellow students in the rest of the university, benefit from these contacts, and not become insular in their preoccupation with their profession. It is apparent from reading this address, that once again McEachran had succeeded in obtaining for his students a man of wide intellectual horizons, who would provide education rather than training, a physician, who like his two predecessors, Johnston and Osler, felt that veterinary medicine was an integral part of medicine and spoke to veterinary students with affection rather than condescension. It becomes clear how exposed to teachers exemplifying such lofty aspirations, a seemingly endless array of veterinarians educated at McGill assumed positions of importance and leadership in their profession shortly after graduation.

Adami likewise attended and contributed to the meetings of the Montreal Veterinary Medical Association, and like Osler before him, served for a year as its president.[114–116]

Adami taught pathology to W.R. Blair and C.H. Higgins while they were undergraduates, and to the latter also as a postgraduate. He also did research on Pictou Cattle Disease.[105] His other contributions dealt with tumors,[109,111] actinomycosis,[110] glanders[117] and tuberculosis[118] in which he was especially interested. His paper on the teaching of pathology[94] reveals what a dedicated teacher the veterinary students in Montreal had.

During the period 1840 to 1898, bovine contagious pleuro-pneumonia caused serious losses in Great Britain. It was eventually controlled by prohibiting the import of cattle from countries harboring the disease. It had been stamped out in North America earlier than in Britain, in 1892, but the British embargo still remained. At a meeting of the Montreal Veterinary Association, in December 1893, Duncan McEachran spoke of the unfairness of continuing the embargo on Canadian cattle, which he said was based on "errors of judgment of officials of the Imperial Government."[119] He advocated the appointment of a scientist in England who would find "reliable means of arriving at a correct diagnosis." He stated that he and Professor Adami had examined microscopically tissues from the lungs of two cattle which the British inspectors had suspected of having pleuro-pneumonia, and in their opinion it was not that disease. Adami described the gross and histologic lesions of contagious pleuro-pneumonia, and stated that ". . . what the British veterinary inspectors call 'Canadian lung', but which Professor McEachran states would be more appropriately named transient pneumonia, . . . is only seen in animals traveling by railroads or an ocean journey."

It is apparent that the British inspectors at the ports of entry were not familiar with what was later called "shipping fever" in North America, and attributed to infection with Pasteurella bacteria. I seriously doubt whether the British inspectors, none of them trained in pathology, could distinguish between the two diseases, or for that matter between any kinds of pulmonary lesions. Although they were required to send tissues to Professor McFadyean in London for confirmation, it is not clear how often they did so. What is clear is that inspectors untrained in pathology would have been selecting which pieces of tissue to send in. The British government remained adamant and kept the embargo.

Some four years later, an editorial by John McFadyean, of the Royal Veterinary College in London, appeared in his own journal on the topic of pleuro-pneumonia.[120] He complained that Adami had raised the subject at the meeting of the British Medical Association in Montreal, and had argued that the British authorities—with one exception—had not done any first class work. McFadyean did not attempt to refute this allegation by submitting evidence that the British diagnostic efforts were scientifically competent and, therefore, really did merit confidence. Rather he wrote: "Professor Adami set a bad precedent for scientific discussions when he resorted to disparagement of his opponents. . .". Perhaps therein lay the seeds of some later acrimony, reported below.

In a recent book, Iain Pattison has reviled Adami, who after World War I, returned to England and became Vice-Chancellor of Liverpool University.[121] I do not know the merits of either side's case in the acrimonious exchange of correspondence between Adami and John McFadyean that began in "The Times" of London in June of 1920. In view of Pattison's attack, however, it is worth noting that no physician, pathologist or other, ever served North American veterinary students, Canadian veterinarians and the Dominion Department of Agriculture with more devotion and more effectiveness than J.G. Adami. He loyally supported the Faculty of Comparative Medicine at McGill until its last graduating class in 1903, and he made sure that the Dominion government would have a talented, Adami-educated pathologist (Higgins) when it opened its first diagnostic and research laboratory.

Nothing comparable to his superlative educational contribution and unwavering moral support can be identified elsewhere in veterinary schools on the North American continent up to 1903. With Adami, who died in Liverpool in 1926, we close the circle of men (Osler, Clement and Johnston) who during the quarter century 1877–1903, established veterinary pathology on this continent as a discipline which was first taught in Canada.

Charles H. Higgins

One of the most promising students to study in the Faculty of Comparative Medicine at McGill, Higgins was one of the numerous Americans who enrolled there. Born in Newtonville, Mass., on February 23, 1875, he was educated at the Massachusetts State College, graduating with a B.Sc. degree in 1893. He came under the influence there of Dr. James Paige, a McGill alumnus, who taught veterinary science.[122] Paige was a good laboratory diagnostician, who some years after this time (together with two colleagues) identified the first cases of sporotrichosis in North America. He induced Higgins to enter McGill University.

Higgins showed his scientific interests early. Thus, the record shows him attending the meetings of the Montreal Veterinary Medical Association in his senior year. In the meeting of December 6,f 1895, he presented a paper on "Bacteriology and its Practical Application," including a historical resumé of the development of this science.[123] At the meeting of December 20, he suggested certain scientific publications be added to the library of the Association. On January 15, 1896, he participated in the discussion of a case and presented one of his own, of a ventral hernia with peritonitis.[124] When he graduated on March 27, 1896, he won the prize of $50, presented by Professor Adami for original pathologic research.[112]

After graduation, Higgins spent some postdoctoral time at McGill studying bacteriology under Wyatt Johnston and pathology under George Adami. He then returned to the United States and was in veterinary practice in Massachusetts for two years.

His eulogist wrote:[122]

"By 1899, the veterinary pathological work carried on by McGill for the Department of Agriculture had assumed considerable proportions. Dr. Adami had to have more staff and consequently induced Higgins to accept an assistantship with him. In this capacity he carried on work at the Outremont Station, which was the first veterinary laboratory in Canada. This had been established by McEachran for the Dominion Department of Agriculture. Here Higgins isolated strains of tubercle bacilli and produced the first tuberculin in Canada."

Higgins was concurrently appointed assistant to the professor of pathology in the Faculty of Comparative Medicine and Veterinary Science at McGill.[125] He did some high-class work on fowl cholera during this appointment.[126]

In 1902, J.G. Rutherford was appointed chief veterinary inspector of Canada, and he decided to move the animal pathology work from Montreal to Ottawa. Dr. Higgins was appointed "Pathologist to the Department of Agriculture" and moved into a temporary laboratory on Queen Street. Later that year, a special building was constructed on the experimental farm and served as headquarters for the pathology work for the next 20 years. This was the first full-time post for a veterinary pathologist in Canada. Its establishment was an historical milestone, for it marked the turning over of responsibility for animal pathology from a series of physicians (Osler, Johnston, Adami and Martin) to a veterinarian.[106]

In 1903, Higgins identified the first cases of actinobacillosis in Canada, i.e. in the same year that Lignieres and Spitz published on the distinction of this disease from actinomycosis.[127] Higgins was obviously alert in keeping up with the scientific literature of his day, and able to apply it immediately to Canadian animal disease problems.[128]

The Dominion Department of Agriculture was conducting feeding experiments in Nova Scotia, in an attempt to discover the cause of Pictou Disease of cattle. Wyatt Johnston had already described the histologic appearance of the characteristic lesion in the spontaneous disease, hepatic cirrhosis.[96] Higgins supplied the vital laboratory support for the research in Nova Scotia; he conducted histologic examination to determine whether or not cirrhosis was present in the livers of the experimental cattle.[129]

Much of the early activity in the Ottawa laboratory was the manufacture of diagnostic and prophylactic biological products, e.g. tuberculin, mallein and vaccines for blackleg and anthrax. Some was diagnostic work, and from specimens submitted for this purpose Higgins commenced a fine pathologic museum. Based on his experience in diagnostic work. Higgins gave a paper on the postmortem and laboratory diagnosis of anthrax and blackleg at the AVMA meeting in 1903.[130] In the discussion, he engaged in a spirited debate with Veranus Moore of Cornell, condemning the latter's suggestion that specimens submitted for anthrax diagnosis should be wrapped in wet rags for shipment.

It became apparent a year or so after the Ottawa laboratory was founded that more help was needed. Dr. Rutherford hired Drs. Hadwen and Watson, but after a brief period in Ottawa, he sent them to head small regional laboratories in Alberta and British Columbia. Not only were they no help to Higgins, but also Rutherford had them report directly to himself rather than to Higgins. His anonymous eulogist, who I presume is Charles Mitchell, wrote: "As a result, the full force of a consolidated laboratory service had to wait for years."[122] One feels that McEachran would have known better. Rutherford showed good strategic sense in setting up a central laboratory for pathology and bacteriology, but tactically, very little sense of knowing what to do with it once he had it. Perhaps a more charitable view is, as Laidlaw explains, that Rutherford's plan of action was to make haste slowly.[131]

In 1909, there was an outbreak of rabies in Canada, and Higgins' laboratory did some of the microscopic examination of the brains of suspect animals, and also rabbit inoculations.[132] Higgins also did the laboratory work on an outbreak of suspected actinomycosis in cattle in Saskatchewan, and was able to establish that it was not that disease. In conjunction with a botanist, he was able to identify the condition as pharyngeal trauma caused by the ingestion of "wiregrass," a variety of rush known as *Juncus balticus*. The swellings which the cattlemen saw were suppurating lymph nodes draining the pharyngeal area. Higgins was able to work out the cause of this condition by applying the knowledge of histologic examination he had learned from Adami. Doing so was no mean feat in an era where veterinary pathologists all too often thought that all diseases were due to infection.[132]

In his eighth report as pathologist, for the year 1910–1911, Higgins noted that his overworked condition was temporarily alleviated by the hiring of Drs. Wickware and Evans to assist him with pathology and bacteriology, respectively. He reported on how he was training them to do the various diagnostic laboratory procedures, and pointed out that they would not be able to undertake any research work on disease problems important to the livestock industry unless more staff were hired. He had received 423 specimens of diseased tissue during the year, some of which were added to the Department's museum.[133]

Rutherford has been described by Smithcors as one of the few great veterinary statesmen in North America.[134] However, we learn (from the eulogist, again) that "Higgins had to fight an uphill and, too often, a losing battle to obtain equipment, personnel and adequate laboratory conditions." ". . . He had visions of organizing an establishment on a much broader scale but even the most modest addition was considered too expensive."[122] Thus, Higgins had to construct incubators and other laboratory equipment with his own hands. It is hard to accept the designation of anyone so penny-wise and pound-foolish as a statesman. It is not clear to me, however, whether Higgins was obliged to endure this lack of support only under Rutherford's administration or also under Fred Torrance, who succeeded him in 1912. Had either of them been worth his salt, he would have induced the Dominion government to part with the money to pipe gas into Higgins' laboratory.

In 1917, i.e. after five years under Torrance, Higgins tired of all these struggles and resigned from the Health of Animals Branch. He was appointed head of the newly established Canadian branch of the Lederle Laboratories Co. As the eulogist puts it, "By this time he had become frustrated by what he deemed lack of support and adequate recognition in official circles." Strangely enough, there is no mention of Higgins' resignation in Torrance's annual report as Veterinary Director General. In a report otherwise full of trivia, this crippling loss is passed over as if it did not matter.[135]

In 1919, Higgins moved to the New York headquarters of the Lederle firm. Unfortunately, his work for them was outside the realm of pathology, and regrettably, a promising individual was lost not only to veterinary pathology but also to veterinary medicine as a whole.

While working as Dominion Animal Pathologist, Higgins was very active in AVMA affairs. Not only did he attend the annual meetings and give papers, but also he was entrusted with the chairmanship of important committees and compiled valuable reports in this capacity.[136–138] He became a prominent figure in North American veterinary medicine.[139] All of this ceased when he left Canada.

Viewed historically, I think Higgins' greatest contribution was in providing a pathologic basis which enabled the government to establish which diseases were prevalent in Canada, and to sort them out from one another. His second contribution was the establishment of the museum of animal pathology in the Department of Agriculture in Ottawa, a valuable teaching aid for the Meat Inspection Branch, and one from which educational exhibits were mounted at agricultural and veterinary conventions. His third contribution was in training some of the scientific staff of the Division of Pathology, which he was well equipped to do. If he did not do much original research, it was through failure of two Veterinary Director Generals to give him support, moral and financial; worse, failure to support the very idea of research. Thus, Canada lost an expatriate American to the United States in what might be termed a "reverse brain-drain"—an American leaving because the milieu north of the border was inhospitable to a life of the intellect. In his last paper dealing with pathology, one on tuberculosis, Higgins gave as one of his goals in presenting his work at the A.V.M.A. meeting, ". . . to stimulate greater care in the performance of autopsies. . ."[140] The McGill stamp—in his case the training under Adami—had impressed itself deeply upon him.

Sometime during his sojourn in Canada, Higgins was commissioned in the Canadian Army Veterinary Corps. He appears in the Militia List of the Dominion of Canada, 1925, as a major with date of rank of September 21,

1916, and date of transfer to the Reserve of Officers of January 15, 1921.[141] I have found no other information on his military service.

Higgins died in New York on November 22, 1954.[142]

W. Reid Blair

William Reid Blair was born in Philadelphia on January 17, 1875, educated in that city, and after the age of ten in Massachusetts.[143-145] He entered McGill University in 1899 and graduated as a veterinarian in 1902.[146] Shortly thereafter he became pathologist to the recently established New York Zoological Park, the first American zoo to employ one on a full time basis. By the following year, Blair was publishing the results of his autopsies at the zoo, antedating similar publications from the National Zoo in Washington and the Philadelphia Zoo by several years.[147,148]

In conjunction with a part-time colleague, Dr. H. Brooks, Blair published a classical paper entitled "Osteomalacia of Primates in Captivity" in 1905. This identified the osseous lesion and correlated it with the clinical signs, in an enigmatic disesase long known as "cage paralysis" which afflicted wild primates after a period of captivity in many zoos.[149]

Concurrent with his major job at the zoo, Blair also served between 1905 and 1917 as professor of comparative pathology in the veterinary department of New York University, providing education to the undergraduates in this subject.[143] In 1906, Blair mounted a large exhibit of pathologic tissue specimens at the 43rd annual meeting of the A.V.M.A. in New Haven, Connecticut.[150]

Blair published a considerable number of reports on diseases of the captive animals until World War I.[151-156] These dealt with the pathological effects of captivity on wild animals, with the pathology of parasitism, and with that of tuberculosis and other infectious diseases. In 1913, Blair was appointed to the editorial board of the American Veterinary Review. This activity as well as his autopsy work and teaching ended when he volunteered for service in 1917, and was commissioned as a major.

Blair had a distinguished military career as corps veterinarian for the U.S. IVth Army Corps in France.[157] Following demobilization in 1919, he remained in the Veterinary Corps Reserve, reached the rank of colonel in 1923 and retired in 1928.[158] The administrative talents he had shown as commander of a large field hospital were recognized when he returned to the zoo, and he was appointed as Assistant Director of it in 1922. He assumed duties of a clinical nature after his return. With his promotion to Director in 1926, he was lost to pathology.

He made many valuable contributions to the New York Zoological Park. Some were in the realm of preventing the extinction of rare animal species, others in providing outdoor, natural settings rather than cages for the exhibit of animals.[144] He published a book covering a quarter century of his medical and surgical experiences with captive wild animals.[159] When he joined the zoo in 1902 it had 205 specimens, representing 106 species of animals.[160] When he retired in 1940, he had built what the New York Times termed the "most varied zoological collection in the world," comprised of 2600 specimens representing 1000 species. His alma mater, McGill University, recognized his achievements by the award of an honorary LL.D. degree in 1928.[161]

As luck would have it, both Blair and his fellow McGill alumnus Higgins were essentially lost to veterinary pathology in the same year, 1917. But each left behind him functioning pathology laboratories, which even if they were not continued on the same plane by others, exemplified what could be done by talented men provided with fine professional education and imbued with high aspirations. During the first two decades of this century, Blair and Higgins were recognized leaders in North American veterinary medicine as well as in veterinary pathology.[162] Again, Duncan McEachran had done his work superbly in Montreal, in selecting his students as well as his teachers!

Blair died in New York on March 1, 1949.

W.L. Williams

The numerous biographical writings on Osler indicate that he left deep and lasting impressions on his students. Few were deeper, and none could have been more lasting than the one he made on Walter L. Williams, born in 1856 in Argenta, Illinois.

A member of the original faculty which founded the New York State Veterinary College at Cornell University in 1895, Williams was educated at the Illinois Technical University (later known as the University of Illinois).[163] He attended the Montreal Veterinary College from 1878 until 1879, where he was taught pathology and physiology by William Osler. He won the silver medal awarded by the province of Quebec to the leading student in the class.[20]

After graduation Williams was in practice in Illinois and in 1887 was the first to recognize the disease dourine in the United States.[164] In 1891 his health broke down, and he joined the faculty first of Purdue University and later of Montana State College. A careful investigator and a prolific writer, he published on pathology while still a large animal practitioner.[165–168] In Montana, he issued a bulletin in which the gross lesions of glanders were clearly and expertly illustrated.[169] His publications, before he joined Cornell University, are too numerous to list here, but one of them requires attention because it reveals Williams' Oslerian heritage.[170]

In 1887 Williams had published a paper on invasion of the mesenteric arteries by nematodes in the horse.[168] In 1895, in a paper on the therapeutics of colic in the horse, he demonstrated at once his ability to learn from experience, his knowledge of the German literature, and the lesson learned from Osler that if one understood the pathology of a disease one would be disinclined to overtreat it.[170]

Williams reflected on the poor results he had obtained from treating equine colic by medication, and on a body of German literature which indicated that a greater percentage of cases recovered without treatment than with it. He wrote that early in his practice, when he medicated such cases:

> "... my losses from colic were appalling, costing me many anxious hours and valued patrons, but as necessity and reason drove me further from what I thought classic methods, and taught me a higher appreciation of nature's powers and her abhorrence of unnecessary meddling in disease, my losses became much less."

Pointing out that among the causes of colic was interruption of the gastro-intestinal blood supply by thrombi, he stated:

> "The application of rational therapeutics to this group of pathological conditions renders it necessary that our first law shall be to rigidly avoid the use of any medical agency which would tend to aggravate any pathological conditions present, whether recognizable or not; or to pursue, as far as possible, an expectant line of treatment."

In Williams' words, one can clearly discern the Oslerian approach to diagnosis and treatment; in fact, one can easily imagine Osler—equally familiar with the German literature on verminous mesenteric arteritis in horses—speaking or writing the same words.

At Cornell, Williams was professor of surgery and later of obstetrics, breeding diseases and ethics. His textbooks on the first three of these subjects remained the standard ones for 50 years and were translated into foreign languages.[171–173]

Williams was an inspired teacher, gifted with keen intellect, lifelong curiosity, enthusiasm for his subject, the highest scientific and ethical ideals, and a superlative command of his written and spoken language. Williams' books, papers,[174–180] lectures and demonstrations at meetings on breeding diseases at veterinary conventions moved him into a position of undisputed leadership in this field, which he held for decades. No American or Canadian veterinary school in the first quarter of the 20th century had any clinical teacher remotely approaching his erudition, knowledge of the domestic and foreign literature, pedagogic ability and research productivity.

His distinguished career at Cornell brought him worldwide recognition. To an extent that none of his contemporaries even remotely approached, Williams' clinical work was always based on a solid foundation of pathology. He had acquired this cast of mind from Osler, and it stamped him for life, as it had so many of Osler's students.

Although Williams retired from teaching at Cornell in 1922, he remained active in research and writing for almost a quarter of a century thereafter, during which he could be found on the campus almost every day. In 1944, sixty-five years after he had graduated from the Montreal Veterinary College, Williams gave a lecture on his professional career which spanned this period.[181] Here in his own words, is the recollection of his student day under Osler, shining forth undimmed more than half a century later.

> "The physiology-pathology was a lecture course by Dr. William Osler. He was the greatest, most inspiring teacher I had known, and since that time I have not consciously met his equal. Then a young man, seven years my senior, he came upon the rostrum at a brisk walk at the minute due, began his lecture without delay, and rapidly and clearly discussed the subject under consideration. As I now recall, he never emphasized what he knew, and never intimated that he knew very much. He placed great emphasis upon the interesting and important things which a student might learn. But it remained for the student to do the learning. He did not resort to the pumping process so profusely used by some professors in an effort to inject knowledge into registrants in his classes. In the opening address to the students in the veterinary college, Dr. Osler defined pathology as the 'physiology and microscopical anatomy of disease.' His lectures, as I understood them, were devoted to the development of this theme and the 'inseparability of physiology and pathology' emphasized. His abundant illustrations were largely the tissues and organs freshly obtained from autopsies in the Montreal General Hospital."

Hearing this, can anyone doubt that Osler left an indelible imprint on Williams? Can you imagine especially those of you who are teachers, having such an impact on a student that he recalls it in vivid prose 65 years later? Have you ever read admiration for a mentor expressed more eloquently? And lest anyone think that what I have cited here is the product of some senile musing, here (Figure 6) is a picture of "Uncle Billy", as he was fondly known at Cornell, as active as a cricket in his 88th year! And what is this activity? He is doing what Osler did—a brilliant clinician sitting at the autopsy table and dissecting, a bright sparkle in his eye and an intent and child-like curiosity in his mien. He is also practicing what he has been "preaching" at least since 1888, when he advocated to his fellow veterinary practitioners:

> "The post-mortem study of disease is far more available to us than to the medical practitioner, there being no adverse sentiment in our way; so that we should make a careful post-mortem study of most of our fatal cases, and should allow nothing but the most urgent duties to interfere with our plans."[182]

Like A.W. Clement, who likewise bore the stamp of Osler's teaching all of his professional life, Williams took the principle of applying a knowledge of

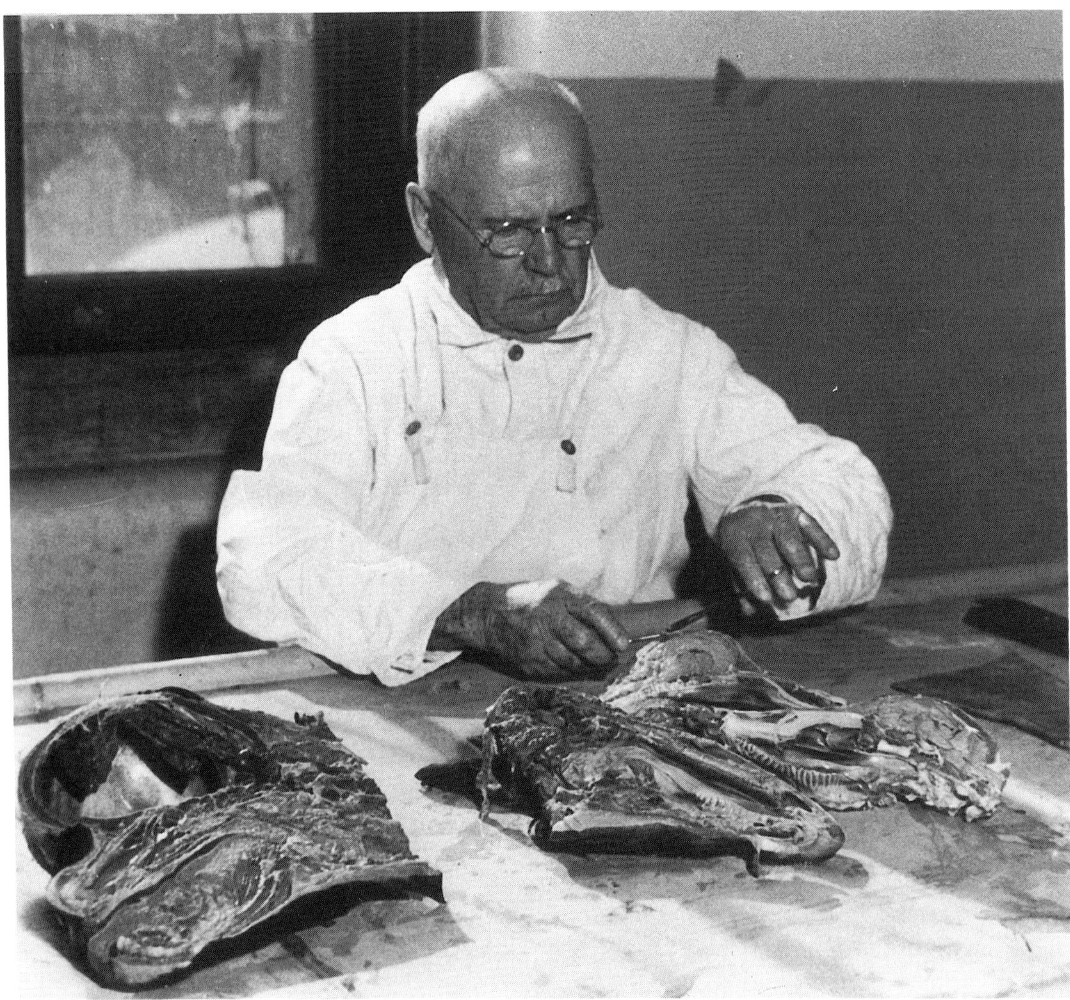

FIGURE 6.   Walter L. Williams, dissecting a pathological specimen at Cornell University in 1944. (Courtesy of Dr. Lennart Krook, Cornell University).

pathology to clinical practice with him from Montreal. In the earlier part of his career at Cornell, Williams concentrated on surgery. Later his interests shifted to obstetrics and reproductive diseases. As one reads his papers and books, some now 95 years old, one repeatedly encounters pathology, both as pathogenesis and as pathologic anatomy in work after work. Whether in surgery or in obstetrics, the basic emphasis on altered function, altered structure, embryology or etiology is ever present, and always in a logical sequence, preceding surgical or medical treatment.

It is there to an extent that one does not expect from a veterinary clinician before the turn of the century, or get from some clinical teachers even in 1984! Moreover, Williams' descriptions of genital lesions or surgical conditions in horses and cattle are often better than we can find from some of his contemporaries who professed to teach pathology, either at Cornell or elsewhere. Better is perhaps the wrong word when comparing the output of a clinician who was doing pathologic investigation with that of pathologists who were not.

It does not diminish Williams' stature in the slightest, to point out that the stimulus of Osler's teaching, the example which showed that a clinician can ask and answer basic questions, can be unmistakably recognized in the pupil. In fact Williams had already acknowledged his professional heritage publicly on an earlier occasion, when he stated at the A.V.M.A. convention in 1940, relative to the founding of the veterinary college at Cornell in 1895: "The clinics initiated by Professor Law and myself. . . constitute, in a large measure, *an adaptation of Osler's ideals* to the teaching of veterinary medicine." (italics mine).[134] Williams, of course, provided a fruitful soil in which Osler's influence could germinate.

Williams' contributions to veterinary pathology were so extensive that he merits inclusion in any historical list of veterinary pathologists. Unlike Clement, Williams did not study in Virchow's institute. But through the teaching of Osler, one of Virchow's most ardent admirers, Williams was exposed to Virchow's ideas secondhand; thus he was molded by the thinking of two of the best minds in nineteenth century pathology. He had learned German at the Illinois Technical University before enrolling at Montreal, sufficiently well that he later translated a German book on veterinary surgery into English. Mastery of German gave him access to the work of German veterinary pathologists, whose publications dominated veterinary literature in the nineteenth century. Of course, Williams' accomplishments were chiefly the product of his own curiosity, intellect, energy and drive. But one may still ask, given such a mentor, could Williams have done anything other than succeed brilliantly?

Williams' death in Ithaca on October 23, 1945, in his ninetieth year, marked the end of an academic career unparalleled in North American veterinary medicine. It also marked the demise of the last of Osler's students at the Montreal Veterinary College. Never had McEachran and Osler's judgment been better vindicated than in their selection of the silver medallist from the class of 1879.

The Enduring Osler

Tenuous though it may seem, Osler's influence can be traced to the lives of several contemporary veterinary pathologists, through their mentor, Peter

Olafson (1897–1985). The latter had studied at the North Dakota Agricultural College, and sought advice from Dr. A.F. Schalk, a research veterinarian there, as to where he might best go to veterinary school. Schalk advised Olafson to go to Cornell because W.L. Williams was teaching there. When Olafson arrived at Cornell in 1924, Williams was already retired, but (as mentioned earlier) he continued to work for another 25 years and to influence all who came in contact with him. After graduation, Olafson remained at Cornell as a teacher.

Almost sixty years later, in October of 1983, I told Dr. Olafson that in studying Dr. Williams' career, it seemed to me that he had become a renowned clinician because he was not merely treating disease, but had acquired from Osler a mind set to learn the pathology of what he was treating. Further, I thought that Williams had contributed enough to veterinary pathology to merit inclusion in a biographical history of this discipline which I was writing. He had even had the audacity, as a clinician, to review a German book on veterinary pathology![183] Olafson replied that Williams indeed merited such historical treatment. He then surprised me by relating that he had chosen to study at Cornell because Williams was there, something he had not mentioned in the 35 years I had known him! [This had been documented by Leonard in 1982,[184] but at the time I spoke with Olafson I had not yet read it.]

As we have seen, Osler's teaching and example helped to shape Williams into the outstanding veterinarian that he became. Although their lives followed different paths, Olafson learned a lot from Williams, who served as a role model of lofty ethical and intellectual standards and a lifelong example of remaining curious, always thinking and always investigating.

Olafson also learned from Williams that clinical medicine and surgery were only one side of the coin of disease; he consequently taught pathology not in isolation, but correlated with the other, clinical side of the coin. By mid-twentieth century Olafson had achieved great distinction as an undergraduate and graduate teacher and as a research worker.[185] His famous ''show and tell'' method of teaching at the autopsy table, rivetted the attention of students. It was a counterpart of Osler's teaching, of which Thomas McCrae had written: ''William Osler was a great morbid anatomist and his 'clinics' in the autopsy room were if anything more interesting than those by the bedside . . . [He] reconstructed the history of events from the specimens.''[186]

In my D.L.T. Smith Lecture earlier this year. I said: ''Certainly Larry Smith went to Cornell solely because he wanted to work with Olafson; and so the thread remains unbroken, between William Osler and his veterinary students in Montreal and Larry Smith and his veterinary students, first in Guelph and later in Saskatoon.'' It remains unbroken also between Peter Olafson and his other students: Frank Bloom, Donald Cordy, Leonard Goss, Kenneth Jubb, Peter Kennedy, John King, Kenneth McEntee, William Monlux, and William Sippel to name but a few who have enriched North American veterinary pathology. All are professional descendents, through Walter Williams, of William Osler.

It is a thread of hard work, clear thinking, concern for one's patients or charges rather than for oneself, and a vision of the future—that one can make it better by dedication to the pursuit of excellence in service to the public. William Osler has left us an enduring legacy, in a tradition now exactly one hundred years old—roots of which we veterinary pathologists may all be proud. He was a devout believer in continuing education and constantly proclaimed its virtues. He showed specimens and gave talks at innumerable

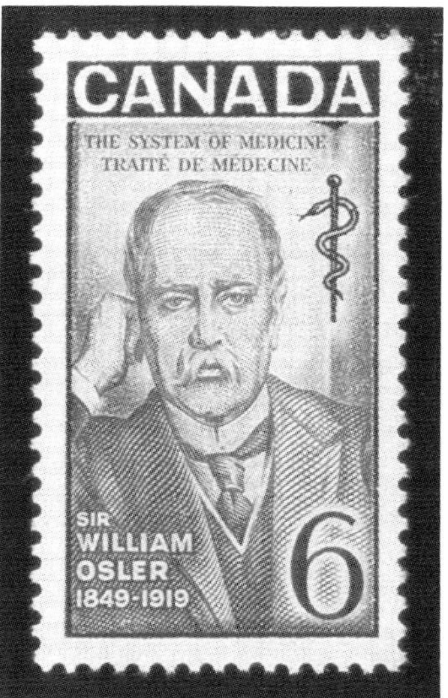

FIGURE 7. Postage stamp portraying Sir William Osler, issued by the Canada Post Office in 1969, on the 50th anniversary of his death. (By permission of Canada Post Corporation).

medical society and veterinary medical society meetings in Montreal and Philadelphia.

His Canadian compatriots have expressed their affection for and pride in Osler in many ways; a few years ago by the issuance of a postage stamp (Figure 7).[187] As we look at it, it is easy to imagine that Sir William, the inspired teacher, has returned to Toronto and is here with us in spirit today. If so, he would surely be pleased at how the discipline of pathology which he introduced in our North American veterinary schools is flourishing on the continent which gave him birth. And he would surely find it heartening to view the unrivalled annual participation in continuing education by our North American veterinary pathologists, in keeping with one of his most cherished goals.

In introducing the spirit of William Osler to a group of his professional descendants, gathered near his birthplace for the purpose of continuing their education, I can think of no more apt citation from his writings than this:

> "This higher education so much needed today is not given in the school, is not to be bought in the market place, but it has to be wrought out in each one of us for himself; it is the silent influence of character on character and in no way more potently than in the contemplation of the lives of the great and good of the past, in no way more than in 'the touch divine of noble natures gone'[188]."

Ladies and gentlemen, mesdames et messieurs, I have heeded Sir William's advice, and have indulged in the contemplation he advocated, of "the lives of the great and good of the past." The result of this contemplation, which you have graciously allowed me to share with you today, is that if veterinary pathology in North America is thriving in 1984, it is in no small measure due to the man who had given it such a fine start by 1884.

Thank you very much, my friends. Merci beaucoup, mes amis.

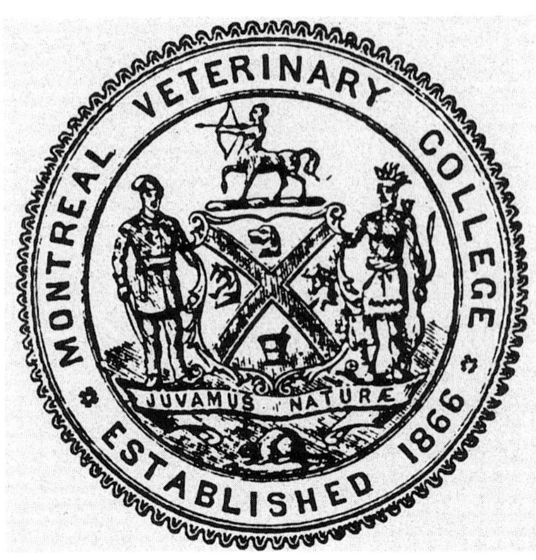

FIGURE 8. Coat of arms of the Montreal Veterinary College, from the McGill University catalog of 1901.

Acknowledgements

This essay is dedicated to the memory of Nathan I. Dubin, MD, ChM (McGill), late chairman and professor of pathology at the Woman's Medical College in Philadelphia. He shared Osler's interests in comparative pathology and medical history, and introduced me to the importance of his alma mater in both of these fields.

I am grateful to Charles G. Roland, MD, Jason A. Hannah Professor of the History of Medicine at McMaster University, for taking the time during an academic leave of absence to review an earlier version of the manuscript and make helpful suggestions. I thank Philip Teigen, PhD, formerly the Osler Librarian at McGill University, for help in locating the only existing portrait of A.W. Clement, and Lennart Krook, DVM, professor of veterinary pathology at Cornell University, for finding a portrait of W.L. Williams. I am grateful to Mrs. Margaret Covatta for her meticulous work on the bibliographic aspects of this paper. I appreciate very much the sustained interest in and encouragement of my historical endeavours of R.G. Thomson, DVM, Dean of the Atlantic Veterinary College.

References

1. Saunders LZ, Barron CN: A century of veterinary pathology at the AFIP. 1870–1970. Path Vet 1970; 7: 193–224.
2. Jones, TC, Saunders LZ: A tribute to Colonel James Earle Ash, MC U.S.A. (Retired) on the occasion of his 100th birthday September 8, 1984. Vet Path 1984, 21: 367–369.
3. Cushing H: The life of Sir William Osler. Vols 1 & 2. Oxford: Clarendon Press, 1925. (Unsatisfactory single volume edition. on cheap paper, with

36 of the original 47 illustrations omitted, New York: Oxford University Press, 1940).

4. Gattinger FE: A century of challenge. Toronto: University of Toronto Press, 1962: 25–32.

5. Mills TW: The Montreal Veterinary College and its founder and principal. J Comp Med Vet Arch 1888; 9: 74–84.

6. Mitchell CA: Duncan McEachran. Can J Comp Med 1939; 3: 255–258.

7. Vokaty S: The adventures of Dr. Duncan McNab McEachran in Western Canada. Can Vet J 1979; 20: 149–156.

8. Todd JL, Wolbach SB: The swamp fever of horses. Rep Vet Dir Gen for yr ending Mar 1911. Ottawa, 1911; 157–177.

9. Houck UG: The Bureau of Animal Industry of the US Department of Agriculture. Washington: Published by the Author, 1924: 59–60.

10. Christiansen GC: Veterinary medical education, a rapid revolution. In: Smithcors, JF. The American veterinary profession. Ames: Iowa State University Press, 1963: 641–665.

11. Anonymous: Veterinary colleges of North America. Amer Vet Rev 1895; 18: 432–435.

12. French C: Intestinal parasitism in the dog. J Comp Med Vet Arch 1896; 17: 441–452.

13. Gill HD: Defective development of the central nervous system in a cat. J Comp Med Vet Arch 1895; 17: 393–394.

14. Huddleston JH: Tumors from the choroid plexus of a horse. Proc Path Soc NY 1895; 29–30.

15. Saunders LZ: Veterinary pathology in Russia 1860–1930. Ithaca: Cornell University Press, 1980.

16. Merillat LA, Campbell DM: Veterinary military history of the United States. Kansas City, Mo: Haver-Glover Laboratories, 1935: 238.

17. Knopf SA: Dr. John Henry Huddleston. In memoriam. Med Rec 1915; 88: 839–840.

18. Smith DK: Practical hints in pathology. J Comp Med Vet Arch 1902; 23: 228–230.

19. Smith DK: Malignant tumors. Proc 40th Ann Mtg A.V.M.A. 1903; 314–315.

20. Leonard EP: A Cornell heritage: veterinary medicine 1868–1908. Ithaca, N.Y. State Coll. Vet. Med., 1979; 194–195.

21. Stange CH: History of veterinary medicine at Iowa State College. Ames: Iowa, Iowa State College, 1929: 15–17.

22. Satterthwaite TE: Some of the recent contributions to the literature of comparative medicine. J Comp Med Surg 1880; 1: 185–192.

23. Satterthwaite TE: The study of comparative pathology: Introductory lecture of a course, delivered at the Columbia Veterinary College in 1881–1882. J Comp Med Surg 1882; 3: 1–13.

24. Schrady J: ed. The College of Physicians and Surgeons in New York, Vol 1: New York, 1903, 550–554.

25. Long ES: A history of American pathology. Springfield: Charles C Thomas, 1960: 178, 229–230.

26. Nielsen NO: Schofield lecture 1982. Comparative medicine. Can Vet J 1983; 24: 269–277.

27. McEachern D: Osler and the Montreal Veterinary College. Can Med Assoc J 1920; 20: (Osler Memorial Number) 35–37.

28. Murphy DA: Osler, now a veterinarian. Can Med Assoc J 1960; 83: 32–35.

29. McEachran D: "Be gentlemen." Am Vet Rev 1890; 14: 109–114.
30. McEachran D: Contagious pleuro-pneumonia. p. 222. In: Annual report on the cattle quarantines. In: Canada, Dept. of Agr., Chief Veterinary Inspector. Ottawa, 1886: 195–235.
31. Anonymous: Montreal Veterinary College. Vet J 1881; 13: 455–456.
32. Mitchell CA: A note on the early history of veterinary science in Canada. Can J Comp Med 1939; 3: 276–281.
33. Eby CH: Sir William Osler and veterinary medicine—a biographical sketch. J Small Anim Pract 1960; 1: 273–276.
34. Roland CG: The palpable Osler: A study in survival. Persp Biol Med 1984; 27: 299–313.
35. Cameron TWM: Sir William Osler and parasitology. J Parasit 1950; 36: 93–102.
36. Talbott JH: A biographical history of medicine. New York: Grune & Stratton, 1970: 1138–1141.
37. Barker CAV: The Ontario Veterinary College: Temperance Street era. Can Vet J 1975; 16: 319–328.
38. Ware J, Hunt H: The several lives of a victorian vet. London: Bachman & Turner, 1979: 99.
39. Osler W: Berlin correspondence. Can Med Surg J 1873–1874; 2: 231–233; 308–315.
40. Osler W: Allgemeines Krankenhaus. Can Med Surg J 1873–1874; 2: 451–456.
41. Osler W: Rudolf Virchow, the man and the student. Boston Med Surg J 1891; 125: 425–427.
42. Opie EL: Osler as a pathologist. Bull Hist Med 1949; 23: 321–324.
43. Bean WB: Foreword (pp. xiii–xv) In: Rodin AE. Oslerian pathology. An assessment and annotated atlas of museum specimens. Lawrence, Kansas: Coronado Press, 1981; 194–195.
44. Anonymous: Society proceedings. Medico-Chirurgical Society of Montreal. Pneumo-enteritis of the hog. Can Med Surg J 1884; 12: 429.
45. Anonymous: Society proceedings. Medico-Chirurgical Society of Montreal. Portions of muscle, intestine and kidney from horse dying of toxic haemoglobinuria or azoturia. Can Med Surg J 1884; 12: 545–546.
46. Anonymous: Society proceedings. Medico–Chirurgical Society of Montreal. Actinomykosis(cow). Can Med Surg J 1884; 12: 599.
47. Anonymous: Montreal Veterinary College. Vet J 1876; 3: 465–466.
48. Anonymous: Opening of the Montreal Veterinary College. Vet. J. 1878; 7: 405–408.
49. Osler W: The master-word in medicine. Brit Med J 1903; ii: 1196–1200.
50. Osler W: Verminous bronchitis in dogs. The Veterinarian 1877; 50: 387–397.
51. Osler W: On the pathology of so-called pig typhoid. Vet J Ann Comp Path 1878; 6: 385–402.
52. Saunders LZ: Schofield memorial lecture. Some pioneers in comparative medicine. Can Vet J 1973; 14: 27–35.
53. Osler W: On echinococcus disease in America. Am J Med Sci 1882; 84: 475–480.
54. Osler W, Clement AW: Parasites in the pork supply of Montreal. Can Med Surg J 1883; 11: 325–326.
55. Osler W, Clement AW: Diffuse purulent bronchiestasy in a calf, with morbid anatomy notes. J Comp Med Surg 1882; 3: 317–319.

56. Osler W, Clement AW: Chronic bronchitis—spurious melanosis of lungs in a dog. J Comp Med Surg 1882: 3: 319–320.

57. Osler W, Clement AW: Haemato-pyo-metra in a bitch. J Comp Med Surg 1882; 3:320–321.

58. Osler W, Clement AW: Cestode tuberculosis. A successful experiment in producing it in the calf. Am Vet Rev 1882; 6: 6–10.

59. Osler W. Report on Pictou Cattle Disease investigations. Rep. Min. Agr. Dominion of Canada for 1882, Ottawa, Queen's Printer, 1883; 289–293. (Reprinted in: The Veterinarian 1883 56: 478–485).

60. Anonymous: Montreal Veterinary Medical Association. Vet J 1880; 11: 431–432.

61. Anonymous: Montreal Veterinary Association. Vet J 1877; 5: 457.

62. Anonymous: Montreal Veterinary Medical Association. Vet J 1878; 6: 62–63.

63. Teigen PM: William Osler and comparative medicine. Can Vet J 1984; 25: 400–405.

64. Anonymous: Necrology. Albert W. Clement. J Comp Med Vet Arch 1901; 22: 178–180.

65. Martenet WH: Obituary. Albert W. Clement, D.V.S. Am Vet Rev 1901; 25: 65–66.

66. Rodin AE: Oslerian pathology. An assessment and annotated atlas of museum specimens. Lawrence, Kansas: Coronado Press. 1981: 194–195.

67. Osler W, Clement AW: Lungs of a horse which had died of pneumonia. Can Med Surg J 1883; 11: 498.

68. Anonymous: Montreal Veterinary College. Vet J 1884; 18: 460–461.

69. Clement AW: Acute parenchymatous nephritis. J Comp Med Surg 1885; 6: 308–315.

70. Jones TC, Hunt RD: Veterinary pathology. 5th ed. Philadelphia: Lea & Febiger, 1983: 1145–1148.

71. Clement AW. A few notes on some of the principal centers of veterinary education in England and on the Continent. J Comp Med Surg 1887; 8: 144–149.

72. Saunders LZ: Albert W. Clement, the first president of the A.V.M.A. (In preparation) 1987.

73. Clement AW: Veterinary post-mortem examinations. In: Buck AH. ed. Reference handbook of the medical sciences. Vol 7. New York: William Wood, 1889: 641–653. (Also published as separate book with the same title. New York: Sabiston & Murray. 1891).

74. Conklin WA: Review of Clement AW. Veterinary Post-Mortem Examinations. J Comp Med Vet Arch 1891: 12: 409.

75. Clement AW: Discussion on hog cholera. Proc U.S.V.M.A. 28 Ann Meet 1891. Philadelphia; 1893; 154.

76. Clement AW: Case reports: Rupture of mesenteric artery; Hemorrhage at the base of the brain; Rupture of the coronary artery. J Comp Med Surg 1886; 7: 186–188.

77. Welch WH: Preliminary report of investigations concerning the causation of hog cholera. Bull Johns Hopkins Hosp 1889; 1: 9–10.

78. Welch WH, Clement AW: Remarks on hog cholera and swine plague. Proc 30th Ann Meet, US Vet Med Assoc. Oct. 16–20, Chicago, 1893; 206–214. Philadelphia, U S Vet Med Assoc (Reprinted In: Vol 1, 86–96 In: *Welch, WH.* Papers and addresses. Baltimore: Johns Hopkins Press, 1932 also Historiae Med Vet 1980; 5: 1–37.).

79. Clement AW: Description of some specimens of pleuro-pneumonia contagiosa. J Comp Med Surg 1888; 9: 151–155.

80. Clement AW: "So-called" spinal meningitis. J Comp Med Vet Arch 1892: 13: 486–488.

81. Clement AW: Record of a case of glanders in man with history of infection from a horse, together with a clinical and post-mortem record of the case in the suspected animal. J Comp Med Vet Arch 1893; 14: 65–69.

82. Clement AW: Dislocation between the second and third cervical vertebrae in a horse. J Comp Med Vet Arch 1894; 15: 455–456.

83. Clement AW: Some of the more prevalent diseases affecting animals. J Comp Med Vet Arch 1898; 19: 6–12.

84. Clement AW, Stokes WR: Rabies in sheep. J Comp Med Vet Arch 1897; 18: 271–274.

85. Stokes WR, Clement AW: An epidemic of purulent inflammation of the milk ducts, affecting seventy cows. J Comp Med Vet Arch 1897; 18: 135–138.

86. Clement AW: Review of Jahresbericht der K. Central Thierarznei-Schule in München 1886. J Comp Med Surg 1888: 9: 205–206.

87. Clement AW: President's address. Proc. 36th Ann Meet Am Vet Med Assoc 1899; 1–8.

88. MacCallum WG, Clement AW: Pulmonary tuberculosis with diffuse pneumonic consolidation in a lion. Bull Johns Hopkins Hosp 1900; 2: 85–86.

89. Clement AW: State examinations. Proc. Am Vet Med Assoc 36th Ann Meet 1899; 270–274.

90. Clement AW: The inspection of meat and milk with special reference to tuberculosis. Am Vet Rev 1890; 14: 76–86, 114–124.

91. Anonymous: McGill University. J Comp Med Vet Arch 1896; 17: 428–429.

92. Abbot M: History of medicine in the province of Quebec. Montreal: McGill University, 1931; 87.

93. Anonymous: Obituary. Professor Wyatt Galt Johnston. Montreal Med J 1902; 31: 554–560.

94. Adami JG: On the teaching of pathology. Phila Med J 1900; 6: 399–402.

95. Johnston W: Preliminary report on the pathology of the Pictou cattle disease. Rep Min Agr Dominion of Canada, for 1892; 41–47. Ottawa, Queen's Printer 1893.

96. Johnston W: Biliary cirrhosis of the liver in cattle (Pictou cattle disease). Proc 30th Ann. Conv. US Vet Med Assoc Chicago 1893; 120–126. Philadelphia US Vet Med Assoc 1894.

97. Anonymous: Montreal Veterinary Medical Association. Am Vet Rev 1891; 15: 56–57.

98. Anonymous: Montreal Veterinary College. J Comp Med Surg 1888; 9: 237–238.

99. Johnston W: Local tuberculous abscess in a bull. Proc. 29th Ann. Meet. U S Vet Med Assoc, Boston 1892; 347–350. Philadelphia, US Vet Med Assoc 1893.

100. Abbot M: The Wyatt Johnston descriptive classification of museum specimens, as applied in the pathology museum of McGill University. Bull Int Assn Med Museums 1925; 11: 78–89.

101. Douglas AJ: et al. Wyatt Galt Johnston. Am J Publ Health 1931; 21: 1243–1245.

102. Osler W: Obituary. Dr. Wyatt Johnston. Med. News (N.Y.) 1902; 80: 1233.

103. Adami JG: J. George Adami, A memoir. London: Constable. 1930.

104. Adami JG: Principles of pathology. Philadelphia: Lea & Febiger, Vol. 1, 1908, Vol. 2, 1909.

105. Adami JG: Pictou cattle disease. Montreal Med J 1902; 31: 105–117.

106. Adami JG, Martin CF: Report on observations made upon the cattle at the experimental station at Outremont, recognized to be tuberculous by the tuberculin test. Ottawa, 1899.

107. Adami JG: On the significance of bovine tuberculosis and its eradication in Canada. Can J Med Surg 1899; 6: 391–405.

108. Adami JG: On the relationship between human and bovine tuberculosis. Phila Med J 1902; 9: 356–365.

109. Adami JG: Secondary enchondroma in a bitch. Can Med Rec 1895; 23: 105.

110. Adami JG: Certain points in connection with the development of our knowledge of actinomycosis and its causation. Montreal Med J 1905; 34: 88–93.

111. Adami JG: On a giant-celled rhabdomyosarcoma from the trout. Montreal Med J 1908; 37: 163–165.

112. Anonymous: Commencement exercises at the veterinary department, McGill University. Vet Mag 1896; 3: 390–391.

113. Adami JG: "On this side Jordan": Inaugural lecture in the faculty of comparative medicine, McGill University, October 1894. Montreal Med 1895; 23: 256–270.

114. McGregor J: Montreal Veterinary Medical Association. J Comp Vet Med Arch 1898; 19: 832–834.

115. Lehnert EH: Montreal Veterinary Medical Assn. Vet Mag 1895; 2: 63–65.

116. Dell, HH: Montreal Veterinary Medical Assn. Vet Mag 1895; 2: 648–649.

117. Adami JG, Bell J, Robbins GD: Chronic human glanders. Montreal Med J 1905: 34: 538–540.

118. Adami JG: On tuberculosis in relation to the live-stock industry. Boston Med Surg J 1902; 146: 619–624.

119. Anonymous: Pleuro-pneumonia. The subject of an interesting discussion by the Montreal Veterinary Medical Assn. Vet Mag 1894; 1: 71–72.

120. McFadyean J: The discussion on pleuro-pneumonia at the Montreal meeting of the British Medical Assn. J Comp Path Therap 1897; 10: 349–350.

121. Pattison I. The British veterinary profession 1791–1948. London: JA Allen, 1983: 156–157.

122. Anonymous: Obituary. Charles H. Higgins. Can J Comp Med 1955; 19: 2–5. (Author is probably CA. Mitchell).

123. Dell, H: Montreal Veterinary Medical Assn. Vet Mag 1896; 3: 128, 202–203.

124. Dell, H: Montreal Veterinary Medical Assn. Vet Mag 1896; 3: 256.

125. Anonymous: Veterinary department of McGill University. J Comp Med Vet Arch 1901; 22: 256–258.

126. Higgins CH: Notes upon an epidemic of fowl cholera. J Exp Med 1898; 3: 651–671.

127. Higgins CH: Actinobacillosis. In: Rpt Vet Dir Gen Dominion of Canada for 1904. Ottawa 1905; 146–151.

128. Higgins CH: Actinobacillosis. In: Proc 41st Ann Meet Am Vet Med Assoc 1904; 131–134.

129. Rutherford JG: Special report on Pictou cattle disease: Part 1. (Reprinted from Rep. Vet. Dir. Gen. 1906.) In Can. Vet J. 1982; 23: 361–364.

130. Higgins CH: Anthrax and blackleg. In: Proc 40th Ann Meet Am Vet Med Assoc 1903; 292–300.

131. Laidlaw C: Dr. J.G. Rutherford and bovine tuberculosis. Bull Can Tuberc Assoc (suppl.) 1930; 1–4.

132. Higgins CH: Report of pathologist. In: Rep Vet Dir Gen for 1910. Ottawa, 1911; 40–42; 53–57.

133. Higgins CH: Report of pathologist. In: Rep Vet Dir Gen Dominion of Canada 1911. Ottawa. 1912; 123–127.

134. Smithcors F: The American veterinary profession. Ames: Iowa State University Press, 1963; 606.

135. Torrance F: Pathological division. In: Rep Vet Dir Gen Dominion of Canada for yr ending Mar 1819. Ottawa 1919; 15–17, 39.

136. Higgins CH: Canadian chicken cholera. In: Proc 36th Ann Meet Am Vet Med Assoc, Ithaca, 1899; 227–233.

137. Higgins CH: Laboratory aids. In: Proc 43rd Ann Meet Am Vet Med Assoc 1906; 138–144.

138. Higgins CH: Discussion of methods of mounting museum specimens. In: Proc 50th Ann Meet Am Vet Med Assoc, 1913. Philadelphia, 1914; 759.

139. Higgins CH: Human and comparative medicine. Am Vet Rev 1905; 29: 450–457.

140. Higgins CH: Channels of infection and localization in tuberculosis. J Am Vet Med Assoc 1917 52: 299–308.

141. Canada: Department of National Defence. The Militia List. Part II. 1925; 130.

142. Anonymous: Death of Dr. Charles H. Higgins. J Am Vet Med Assoc 1955; 126: 254.

143. Anonymous: W. Reid Blair, D.V.Sc., 1875–1949. J Am Vet Med Assoc 1949; 114: 345.

144. Anonymous: Dr. W, Reid Bair, Zoo Head 14 Years. Obituary, N.Y. Times March 2, 1949; 25.

145. Crandall LS: W. Reid Blair, in Memoriam. Animal Kingdom April, 1949; 52(2): 59–60.

146. Anonymous: McGill University. J Comp Med Vet Arch 1902; 23: 316–317.

147. Blair WR: Cysticerci in wild ruminants. Am Vet Rev 1903; 27: 386–395.

148. Blair WR: Autopsy summaries of wild animals. Am Vet Rev 1903; 27: 526–529.

149. Brooks H, Blair WR: Osteomalacia of primates in captivity. A clinical and pathological study of "cage paralysis." Rep NY Zool Soc 1904; 9: 135–175.

150. Blair WR: Pathological exhibit. Proc. 43rd Ann Meet Am Vet Med Assoc. New Haven: 1906: 391.

151. Blair WR: Filariae. Am Vet Rev 1905; 28: 1147–1153.

152. Blair WR: Five lambs at one parturition. Am Vet Rev 1906; 30: 224.

153. Blair WR: Correspondence. Am Vet Rev 1906; 30: 603–604.

154. Blair WR: Osteomyelitis in a dog. Am Vet Rev 1906; 30: 696–698.

155. Blair WR: Modes of tubercular infection in wild animals in captivity. Am Vet Rev 1906; 30: 1299–1306.

156. Blair WR: The pathological effects of captivity on wild animals. Proc. 45th Ann Meet Am Vet Med Assoc, New Haven: 1906: 391.

157. Merillat LA, Campbell DM: Veterinary military history of the United States. Vol. 2, Kansas City, Mo: Haver-Glover Laboratories, 1935: 737.

158. Anonymous: Army veterinary service. Changes relative to veterinary officers. Reserve Corps. North Am Vet. 1928; 9(12): 72.

159. Blair WR: In the zoo. New York: Scribner, 1931.

160. Blair WR: The New York zoological park. J Am Vet Med Assoc 1938; 92: 752–759.

161. Miller FH: Academic honors for Wm. Reid Blair. North Am Vet 1928; 9(8): 70.

162. Blair WR: Veterinary medical society of New York county. Am Vet Rev 1906; 30: 1478–1480.

163. Frost JN: Walter L. Williams. Cornell Vet 1946; 36: 100–103.

164. Williams WL: Horse syphylis or maladie du coit (dourine). Am Vet Rev 1888–1889; 12: 295–303; 341–349; 402–410; 445–450.

165. Williams WL: A clinical study of odontomes. Am Vet Rev 1891; 15: 1–17; 64–74.

166. Williams WL: Contagious pleuro-pneumonia of the horse. Am Vet Rev 1892; 16: 301–317.

167. Williams WL: The pathology of azoturia. Am Vet Rev 1890; 14: 172–181.

168. Williams WL: Invasion of the mesenteric arteries of the horse by Strongylus armatus. Vet J Ann Comp Path 1887; 24: 159–164, 234–240.

169. Williams WL: Glanders. Am Vet Rev 1895; 18: 6–23.

170. Williams WL: The therapeutics of colic. Amer Vet Rev 1894; 19: 457–473.

171. Williams WL: Veterinary obstetrics, including the diseases of breeding animals and of the newborn. Ithaca, the Author, 1909.

172. Williams WL: Veterinary obstetrics. Ithaca: the Author, 1917. 2nd ed. 1931; 3rd ed. 1940; 4th ed. 1943.

173. Williams WL: Diseases of the genital organs of domestic animals. Ithaca: the Author, 1921. 2nd ed. 1939; 3rd ed. 1943.

174. Williams WL: Parasitic ictero-hematuria of sheep. Vet Mag 1895; 2: 497.

175. Williams WL: Teratology of the hyo-mandibular gill slit in the horse. Am Vet Rev 1904; 28: 2202–255.

176. Williams WL: The problem of teratology in clinical veterinary practice. Cornell Vet 1936; 26: 1–33.

177. Williams WL: The air sac mite of the fowl. Amer Vet Rev 1898; 22: 8–25.

178. Williams WL, Fisher CW, Udall DH: The spavin group of lameness. Proc 42 Ann Meet AVMA 1906; 283–333.

179. Williams WL: Enzootiac ccrebro-spinal meningitis in horses. Fourteenth Ann Rep Bureau Animal Ind for 1897; 179–184.

180. Lagerlöf N, Williams WL: Researches concerning the morphologic changes in the testicles of sterile and subnormally fertile bulls. Cornell Vet 1934; 24: 361–384.

181. Williams WL: Recollections of and reflections upon sixty-five years in the veterinary profession. Cornell Vet 1945; 35: 166–190, 231–269.

182. Williams WL: The veterinary profession: its opportunities and needs for the future. Amer Vet Rev 1888; 12: 153–160.

183. Williams WL: Book review of Ernst Joest's Spezielle pathologische Anatomie der Haustiere. Cornell Vet 1926; 16: 310–316.

184. Leonard EP: In the James Law tradition, 1908–1948. Ithaca, N.Y. State Coll. Vet. Med., 1982; 222.

185. Saunders LZ: Peter Olafson 1897–1985. A eulogy. Cornell Vet 1986; 76: April, unnumbered 1–4.

186. McCrae T: The influence of pathology on the clinical medicine of William Osler. Bull Int Assn Med Museums (Osler memorial no.) 1926; No. 9: 37–41.
187. Scarlett EP: Philatelic Osler. Group Pract 1969; 18: 60–61.
188. Bean RAB, Bean WB: Sir William Osler. Aphorisms from his bedside teachings and writings. New York: 1950; 79.

James Barry, M.D.
Inspector General of Hospitals
Man or Woman?

 Earl F. Nation, M.D.

In the *Bibliotheca Osleriana*,[5] the great annotated bibliography of Sir William Osler's library housed at McGill University, there appears what seems to be an unlikely entry, number 5384: "Roger, E., 'A Modern Sphinx. A Novel. London, 1895' ". There are precious few novels in this library of medical and scientific rareties. The cryptic notes which follow this entry add to the intrigue, occupying as they do most of a column in this huge tome.

The first note describes the book and adds an interesting statement: "—— including portraits and an account of the woman army surgeon, James Barry (d. 1865) whose career in the character of 'Fitzjames', is the subject of this novel".

There are also notes relating to correspondence by Osler with the author and others about the book and its subject. This material is pasted into the back of Osler's copy of the book.

Osler goes on in the *Bibliotheca* to add: "I became interested in her from having heard the stories and gossip current in Montreal in the seventies. She lived in the house on the N.W. corner of Sherbrooke and Durocher Sts., leading a very secluded life, so Campbell, our old Dean said. He knew her well and attended her professionally without any suspicion of her sex, though her features and ways were feminine".

Among the letters pasted in the novel is one from Olga Racster, coauthor of a play about Barry,[6] which was produced in London. She later wrote a novel about Barry.[7] The letter pertains to restoration of the grave of Barry, an activity in which Osler was interested. The letter is dated August 14, 1919, just four months before Osler's death.

Who was this enigmatic individual who so interested Osler? How could a woman have gone through medical school at Edinburgh sixty years before women were admitted to medicine in Great Britain,[1] have served in the British

Read at the annual meeting of the American Osler Society, April 12, 1986.

Reprinted with permission from *Urology,* *31*:184, 1988

army for forty-six years and have risen to the second highest position in the army medical service without being discovered? (Fig 1)

The same question plagued everyone at the time of her death as shown in this extract from the *Manchester Guardian* of August 21, 1865.

> An incident is just now being discussed in military circles so extraordinary that were not the truth capable of being vouched for by the official authority, the narration would be deemed absolutely incredible. Our officers quartered at the Cape between 15 and 20 years ago may remember a certain Dr. Barry attached to the medical staff there, and enjoying a reputation for considerable skill in his profession, especially for firmness, decision and rapidity in difficult operations. This gentleman had entered the army in 1813, had passed, of course, through the grades of assistant surgeon and surgeon in various regiments, and had served as such in various quarters of the Globe. His professional acquirements had procured for him promotion to the staff at the Cape. About 1840 he became promoted to be Medical Inspector, and was transferred to Malta. He proceeded from Malta to Corfu where he was quartered for many years . . . . He there died about a month ago, and upon his death was discovered to be a woman. The motives that occasioned, and the time when commenced this singular deception are both shrouded in mystery. But thus it stands as an indubitable fact, that a woman was for 40 years an officer in the British service, and fought one duel and sought many more, had pursued a legitimate medical education, and received a regular diploma, and had acquired almost a celebrity for skill as a surgical operator.

While this was not a hoax in the true sense (Webster defines a hoax as "A deception for mockery or mischief") it was a supreme deception. How could it happen?

Because of early subterfuges the date and details of Barry's birth are clouded.[3,4,5] She juggled her own age to suit her vocational needs. She said she was born in 1799 when she entered Edinburgh in 1809. The army lists said she was born in 1795, probably nearer the truth. However, being barely five feet tall, pale, delicate, with high cheek bones, tiny hands and feet, high shrill voice, large blue eyes, sandy curls and a long Ciceronian nose (her only masculine feature), she could better pass as a younger boy than a boy of her true age. Thus, at the stated age of 10 years she entered the University of Edinburgh. There was then no lower age limit for entry into the University. A small fee for a ticket to the library was the only requirement for matriculation. (Sir Walter Scott and David Hume had entered Edinburgh at age 12.)[8,10]

Barry probably came of an Irish Catholic family although there is conflicting information about whether she was born in Ireland or London.[3,4,8,10,12] She first "surfaced" as a child in London in the care of a Mrs. Mary Anne Bulkeley, thought to be her mother but always referred to as "Aunt" after the masquerade began. Mrs. Bulkeley's brother was James Barry, R.A.[3] an impoverished and somewhat disheveled artist who was a professor of art at the Royal Academy until he was expelled by the membership after a too-heated argument with Sir Joshua Reynolds (despite which he was buried in St. Paul's Cathedral after his death in 1806).[4,8] The father of Barry, the painter, is known to have been John Barry, a shipbuilder, of Cork, Ireland.[8] So young James Barry at least has an identifiable grandfather.

James Barry, the painter, had patrons and friends in high places. Among these were Francisco Miranda, the famous Venezuelan revolutionary and scholar who was living in exile in London while trying to persuade William Pitt to back Venezuela in its effort to gain independence from Spain. Another was David Steuart Erskine, 11th Earl of Buchan.[3,4,8] These two friends of her uncle

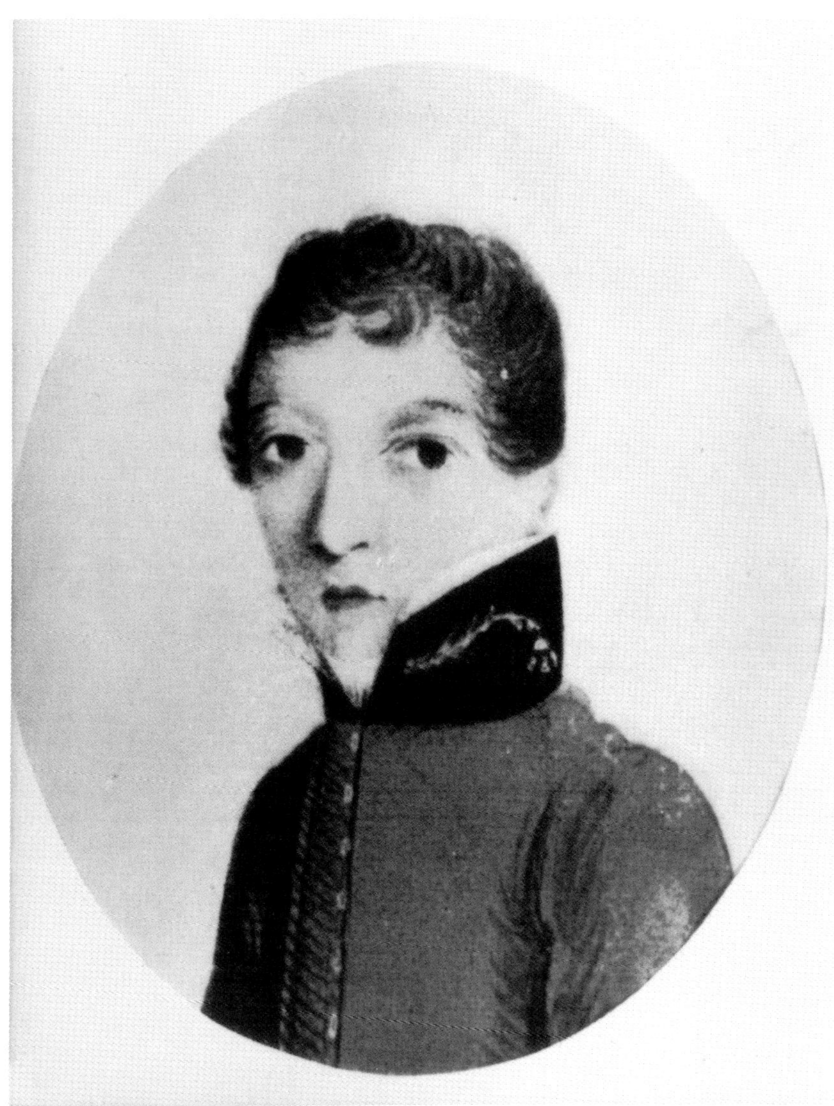

FIGURE 1   Dr. James Barry. A miniature painted on ivory by an unknown artist.

very early took young James Barry under their wings, allowed her the use of their extensive libraries, sponsored her at Edinburgh and in various endeavors for several years afterwards. Whether they were a party to the charade is unclear.

Miranda had even made arrangements for young Barry to join him in Caracas after completion of medical school. This plan was thwarted by Miranda's arrest, imprisonment and eventual death, upon his return to Venezuela.

James Barry signed the matriculation roll at Edinburgh University, the premier center for medical education at the time, in the fall of 1809 as a "literary and medical student."[3,8] During her three years there she had a very heavy academic schedule, enrolling in a number of courses not ordinarily required of a medical graduate. She wrote a thesis on inguinal hernia, defended this and took a stiff oral examination, all in Latin. In 1812 she received the first M.D. degree granted a woman in the British Empire, however unwittingly it was given. Objections to her youth were raised by the examiners but her benefactors prevailed upon her behalf. She prefaced her thesis with a quotation from Menander, the Greek poet: "Do not consider my youth, but consider whether I show a man's wisdom".[4,8,10]

By now Barry had added the names of her two sponsors to her own. She signed herself, "James Miranda Steuart Barry".[4]

After graduation Barry spent one enviable year in London as pupil-dresser under Sir Astley Cooper, England's most distinguised surgeon of the period. One of Cooper's aphorisms for students was "Cultivate the heart of a lion and the hand of a woman." Barry had both.[4]

On joining the army in 1813 Barry was appointed hospital assistant at Plymouth. This was the bottom rung. One wonders about such things as physical examinations. They were cursory at best. Even on the sick, abdominal examinations were often done blindly, under the covers. The army needed doctors with good credentials too badly to look very closely.[3] It has been said that Barry probably had to bare nothing but her teeth, if that. The commanding officer, Dr. Skey, raised objections again to Barry's youth but was advised by Earl Buchan, who had recommended Barry to Skey, "not to agitate the question."[8]

Two years later, six months after Waterloo, Barry was gazetted Assistant Surgeon to the Forces and was sent to the Garrison of Cape Colony. Here Barry was soon in the social whirl and became the personal favorite and family physician of the Governor of Capetown, Lord Charles Somerset, son of the Duchess of Beaufort. Barry, with plumed hat, three inch false soles, high heeled boots, and unwieldy sword, cut a strange figure as she went about, always accompanied by a black body servant and a small dog named Psyche. Both remained with Barry to the end; with renewal of dogs, of course. Psyche always slept on the foot of Barry's bed, perhaps to protect her secret.

Barry's medical and surgical brilliance was no affectation. She soon made a name for herself by repeated diagnostic and therapeutic triumphs.

An interesting observation was made by Count De Las Casas, who had gone into exile with Napoleon and was a virtual prisoner in an old castle on the Cape. Barry was sent to care for the Count and his son who were ill. Las Casas recorded in his eight volume, *Private Life and Conversations of the Emperor Napoleon at St. Helena,* the following: "The grave Dr. was a boy of 18 with the form, the manner, and the voice of a woman. But Dr. Barry (such was his name) was described to be an absolute phenomenon. I was informed that he had saved the life of one of the Governor's daughters after she had been given up"; later, "I found his company very agreeable". Barry was vindicated by helping Las Casas and his son regain their health.

Barry was not one to brook criticism and took umbrage quickly. She fought a pistol duel with Major (later Captain, then Sir) Josias Cleote over remarks made by Barry which led Cleote, as he later stated, to pull Barry's "long ugly nose". Neither dueler was struck, so no harm was done. However, after Barry's true sex was disclosed following death, Cleote was derided as the only British officer ever to have fought a duel with a lady. Incidentally, Barry and Cleote became life-long friends after the duel.

Barry went through various stations and advancements as the years went on. She gained a reputation as a champion of the poor, the prisoners, the common soldier, and others who were underprivileged and mistreated. She

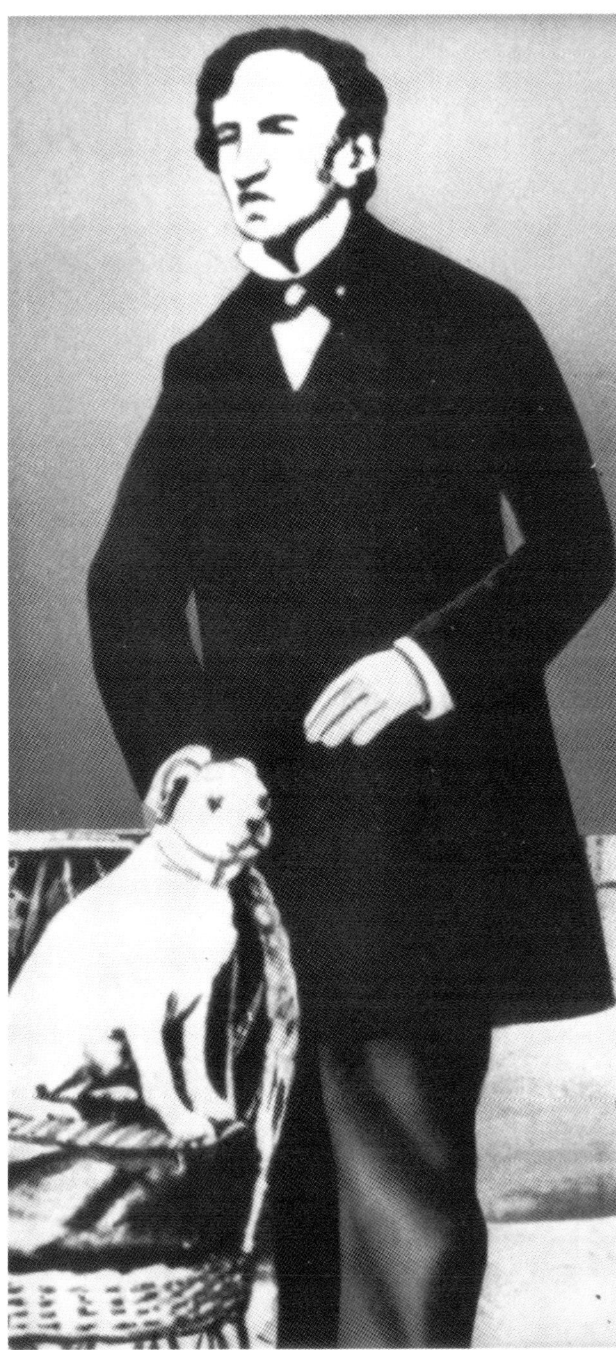

FIGURE 2   Dr. James Barry and dog, Psyche. The photograph probably was taken in Jamaica. In the original photograph Barry's life-long black body servant stood beside her.

made many enemies in the process but was unrelenting. She was reprimanded, arrested, court martialed, demoted, sent home and otherwise disciplined but was never stopped. She progressed in grade in spite of resistance from above.

She had many triumphs.[2,3,4,8] In 1826, she achieved the greatest while stationed at the Cape. A lady was dying in childbirth. Barry did a Caesarean section, without anesthesia, saving both mother and child. This was the first successful section done in the English speaking world.[3,4,8,12] The child became Barry's godchild and was named James Barry Munnik. His godchild's son became General James Barry Munnik Hertzog who was to become Prime Minister of South Africa.[8] The first-born of the Munnik sons is still named after James Barry. The present James Barry Munnik is a psychiatrist in South Africa.[10]

As Barry grew older she became more and more crotchety and intolerant of criticism and obstructions. Some one wrote of her: "Pernickity, bad-tempered, frail, fastidious—one could call Barry all of these things, and even ludicrous as well. Yet this small, curious person raised the standards of medicine and touched the public conscience about the condition of the most degraded members of society—the prisoners, the blacks and the lunatics—

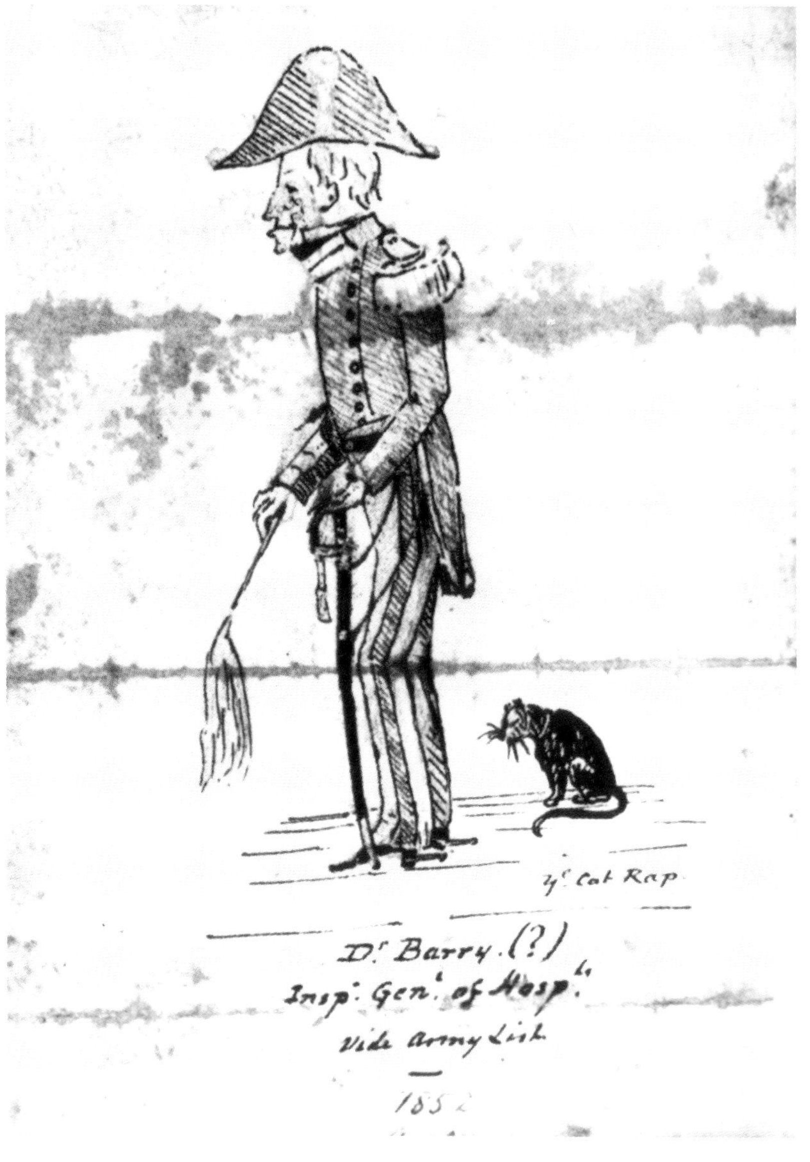

FIGURE 3 Dr. Barry, Inspector General of Hospitals. This satirical cartoon was made in Corfu by an unknown artist.

wherever she went". Barry was also said to "Have been afflicted throughout life by a daemon of a conscience; it drove her to do her duty, as she perceived it, whatever the cost to herself and others. It launched her upon a sea of troubles as Inspector General".[10] One notable individual whose enmity she incurred was Florence Nightingale. After one brief, traumatic encounter in the Crimea Florence Nightingale later wrote, "After she was dead I was told she was a woman. I should say she was the most hardened creature I ever met throughout the army."[4,12]

The title, Inspector General of Hospitals, the equivalent of Major General, finally conferred upon Barry, was the second highest office in the military medical service.

After serving in many tropical stations: the Cape, Mauritius, St. Helena, Malta, the Windward and Wayward islands, Corfu and Jamaica she was shipped off to Canada for two years to inspect and improve hospitals. During this time she nearly froze. She suffered constantly from respiratory problems. It was in this connection that she came under the professional care of Dr. George W. Campbell, Professor of Surgery and later Dean of the Faculty of McGill, while Osler was a student there. Osler recorded Campbell's embarrassed explanations to his students, after Barry's death, of his failure to discover or even suspect her true sex.[4,5,11,12]

Barry was finally returned to England sick and tired. Here she was invalided from the service on half pay over her stiff objections.

Six years later she succumbed to an epidemic of diarrhea in the London district of Marylebone on June 25, 1865 (contrary to the information reported in the *Manchester Guardian* and quoted earlier). Despite her expressed wish to be wrapped in sheets, as clothed, and buried immediately, her final effort to escape detection was spoiled. A Mrs. Sophia Bishop, a charwoman, was delegated to lay her out and made the startling disclosure to the world that Dr. Barry had a perfect female body and, furthermore, bore stretch marks, suggesting that she had borne a child, a matter on which Mrs. Bishop claimed to be an expert since she was a mother of nine.[3,8,12]

The authorities scoffed at such a notion and buried Barry in Kensal Green with a plain sandstone marker without acknowledging the possibility of her ambiguous sex. The death certificate stated that James Barry was a male. (A copy is in Osler's copy of *The Modern Sphinx*.) By the time the story became a sensation in the papers outside London (no obituary was published in the London papers) it was too late to exhume the body for a post-mortem examination. The embarrassed establishment only hoped the stories would go away. A story with such sensational possibilities was not about to be quickly laid to rest, however. Two novels and a play were based on the story in the next few years. Many articles were written about Barry, most without much research and with emphasis on the sexual aspects of the event.

It remained for Isobel Rae, in 1958, to publish a thoroughly researched biography of Barry, based particularly on a large collection of "Barry Papers" which she discovered in the British War Office and Public Records Archives and used for the first time.[8]

A number of analytical medical papers have also explored the sexual aspects of the Barry story, notably two well researched ones by a South African, Professor Percival R. Kirby.[3] Kirby espouses the belief that Barry was a hermaphrodite, perhaps a male variant described by Dr. Harry F. Kleinfelter and his associates in Boston in 1942, and known as Kleinfelter's syndrome. Such an explanation seems plausible. The same suggestion was published in England as early as 1895.[9] The ambiguous genitalia in such cases can sometimes confuse the obstetrician and urologist. A mere charwoman, who attested to her findings on the death certificate with an "X", would not be a reliable witness in such a situation, although one must assume that what Mrs. Bishop saw was more feminine than masculine. This coincided with all other characteristics of the individual, except possibly her irrascible, domineering personality.

Thus, while Kirby and some others would like to consider James Barry a man, everything about her, except her dress, suggested that physically she was a woman; and so the world and most writers would like to believe.

References

1. Greenblatt, Robert B. The secret life of Dr. James Barry 1795–1865. *Contemporary Surgery, 20*:109–111,1982.
2. James, Theodore. Sieketroost: Dr. James Barry's contribution to materia medica. *South African Medical Journal* (Cape Town), *46*:1013–1116 (15 July) 1972.
3. Kirby, Percival R. Dr. James Barry, controversial South African medical figure: a recent evaluation of his life and sex. *South African Medical Journal* (Cape Town), *44*:506–516, 1970.
4. Longford, Elizabeth. James Barry, 1795–1865. *Eminent Victorian Women.* New York; Alfred A. Knopf, 1981, pp. 227–250.
5. Osler, Sir William, Bt. *Bibliotheca Osleriana.* A catalogue of books illustrating the history of medicine and science. Oxford; Clarendon Press, 1929. Also: Montreal, McGill; Queen's University Press, 1969.
6. Racster, Olga and Grove, Jessica. *James Barry*, a play. St. James Theater, London, 1919, starring Sybil Thorndike.
7. Ibid: Dr. James Barry—her secret life, London, 1930.
8. Rae, Isobel, *The strange story of James Barry, Army Surgeon, Inspector General of Hospitals, discovered on death to be a woman.* London, New York; Longmans, Green & Co., 1958.
9. Rogers, E. *A female member of the army medical staff.* Lancet (London), July–December, 1986–1087, 1895.
10. Rose, June. *The perfect gentleman.* London; Hutchinson, 1977.
11. Roland, Charles. James Barry. *Dictionary of Canadian Biography*, pp.33–34.
12. Smith, Kathleen M. Dr. James Barry: military man—or woman? *Canadian Medical Association Journal, 126*:854–857, 1982.

🍎 Appendix

American Osler Society: List of Papers Presented 1982–1991

Billy F. Andrews, "Sir William Osler in Perinatal Perspective," (1983)

Billy F. Andrews, "Sir William Osler in the Neonatal Perspective," (1985)

Billy F. Andrews, "Daniel Drake and William Osler in Rhyme," (1989)

Billy F. Andrews, "Harvey Cushing in Pediatric Perspective," (1990)

Robert Austrian, "Osler, Agnew, and (with apologies) James Thurber," (1984)

Stanley M. Aronson, "The Summer of 1832: Cholera Comes to Providence," (1986)

William B. Bean, "On Brains and Osler's Brain," (1981)

William B. Bean, "Dr. Elisha Kent Kane," (1982)

William B. Bean, "William Osler—Milwaukee Connection," (1983)

William B. Bean, "William Osler: The Milwaukee Connection," (1984)

William B. Bean, "Osler's Last Three Months at Johns Hopkins," (1985)

William B. Bean, "The Friendship of James Herrick and William Osler," (1987)

Edward H. Bensley, "Gertrude Stein as a Medical Student," (1983)

Steven L. Berk, "Sir William Osler, Ageism and 'The Fixed Period': A Secret Revealed," (1989)

Dee J. Canale: "William Osler and the Special Field of Neurological Surgery," (1988)

Dee J. Canale and Lawrence D. Longo, "Harvey Cushing and Pediatric Neurosurgery," (1990)

Richard M. Caplan, "Sherlock Holmes and 'Brain Fever'," (1987)

Richard M. Caplan, "How Fingerprints Came Into Use for Personal Identification," (1989)

John C. Carson, "Biblical Allusions in the Writings of William Osler," (1988)

John C. Carson, "Henry Barton Jacobs: Baltimore Latchkeyer Without a Biography?" (1989)

John C. Carson, "The Message of the Life Above the Message of the Pen," (1990)

G.S.T. Cavanagh, "The Four Seasons, a Series of Anatomical Engravings," (1985)

Eugene H. Conner, "Osler and Anesthesia: Scholarship and Devotion," (1988)

Eugene H. Conner, "Daniel Drake: Another Hero of Sir William Osler's," (1988)

Eugene H. Conner, "The Marcets, Nineteenth Century Teachers of Chemistry," (1990)

Dykes Cordell, "Sir William Osler, Maude Abbott, and the Study of Congenital Heart Disease," (1985)

Nicholas E. Davies and Mark E. Silverman, "Did Osler's Ghost Write the 'GPEP' Report?" (1987)

Nicholas E. Davies, "The S.S. William Osler and Her Sister Ships," (1990)

Nicholas Dewey, "William Osler & Walt Whitman: a Philadelphia Story," (1982)

Nicholas Dewey, "The Open Arms: Myth and Reality," (1987)

Nicholas Dewey, "Osler and Burton: Birds of a Feather," (1989)

Paul G. Dyment, "John McCrae: Physician, Poet, and Soldier," (1984)

Paul G. Dyment, "Father Johnson and Willie Osler," (1987)

George C. Ebers, "Osler and Neurology," (1984)

George C. Ebers, "The History of Multiple Sclerosis: A Revision," (1989)

Richard Eimas, "Paolo Mascagni's Contributions to Anatomy," (1985)

Richard Eimas, "The Osler Connection with Iowa—Men and Books," (1987)

Richard Eimas, "The Influence of Sir Thomas Browne on Sir William Osler," (1988)

Richard Eimas, "Who's Who in the Title Page Woodcut of Andreas Vesalius' De Humani Corporis Fabrica Libri Septem," (1989)

William Feindel, "The Penfield Papers: Pitfalls and Priorities," (1981)

William Feindel, "Biographical Notes on Wilder Penfield: Sir William Osler and the Oxford Period (1915–1919)," (1987)

William Feindel, "Osler's Brain Again," (1990)

Palmer H. Futcher, "William Osler and Marjorie," (1990)

W. Bruce Fye, "S. Weir Mitchell: Philadelphia's 'Lost' Physiologist," (1982)

W. Bruce Fye, "First Physiologist and Patient of William Osler," (1984)

W. Bruce Fye, "Osler and Cardiovascular Disease," (1987)

W. Bruce Fye, "The Goals and Future of the American Osler Society: The Members Speak," (1990)

James T. Goodrich and Lawrence C. McHenry, Jr., "Sir William Osler and the Investigation of Cerebral Localization," (1984)

James T. Goodrich, "A New View on the Illustrations of Vesalius' De Humani Corporis Fabrica (1543)," (1988)

George T. Harrell, "The Tudor and Stuart Club," (1983)

George T. Harrell, "The Osler Tradition at Duke," (1987)

George T. Harrell, "Osler's Use of 'Ike' for Revere," (1990)

H. Alexander Heggtveit, "William Osler and Tait McKenzie," (1981)

William H. Helfand, "The Physician in Political Prints," (1989)

Shigeaki Hinohara, "How Osler Came to Japan," (1984)

Shigeaki Hinohara, "Doctor Wm. Osler's Theory on Habits—How it Originated," (1986)

Shigeaki Hinohara, "Philosophy on Death: Through The Works of Sir William Osler," (1990)

Thomas A. Horrocks, " 'A copy I Send With Pleasure': Sir William Osler, Charles Perry Fisher, and the Library of the College of Physicians of Philadelphia," (1987)

Thomas A. Horrocks and Richard L. Golden, "Osler, Gowers, and Medical Phonography" (1989)

R. Palmer Howard, "Osler's Relations with William Peterson, Principal of McGill University, 1898–1919," (1981)

R. Palmer Howard, "Studies on Pernicious Anemia by R. Palmer Howard and William Osler in the 1870s," (1984)

R. Palmer Howard, "The Foundation of Sir William Osler's Eminent Career: Pathological Reports at the McGill Medical College from 1871–1877," (1990)

Robert P. Hudson, "The Clendening-Knopf Correspondence," (1981)

K. Garth Huston, "Sir Thomas Browne after 300 Years," (1982)

K. Garth Huston, "Sir Kenelm Digby's Library," (1983)

Richard J. Kahn, "The Osler-Jewett Connection," (1983)

Elton R. Kerr, "A presentation regarding Osler's paper of 1919, 'Observations on the Severe Anemias of Pregnancy and the Post Partum State'," (1987)

Jack D. Key and Alvin E. Rodin, "William Osler and Arthur Conan Doyle Versus the Antivivisectionists," (1983)

Robert C. Kimbrough III, "The Didactic Teaching of Medical Students at Vanderbilt University 1915–1916: A Comparison of Fourth Year Classroom Notes to Sir William Osler's Textbook of Medicine," (1990)

Mary E. Kingsbury, "The Critical Reception of Osler's Books in the non-Medical Press," (1986)

Paul D. Kligfield, "A Bicentennial Search for Laennec," (1981)

Paul D. Kligfield, "The Frustrated Benevolence of Dr. Anonymous," (1989)

James A. Knight, "Would Sir William Osler Have Liked a Jazz Funeral New Orleans Style?" (1988)

Richard Lampert, "Osler and his Publishers," (1982)

E. Carwile LeRoy, Faith Wallis, and Warren A. Sawyer, "A Student's Ode to Osler's Text Republished with Notes," (1988)

Lawrence D. Longo, "Dear Uncle 'Willie' and My Dear 'Willum': The Correspondence of Sir William Osler and W.W. Francis," (1984)

Lawrence C. McHenry, "Dr. Samuel Johnson and Dr. Benjamin Rush," (1982)

David M. Mumford and John P. McGovern, "Sir William Osler (1849–1919): A Product of, or Exception to, His Historical Times?" (1987)

Earl F. Nation, "James Barry, M.D. Inspector General of Hospitals: Man or Woman?" (1986)

Earl F. Nation, "The Busts of Osler," (1988)

Donald S. Pady, "John Dryden's Medical Allusions," (1985)

G.R. Paterson, "People Will Ask for Almost Anything," (1987)

Edmund D. Pellegrino, "Scribonius Largus and the Origins of Medical Humanism: Philosophical and Historical Aspects," (1983)

Edmund D. Pellegrino, "Percival's Ethics: The Ethics Beneath the Etiquette," (1985)

Claus A. Pierach, Sarah Wangensteen, and Howard B. Burchell, "The Spa Craze—circa 1900," (1990)

Samuel X. Radbill and Ronald Kotrc, "Osler-Packard Letters at the College of Physicians of Philadelphia," (1981)

Robert E. Rakel, "Literary Favorites of American Osler Society Members: A Modern Version of Osler's Bedside Library," (1985)

Alastair H.T. Robb-Smith, "Osler's Influence on British Orthopaedics," (1988)

Alvin E. Rodin and Jack D. Key, "Conan Doyle's M.D. Thesis: An Example of Fallacious Medical Reasoning," (1981)

Alvin E. Rodin and Jack D. Key, "Assessment and Significance of Conan Doyle's Medical Writings," (1982)

Alvin E. Rodin and Arnold G. Rogers, "Concordance Between Osler's and Strumpell's Textbooks," (1985)

Alvin E. Rodin and Jack D. Key, "Sir William Osler and Sir Arthur Conan Doyle: A Comparison of Two Humanistic Physicians," (1987)

Alvin E. Rodin and Jack D. Key, "Osler's Brain and Related Mental Matters," (1988)

Alvin E. Rodin and Jack D. Key, "Kindred Spirits: Some Interfaces Between John McCrae and William Osler," (1989)

Alvin E. Rodin and Jack D. Key, "Humanizing Medicine Through Literary Medical Eponyms," (1990)

Alex Sakula, "Sir William Osler and the Royal Society of Medicine, London," (1989)

Leon Z. Saunders, "From Osler to Olafson: The Evolution of Veterinary Pathology in North America," (1987)

Leon Z. Saunders, "In Ever Widening Circles: Osler's Influence on Veterinary Medicine in Sweden," (1990)

Mark E. Silverman and Nicholas E. Davis, "William Osler at the Bedside: A Demonstration for the American Osler Society," (1989)

William B. Spaulding, "Osler's Roots in Dundas," (1981)

William B. Spaulding, "Abraham Groves: A Pioneer Ontario Surgeon— Sufficient Unto Himself," (1983)

William B. Spaulding and Charles G. Roland, "Osler's Impact on Two Continents," (1988)

Marvin J. Stone, "Osler's Aphorisms Revisited," (1990)

Philip M. Teigen, "William Osler as Historian of Medicine," (1984)

Philip M. Teigen, "Mirror or Lamp? Forty Years of the Garrison Lectures," (1987)

Fernando G. Vescia, "Sydenham, Rush and Osler: Differences and Similarities," (1990)

Frederick B. Wagner, Jr., "Lady Grace Revere Osler: Relationships, Legacy, and Professorship at Jefferson Medical College," (1982)

Frederick B. Wagner, Jr., "The Physician's Gold-Headed Cane," (1983)

Frederick B. Wagner, Jr., "The Jefferson Medical College Connection: A Letter from Sir William Osler," (1986)

Frederick B. Wagner, Jr., "The Osler-J.C. Wilson Connection," (1988)

Frederick B. Wagner, Jr., "Samuel W. Gross and William Osler: More Than a Friendship," (1989)

Frederick B. Wagner, Jr., "Thomas McCrae: A Life Patterned After Osler," (1990)

James V. Warren, "William Osler: 11:59 PM or 12:01 AM," (1986)

Thomas A. Warthin, "Three Connecticut Yankees and WO," (1985)

Thomas A. Warthin, "Sir William Osler's Siblings—Heights and Valleys," (1989)

Stewart Wolf, "Charles Richet, Physiologist, Playwright, and Rival of the Wright Brothers," (1981)

Charles F. Wooley, "Functional Heart Disease: The Role of Military Medicine and the Development of Speciality Hospitals," (1986)

Charles F. Wooley and John M. Stang, "Samuel A. Levine: 1917—The British

Heart Hospital and His Encounters with Allbutt, Osler, Mackenzie, and Lewis,'' (1987)

Charles F. Wooley, "William Osler, The British Heart Hospital, Samuel Levine, and 'The Picture','' (1989)

Presidential Addresses

Jeremiah A. Barondess, "Osler's Biographer: Notes on the Friendship of William Osler and Harvey Cushing,'' (1984)

W. Bruce Fye, "Osler's Departure from Johns Hopkins: The Price of Success,'' (1989)

William C. Gibson, "Osler's Influence in British Columbia,'' (1982)

Richard L. Golden, "Osler's Legacy: The Principles and Practice of Medicine,'' (1990)

R. Palmer Howard, "A Collection of Artifacts from the William Osler Family,'' (1983)

Robert P. Hudson, "Oslerian Formes Frustes: A Clendening Sampler,'' (1988)

K. Garth Huston, "Sir Geoffrey Keynes and the Oslerian Tradition,'' (1985)

Peter D. Olch, "Osler's Clinical Prig: William S. Halsted,'' (1981)

Charles G. Roland, "On the Need for a New Biography of Osler,'' (1987)

William B. Spaulding, "William Osler's Experience with Smallpox,'' (1986)

McGovern Lectures

Edward J. Huth, "To Humane Medicine: Back Door or Front Door?'' (1987)

Albert R. Jonsen, "Our Lords, the Sick,'' (1986)

Joanne Trautmann Banks, "Thalia and the Doctors,'' (1988)

E.A. Vastyan, "Rx: Hope,'' (1990)

Sir John Walton, "The 'Open Arms' Reviving?: Can We Rekindle the Osler Flame?'' (1989)

A.O.S. Research Studentship Lectures

Cary David Alberstone, "Sickness and Sin: Elizabethan Melancholy and Reformation Thought,'' (1989)

Lawrence B. Berk, "Polio Vaccine Trials of 1935'' (1988)

D. Branch Moody, "Medical Miracles in Medieval Bavaria,'' (1990)

❦ Index